Management of Breast Cancer

Editor

CATHERINE C. PARKER

SURGICAL CLINICS
OF NORTH AMERICA

www.surgical.theclinics.com

Consulting Editor
RONALD F. MARTIN

August 2018 • Volume 98 • Number 4

ELSEVIER

1600 John F. Kennedy Boulevard • Suite 1800 • Philadelphia, Pennsylvania, 19103-2899

http://www.surgical.theclinics.com

SURGICAL CLINICS OF NORTH AMERICA Volume 98, Number 4
August 2018 ISSN 0039–6109, ISBN-13: 978-0-323-61351-4

Editor: John Vassallo, j.vassallo@elsevier.com
Developmental Editor: Meredith Madeira

Surgical Clinics of North America (ISSN 0039–6109) is published bimonthly by Elsevier Inc., 360 Park Avenue South, New York, NY 10010-1710. Months of publication are February, April, June, August, October, and December. Business and Editorial Offices: 1600 John F. Kennedy Blvd., Suite 1800, Philadelphia, PA 19103-2899. Periodicals postage paid at New York, NY and additional mailing offices. Subscription prices are $350.00 per year for US individuals, $802.00 per year for US institutions, $100.00 per year for US students and residents, $420.00 per year for Canadian individuals, $1015.00 per year for Canadian institutions, $475.00 for international individuals, $1015.00 per year for international institutions and $225.00 per year for Canadian and foreign students/residents. To receive student/resident rate, orders must be accompanied by name of affiliated institution, date of term, and the *signature* of program/residency coordinator on institution letterhead. Orders will be billed at individual rate until proof of status is received. Foreign air speed delivery is included in all *Clinics* subscription prices. All prices are subject to change without notice. POSTMASTER: Send address changes to *Surgical Clinics*, Elsevier Health Sciences Division, Subscription Customer Service, 3251 Riverport Lane, Maryland Heights, MO 63043. **Customer Service (orders, claims, online, change of address): Telephone: 1-800-654-2452 (U.S. and Canada); 314-447-8871 (outside U.S. and Canada). Fax: 314-447-8029. E-mail: journalscustomerservice-usa@elsevier.com (for print support); journalsonline support-usa@elsevier.com (for online support).**

Reprints. For copies of 100 or more, of articles in this publication, please contact the Commercial Reprints Department, Elsevier Inc., 360 Park Avenue South, New York, New York 10010-1710. Tel. 212-633-3874, Fax: 212-633-3820, E-mail: reprints@elsevier.com.

The Surgical Clinics of North America is also published in Spanish by McGraw-Hill Interamericana Editores S.A., P.O. Box 5-237 06500 Mexico D.F. Mexico; and in Portuguese by Interlivros Edicoes Ltda., Rua Comandante Coelho 1085, CEP 21250, Rio de Janeiro, Brazil; and in Greek by Paschalidis Medical Publications, Athens Greece.

The Surgical Clinics of North America is covered in *MEDLINE/PubMed (Index Medicus), EMBASE/Excerpta Medica, Current Contents/Clinical Medicine, Current Contents/Life Sciences, Science Citation Index,* and *ISI/BIOMED.*

Contributors

CONSULTING EDITOR

RONALD F. MARTIN, MD, FACS
Colonel (ret.), United States Army Reserve, Department of Surgery, York Hospital, York, Maine, USA

EDITOR

CATHERINE C. PARKER, MD, FACS
Assistant Professor, Department of Surgery, Division of Surgical Oncology, The University of Alabama at Birmingham, Birmingham, Alabama, USA

AUTHORS

DREXELL HUNTER BOGGS, MD
Assistant Professor, Department of Radiation Oncology, The University of Alabama at Birmingham, Hazelrig-Salter Radiation Oncology Center, Birmingham, Alabama, USA

ABIGAIL CAUDLE, MD, MS
Associate Professor, Department of Breast Surgical Oncology, Division of Surgery, The University of Texas MD Anderson Cancer Center, Houston, Texas, USA

JENNIFER F. DE LOS SANTOS, MD
Professor, Department of Radiation Oncology, The University of Alabama at Birmingham, The Kirklin Clinic at Acton Road, Birmingham, Alabama, USA

KATERINA DODELZON, MD
Assistant Professor of Radiology, Weill Cornell Medical Center, NewYork-Presbyterian, New York, New York, USA

MALLORY A. DUNCAN, MD
Department of General Surgery, UT Health San Antonio, San Antonio, Texas, USA

ASHLYN S. EVERETT, MD
Resident, Department of Radiation Oncology, The University of Alabama at Birmingham, Hazelrig-Salter Radiation Oncology Center, Birmingham, Alabama, USA

MEAGAN FARMER, MS, CGC, MBA
Department of Genetics, The University of Alabama at Birmingham, Birmingham, Alabama, USA

ANDRES FORERO-TORRES, MD
Professor, Department of Medicine, Division of Hematology Oncology, The University of Alabama at Birmingham, Birmingham, Alabama, USA

TAMER M. FOUAD, MD
Morgan Welch Inflammatory Breast Cancer Research and Clinic Program, The University of Texas MD Anderson Cancer Center, Houston, Texas, USA; Department of Medical Oncology, The National Cancer Institute, Cairo University, Cairo, Egypt

FANGMENG FU, MD
Fujian Medical University Union Hospital, Fuzhou, Fujian, China

KRISTALYN K. GALLAGHER, DO, FACOS
Assistant Professor of Surgery, Division of Surgical Oncology, Lineberger Comprehensive Cancer Center, The University of North Carolina at Chapel Hill, Chapel Hill, North Carolina, USA

RICHARD C. GILMORE, MD
Johns Hopkins Hospital, Johns Hopkins University School of Medicine, Baltimore, Maryland, USA

HEATHER I. GREENWOOD, MD
Assistant Professor of Radiology and Biomedical Imaging, University of California, San Francisco, UCSF Medical Center at Mount Zion, San Francisco, California, USA

KELLY K. HUNT, MD
Professor, Chair, Department of Breast Surgical Oncology, The University of Texas MD Anderson Cancer Center, Houston, Texas, USA

LISA K. JACOBS, MD, FACS
Johns Hopkins Hospital, Johns Hopkins University School of Medicine, Baltimore, Maryland, USA

CAROLINE JONES, MD, MSPH
Department of Surgery, The University of Alabama at Birmingham, Birmingham, Alabama, USA

JANINE T. KATZEN, MD
Assistant Professor of Radiology, Weill Cornell Medical Center, NewYork-Presbyterian, New York, New York, USA

TARI A. KING, MD
Breast Surgery and Associate Chair for Multidisciplinary Oncology, Department of Surgery, Brigham and Women's Hospital, Boston, Massachusetts, USA

HELEN KRONTIRAS, MD, FACS
Professor and Director, Department of Surgery, Division of Surgical Oncology, The University of Alabama at Birmingham, Birmingham, Alabama, USA

RACHAEL LANCASTER, MD
Department of Surgery, Division of Surgical Oncology, The University of Alabama Birmingham, Birmingham, Alabama, USA

MEEGHAN A. LAUTNER, MD, MSc, FACS
Assistant Professor, Department of Surgery, University at Buffalo, Buffalo, New York, USA

HUONG LE-PETROSS, MD
Morgan Welch Inflammatory Breast Cancer Research and Clinic Program, Breast Diagnostic Imaging, The University of Texas MD Anderson Cancer Center, Houston, Texas, USA

BORA LIM, MD
Morgan Welch Inflammatory Breast Cancer Research and Clinic Program, Breast Medical
Oncology, The University of Texas MD Anderson Cancer Center, Houston, Texas, USA

ANTHONY LUCCI, MD
Morgan Welch Inflammatory Breast Cancer Research and Clinic Program, Breast Surgical
Oncology, The University of Texas MD Anderson Cancer Center, Houston, Texas, USA

KANDACE P. McGUIRE, MD, FACS
Associate Professor of Surgery, Chief, Section of Breast Surgery, VCU Massey Cancer
Center, West Hospital, Richmond, Virginia, USA

ARJUN MENTA
The University of Texas at Austin, Austin, Texas, USA

ELIZABETH A. MITTENDORF, MD, PhD
Robert and Karen Hale Distinguished Chair in Surgical Oncology and Director of
Research, Breast Surgical Oncology, Department of Surgery, Brigham and Women's
Hospital, Boston, Massachusetts, USA

LAKISHA MOORE-SMITH, MD, PhD
Internal Medicine Resident, Department of Medicine, Brookwood Baptist
Health-Princeton, Birmingham, Alabama, USA

APOORVE NAYYAR, MBBS
Division of Surgical Oncology, Post-Doctoral Research Associate, Lineberger
Comprehensive Cancer Center, The University of North Carolina at Chapel Hill, Chapel
Hill, North Carolina, USA

KO UN PARK, MD
Breast Surgical Oncology Fellow, Department of Breast Surgical Oncology, Division of
Surgery, The University of Texas MD Anderson Cancer Center, Houston, Texas, USA

CATHERINE C. PARKER, MD, FACS
Assistant Professor, Department of Surgery, Division of Surgical Oncology, The University
of Alabama at Birmingham, Birmingham, Alabama, USA

HANI SBITANY, MD
Associate Professor of Surgery, Division of Plastic and Reconstructive Surgery, University
of California, San Francisco, San Francisco, California, USA

MICHAEL C. STAUDER, MD
Morgan Welch Inflammatory Breast Cancer Research and Clinic Program, Radiation
Oncology, The University of Texas MD Anderson Cancer Center, Houston, Texas, USA

ERICA STRINGER-REASOR, MD
Assistant Professor, Department of Medicine, Division of Hematology Oncology, The
University of Alabama at Birmingham, Birmingham, Alabama, USA

MEDIGET TESHOME, MD, MPH, FACS
Assistant Professor, Department of Breast Surgical Oncology, The University of Texas
MD Anderson Cancer Center, Houston, Texas, USA

NAOTO T. UENO, MD, PhD
Morgan Welch Inflammatory Breast Cancer Research and Clinic Program, Breast Medical
Oncology, The University of Texas MD Anderson Cancer Center, Houston, Texas, USA

FLORA VARGHESE, MD, MBA, FACS
Department of Surgery, University of California, San Francisco, San Francisco, California, USA

ANNA WEISS, MD
Associate Surgeon in Breast Surgery, Department of Surgery, Brigham and Women's Hospital, Boston, Massachusetts, USA

JULIE WHATLEY, RN, BSN, CRNP
Division of Surgical Oncology, Department of Surgery, The University of Alabama at Birmingham, Birmingham, Alabama, USA

MEREDITH WITTEN, MD
Breast Surgical Oncology Fellow, Division of Surgical Oncology, The University of Alabama at Birmingham, Birmingham, Alabama, USA

JASMINE WONG, MD, FACS
Assistant Professor, Department of Surgery, University of California, San Francisco, San Francisco, California, USA

WENDY A. WOODWARD, MD, PhD
Morgan Welch Inflammatory Breast Cancer Research and Clinic Program, Radiation Oncology, The University of Texas MD Anderson Cancer Center, Houston, Texas, USA

Contents

New emerging breast imaging techniques have shown great promise in breast cancer screening, evaluation of the extent of disease, and response to neoadjuvant therapy. Tomosynthesis allows 3-dimensional imaging of the breast and increases breast cancer detection. Fast abbreviated MRI has reduced time and costs associated with traditional breast MRI while maintaining cancer detection. Diffusion-weighted imaging is a functional MRI technique that does not require contrast and has shown potential in screening, lesion characterization, and also evaluation of treatment response. New image-guided preoperative localizations are available that have increased patient satisfaction and decreased operating room delays.

Ductal carcinoma in situ has been stable in incidence for a decade and has an excellent prognosis. Breast conservation therapy is safe and effective for most patients. Adjuvant whole breast radiation therapy is recommended to reduce the risk of local recurrence. Accelerated partial breast irradiation is a promising alternative to decrease toxicity and improve cosmetic results. Adjuvant hormonal therapy can reduce local recurrence but should be used cautiously. Future directions in management include developing predictive tools for guidance for use of adjuvant therapy and selecting low-risk patients with ductal carcinoma in situ in whom surgery may be safely omitted.

Evaluation of the axillary lymph nodes is critical in the management of breast cancer because it is a key predictor of survival outcome. Surgeons must not only be able to perform sentinel lymph node dissection with high accuracy but also understand the implications of the results. Management of clinically node-negative and node-positive cases can vary significantly, as described in this article. With emerging data, management of the axilla in breast cancer will continue to evolve.

Breast-conserving surgery (BCS) followed by radiation therapy is the current standard of care for early-stage breast cancer. Successful BCS necessitates complete tumor resection with clear margins at the pathologic assessment of the specimen ("no ink on tumor"). The presence of positive margins warrants additional surgery to obtain negative final margins, which has significant physical, psychological, and financial implications for the patient. The challenge lies in developing accurate real-time intraoperative margin assessment techniques to minimize the presence of "ink on tumor" and the subsequent need for additional surgery.

Breast cancer is the second leading cause of cancer-related death in women in the United States. In general, advances in targeted treatment for breast cancer have improved over the last 20 years, except in the triple-negative breast cancer (TNBC) subtype. TNBC is an aggressive breast cancer subtype with limited treatment options as compared with hormone-positive breast cancers. Genomic profiling of TNBC has shown promise in aiding clinicians to develop personalized targeted agents. Prioritizing novel molecular-based therapies in the neoadjuvant setting may help investigators understand mechanisms of resistance and ultimately improve patient outcomes in TNBC.

Inflammatory breast cancer (IBC) is a rare form of breast cancer that accounts for only 2% to 4% of all breast cancer cases. Despite its low incidence, IBC contributes to 7% to 10% of breast cancer caused mortality. Despite ongoing international efforts to formulate better diagnosis, treatment, and research, the survival of patients with IBC has not been significantly improved, and there are no therapeutic agents that specifically target IBC to date. The authors present a comprehensive overview that aims to assess the present and new management strategies of IBC.

Throughout various eras of breast cancer therapy, postmastectomy radiation therapy (PMRT) has played an important role in the treatment of locally advanced breast cancer. PMRT decreases locoregional recurrence and may improve overall survival in patients with tumors over 5 cm or positive lymph nodes. As novel cancer therapies improve survival in breast cancer, the role of radiation therapy is evolving. Individualized recommendations for PMRT dependent on pathologic response after neoadjuvant systemic therapy are under investigation. This article summarizes the role of PMRT during breast cancer therapy and discusses open questions that may change the landscape of future breast cancer treatment.

With increasing life expectancy and growth of the elderly US population, it becomes paramount that breast cancer research focuses more on the prevention, screening, and treatment of these patients. Age is no longer a cut-off for managing breast cancer in the elderly. Studies have shown the current undertreatment of cancer undermines survival, but the tide is turning to provide evidence-based medicine for the elderly. More often, clinicians and surgeons look not only at tumor-specific characteristics of

breast imaging and core biopsy as in breast epithelial carcinoma. Surgical management is often wide local excision in the form of breast conservation if possible for primary breast sarcoma or total mastectomy. Radiation-associated breast angiosarcomas often require total mastectomy with radical excision of skin. Breast sarcomas have a hematogenous spread, so lymph node evaluation is not a part of treatment or staging. Local recurrence rates are high; prognosis remains poor despite ongoing advances in the treatment of epithelial breast carcinoma.

Management of Breast Cancer

SURGICAL CLINICS
OF NORTH AMERICA

ISSUE OF RELATED INTEREST:

Surgical Oncology Clinics
www.surgonc.theclinics.com
Thoracic Surgery Clinics
www.thoracic.theclinics.com
Advances in Surgery
www.advancessurgery.com

THE CLINICS ARE AVAILABLE ONLINE!
Access your subscription at:
www.theclinics.com

Foreword

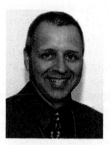

Ronald F. Martin, MD, FACS
Consulting Editor

If there is a disease or group of disease processes that equally captures the minds of clinicians, molecular biologists, philanthropists, and politicians alike more than breast cancer and breast related maladies, I am unaware of it. One can look anywhere for a forum that claims domain over breast disease and will find one. On occasion, facts and data are considered, and other times, not so much. Still, ubiquitous interest is present and is unlikely to decline any time soon.

There are many historical and clinical reasons for the broad development of interest in breast disease. The history of our understanding of breast cancer and the treatments we have suggested for it have been replete with examples of better and worse judgment. Our development has seen some of the best examples of clinical investigation and some of the worst examples of dogma. Still, progress was made and continues to be made on this front. Thankfully, the pace of progress seems to be accelerating.

Despite great advances in our understanding, our ability to provide consistent and good information to patients has been hindered by the very business of patient care itself. The practice of breast care, in particular surgical breast care, has on occasion become a turf battle with clinical, ethical, and economic impacts. I would not suggest that breast care is the only example of this, but it is a glaring example.

The American Board of Surgery includes breast surgery as one of its core components for board certification. I am asked almost daily in my current role if there is some "additional certification" that breast surgeons can get—preferably without having to undergo additional training or fellowship. I always respond, "basically no." Then, I have to explain that there are no other American Board of Medical Specialties boards for breast surgery. I further explain that there are other societies or groups that confer some recognition for breast surgeons and explain what those mean—or don't mean. Still, I get pressed on what can be done to have an organization appear to have "better" breast surgeons than one or more of its competitors. Oddly, I am rarely asked what improved processes or outcomes one could have or what one could do to streamline or expedite care for breast patients initially. Eventually, the latter topics come up and we talk about them, but the appearance or marketing angle seems forever present—at least to me.

Surg Clin N Am 98 (2018) xiii–xv
https://doi.org/10.1016/j.suc.2018.06.009
0039-6109/18/© 2018 Published by Elsevier Inc.

surgical.theclinics.com

I am a big believer in focus and dedication to understanding clinical issues to get the best outcomes. I am also a believer that there are many ways to achieve best outcomes that don't require every institution or organization to look exactly alike. There is now, and there is likely to be for some time, a need to balance surgical generalization and specialization for all institutions. At some places I have worked, the greater need was for hyperspecialization. We had large clinical volumes, a large number of surgeons, and large institutional capacities. Though no matter how hard one tries, even in systems like those, gaps develop when one or two key people are out of town or sick or otherwise unavailable. In other places I have worked, there is a need for substantial cross coverage and redundancy just to keep the doors open. Neither system is intrinsically better or worse than the other—they are just different. They serve different and important needs for the communities and systems they belong to. Even within these very different types of organization, there is always room for an individual to take a lead role in certain clinical areas.

For many decades, we had few or no fellowships. Over the last half-century, the number of fellowships has grown dramatically. The great majority of general surgery residents who are finishing training in general surgery will now pursue fellowship training. Before fellowship training was as common as it is today, most communities had people who self-identified their interests and focused their professional, educational, and clinical activities accordingly. Most of them were regarded, at least locally, as persons with valued expertise. Now, some of those people who have years or decades of clinical focus and experience are being regarded as "not formally trained" because they did undergo fellowship training. This can't be right in all circumstances. I would submit that some of those persons with years of clinical experience and focus have been the trainers of the fellows.

As with many other topics in surgery, we need to find the balance of what the generalist can, should, and must do and what must be given to the domain of the hyperspecialists. The ability to care for all of our citizenry depends on being able to generate the numbers of surgeons to deliver care and the ability to distribute that expertise properly. We cannot pretend that every hospital must be a stand-alone entity in a most austere environment devoid of assistance from other entities. We also cannot decree that patients can only be taken care of by someone with a very specific training path to achieve mastery—especially when other mechanisms to attain clinical excellence exist. Mastery is a level of understanding and capability that is attained; mastery is not necessarily conferred by completing one specific form of training. That said, specific focused training usually accelerates one's path toward mastery and helps to focus the mind on what is important. It is what one does with that focus and how one grows and develops systems to support patients that will lead to developing mastery.

The care of patients with breast diseases, particularly breast cancer, may be one of our better examples of real team-delivered care. When I was younger, there was great emphasis placed on the surgeon being the "Captain of the ship" when it came to breast cancer. There may be some surgeons who disagree with me, but I believe those days are bygone. At least they are bygone to our colleagues in medical oncology, radiation oncology, plastic surgery, genetics, and other disciplines. Surgeons remain valued members of the team and surely have leadership needs, but they do not rule the ship by default. They do need to develop mastery in order to successfully play whatever role on that team they may.

Whether one is a generalist, a specialist, a team member, or would-be captain, one still has to know the basis of knowledge that we all need in order to make good decisions. We are indebted to Dr Parker and her colleagues for providing us with the benefit of their insight and mastery on a wide range of topics related to the care of patients with breast disease.

We surgeons as a group are collegial by nature. Most of us spent our formative years of development as surgeons as members of teams. Most of us played all the positions on those teams from most junior person to leader. We work in teams in the operating room. We mostly understand that we are part of a larger system and that we are not the system itself.

We need to convince those who would take measures to reduce that collegial and cooperative foundation, whether it is one of our own surgeons or someone else, to reconsider that divisive position. We will always do better by cooperating than by fighting. To paraphrase Jefferson, no war, no matter how successfully prosecuted, will pay for itself. In my opinion, that goes for turf wars as well.

Ronald F. Martin, MD, FACS
Colonel (ret.), United States Army Reserve
Department of Surgery
York Hospital
16 Hospital Drive, Suite A
York, ME 03909, USA

E-mail address:
rmartin@yorkhospital.com

Preface

Management of Breast Cancer

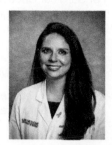

Catherine C. Parker, MD, FACS
Editor

The lifetime risk of developing breast cancer is about 12% for the average woman. Breast cancers are heterogeneous, and the management of breast cancer has evolved due to advances in technology and a better understanding of tumor biology. Screening mammography provides early detection, and improvements in imaging modalities assist with evaluating the extent of disease and identifying additional disease. Genetic testing and prophylactic mastectomy for patients with high-risk breast cancer now offer risk reduction. The American Joint Committee on Cancer breast staging system has acknowledged the importance of tumor biology by incorporating grade, estrogen/progesterone receptor status, HER2 status, and multigene panels in the new 8th edition.

The surgical approach to breast cancer has seen advancements. New localization techniques for lumpectomy are improving patient satisfaction and decreasing operative delays. Historically, all patients with breast cancer underwent axillary lymph node dissection; however, management of the axilla has changed with the utilization of sentinel lymph node biopsy. The evolution of the mastectomy from radical to nipple-sparing techniques along with developments in breast reconstruction provides patients with breast cancer surgical options previously unavailable.

Emerging areas of research include developing a better understanding of ductal carcinoma in situ in an effort to address overtreatment. Improvements in survival have been made for many patients diagnosed with breast cancer; however, patients with inflammatory and triple-negative breast cancer are often still in need of additional treatment options.

These topics and more are covered in this issue of *Surgical Clinics of North America*. I would like to thank my fellow authors who contributed their time and expertise in creating this issue designed to provide an overview of the improvements, management, and challenges of treating breast cancer. I would also like

Surg Clin N Am 98 (2018) xvii–xviii
https://doi.org/10.1016/j.suc.2018.06.008
0039-6109/18/© 2018 Published by Elsevier Inc.

surgical.theclinics.com

to thank the editorial staff at Elsevier for their assistance and commitment. It has been an honor serving as an editor for this issue, and I am grateful for the opportunity.

Catherine C. Parker, MD, FACS
Division of Surgical Oncology
Department of Surgery
University of Alabama at Birmingham
FOT 1138
1720 2nd Avenue S
Birmingham, AL 35294, USA

E-mail address:
ccparker@uabmc.edu

Screening Mammography

Recommendations and Controversies

Meredith Witten, MD*, Catherine C. Parker, MD

KEYWORDS

- Mammogram (MMG) • Screening • Analog • Digital

KEY POINTS

- The focus of screening mammography remains to prevent breast cancer death through early detection and treatment with the goal of increased survival.
- Screening mammography does have associated risks and potential harms.
- Although one perspective is that the value of even one life outweighs anxiety caused by false positives or health care costs, this may not be the perspective of every patient.

INTRODUCTION
Content

Over the past several years, there have been numerous changes in the guidelines for screening mammography. Additionally, different societies have released guidelines with variance in the recommendations. The importance of screening mammography in decreasing breast cancer, however, remains clear. The current recommendations as well as the importance of screening mammography in the disease process, early detection, and survival are discussed.

Breast cancer is a common disease, and the survival has been greatly improved in recent years. Overall, in the United States, the risk of developing breast cancer is 1 in 8 (12%). There are an estimated 252,710 new cases of breast cancer resulting in 40,610 deaths estimated in the United States in 2017. In addition, there are an estimated 63,410 new cases of ductal carcinoma in situ (DCIS). Mortality rates for breast cancer have decreased over the past 50 years. The current 5-year survival rate is now 95% compared with 75% in 1975.[1] Before the mid-1980s the death rate from breast cancer had not changed in more than 4 decades. Since 1990, the death rate has steadily declined by at least 38% through 2014.[2] In addition to improvements in screening, there have also been advances in treatment. However, screening has a greater

The authors have nothing to disclose.
Division of Surgical Oncology, The University of Alabama at Birmingham, FOT 1138, 1720 2nd Avenue S, Birmingham, AL 35294-3411, USA
* Corresponding author.
E-mail address: mwitten@uabmc.edu

reduction in mortality.[3] The improvement in survival has been in large part due to improvements in screening leading to early detection and improved breast cancer treatment (**Table 1**). There are an estimated 3.5 million women in the United States living with breast cancer. The main risk factors for breast cancer include female sex and advancing age.[1]

The history of mammography helps understand its current state and underscores the importance of screening mammography. Reports of radiographs of the breast date back to 1929 in the United States, noting the roentgenographic appearance of tumors and the accuracy of diagnosis. In 1960, Robert Egan[4] published a statistical analysis showing that soft-tissue roentgenography of the breast can provide definitive diagnosis of malignant, benign, and normal conditions of the breast. The article evaluated 1000 consecutive images with an error rate of less than 1%. It also noted the inaccuracy of palpation in detecting breast lesions.[4] Breast cancer is the most common cancer in women other than skin cancer and the second most common cause of cancer death in women. Screening mammography has reduced mortality rates at least 30% for breast cancer through the detection of earlier breast cancer leading to improved survival. Additionally, when breast cancer is diagnosed at the earliest stages, the survival rate is greater than 95%.

There have been significant advancements in the quality of mammographic images. The imaging used for mammography has evolved from analog to digital.[5] In addition to higher-quality imaging with digital mammography, interpretation times are improved, shown through comparison of full-field digital mammography (FFDM) compared with FFDM using analog from priors. The use of FFDM also significantly increased the referral rate as well as the cancer detection rate. However, there is a lower positive predictive value of referral and biopsy. The additional tumors detected by FFDM were mainly low- to intermediate-grade DCIS, smaller invasive tumors, and overall more favorable tumor characteristics.[6] Digital breast tomosynthesis (DBT) creates a 3-dimensional image of the breast and was approved by the Food and Drug Administration in 2011 for breast cancer screening. Studies have shown increased detection rates with DBT with dense breasts as well as a higher average true-positive rate compared with 2-dimensional mammography. The sensitivity and specificity are higher, and the overall recall rate has been shown to be lower. Additionally, there was a higher detection of Breast Imaging Reporting and Data System 5 lesions; however, there was no difference between the detection of benign lesions.[7] The

Table 1
Benefits of recommended screening strategies

Screening Strategy	Examinations per 1000 Women	Percentage Mortality Reduction	Breast Cancer Deaths Averted per 1000 Women	Life Years Gained per 1000 Women Screened	Number Needed to Screen per Death Averted
Annual 40–84 y old	36,550	39.6	11.9	189	84
Annual 45–54 y old, biennial 55–79 y old	19,846	30.8	9.25	149	108
Biennial 50–74 y old	11,066	23.2	6.95	110	144

Data from Monticciolo DL, Newell MS, Hendrick RE, et al. Breast cancer screening for average-risk women: recommendations from the ACR commission on breast imaging. J Am Coll Radiol 2017;14(9):1137–43; and Arleo EK, Hendrick RE, Helvie MA, et al. Comparison of recommendations for screening mammography using CISNET models. Cancer 2017;123(19):3673–80.

amount of digital compression needed during digital mammography versus tomosynthesis has been studied because pain associated with mammography has been a cause of low compliance with screening mammography guidelines. The study showed compression force could be reduced by 50% with DBT without affecting image quality. In addition, there were similar results indicating the same reduction may be possible with digital mammography.[8]

With advances in imaging and increased detection due to more sensitive techniques, controversy about screening guidelines and recommendations has also occurred. Regular screening mammography beginning at 40 years of age reduces the risk of breast cancer mortality in the average-risk woman. However, it also leads to harm because screening may lead to false-positive test results, anxiety, cost, inconvenience, and overdiagnosis of nonmalignant lesions (**Table 2**). Because of the efforts to balance harm and benefit, there have been major differences in guidelines regarding initiation age of screening, termination of screening, and frequency of screening in women at average risk of breast cancer. A summary of the recommendations for initiation of screening mammography, screening interval, and stop age is found in **Table 3**.

Although there are several areas of controversy, there are certain points that are agreed on. The US Preventative Task Force and the American College of Surgeons (ACS) both conducted separate reviews of the evidence for breast cancer mammography screening in the average-risk woman. These reviews, however, are difficult in part because of the number of women needed and the long-term follow-up involved to analyze the benefit and harm of screening. The reviews agreed that screening decreases breast cancer mortality. The US Preventative Task Force also reported results by age finding a reduced risk of advanced breast cancer, stage IIB or greater in women aged 50 years or older. The ACS also concluded that screening mammography increased life expectancy but was unable to quantify the amount of increase.[1]

Overall, there is agreement that a woman at average risk of breast cancer should not begin routine screening earlier than 40 years of age. Additionally, it is agreed on that screening mammography should begin no later than 50 years of age. However, the guidelines have a discrepancy in their recommendations between 40 and 50 years of age. This discrepancy is in part due to the breast cancer incidence and deaths increasing with age beginning in the 40s and continuing through the 50s.[9] Breast cancer in women younger than 40 years is less common; therefore, harms increase with screening in comparison with the benefit of lives saved. The ACS showed that screening is effective for all age groups, but efficiency improves with age.[10] With

Table 2
Risks of different screening strategies with negative recalls and benign biopsies

Screening Strategy	Examinations per 1000 Women	Negative Recalls per 1000 Women	Benign Biopsies per 1000 Women	Life Years Gained per Benign Biopsy
Annual 40–84 y old	36,550	2780	195	1.0
Annual 45–54 y old, biennial 55–79 y old	19,846	1680	116	1.3
Biennial 50–74 y old	11,066	940	96	1.7

Data from Monticciolo DL, Newell MS, Hendrick RE, et al. Breast cancer screening for average-risk women: recommendations from the ACR commission on breast imaging. J Am Coll Radiol 2017;14(9):1137–43; and Arleo EK, Hendrick RE, Helvie MA, et al. Comparison of recommendations for screening mammography using CISNET models. Cancer 2017;123(19):3673–80.

Table 3
Current recommendations for screening mammography

	American Cancer Society	US Preventative Services Task Force	National Comprehensive Cancer Network	American College of Obstetricians and Gynecologists
Mammography initiation	Offer at 40–45 y; recommends at 45 y	Recommend at 50 y; 40–49 y after counseling if patients desire	Recommends at 40 y	Offer at 40 y; initiate at 40–49 y if patients desire; start routine screening at 50 y
Mammography screening interval	Annual for women 40–54 y; biennial with option to continue annual for ≥55 y	Biennial	Annual	Annual or biennial
Mammography cessation	When life expectancy ≤10 y	Current evidence insufficient to evaluate benefits or harms in women aged ≥75 y	When life expectancy ≤10 y	Continue until 75 y; after 75 y, based on shared decision-making

regard to women in their 40s, the US Preventive Services Task Force states that women in their 40s do benefit from starting regular screening mammography. However, that benefit is decreased in comparison with older women. Overall, the benefit outweighs the harms; but preference for starting screening mammograms may be taken into account because the benefit is lessened. The benefit of the relatively rare but important risk reduction in breast cancer deaths must be weighed against harms of overdiagnosis, overtreatment, a potentially unnecessary invasive procedure, and psychological impact. Women should take these factors into account when deciding on when to begin screening mammography.[11] Interestingly, the ACS has qualified their recommendation and splits their viewpoint from 40 to 45 years of age and 45 to 50 years of age. For patients aged 40 to 44 years, the ACS thinks women should be given the opportunity to begin screening. At 45 years of age, the ACS strongly recommends that women begin regular screening mammography. This recommendation was based on disease burden at 5-year intervals. The 5-year risk in women aged 45 to 49 years was noted to be 0.9%, which was comparable with that of women aged 50 to 54 years of 1.1%. The proportion of incident breast cancer cases was also similar at 10% in 45 to 49 years of age and 12% in 50 to 54 years of age. In women aged 40 to 44 years, the 5-year risk was lower at 0.6% and the proportion of incident breast cancer cases was also decreased at 7.0%.[9] Additionally, as women age, mammography reduction in mortality increases.[12] The harms associated with false positives also decrease as women age. The number of biopsies performed stays constant, but there is a higher number of cancer diagnoses in older women.[11]

The frequency of screening mammography is also a point of debate. It is agreed on that women should undergo screening mammography every 1 to 2 years. The ACS and US Preventive Task Force did not identify any randomized trials comparing annual with biennial screening. Both groups reviewed indirect evidence from met-analyses and observational studies showing that shorter screening intervals are associated with improved outcomes. This improvement is greater in women younger than 50 years. It also included more callbacks and biopsies. It is predicted by the Cancer Intervention and Surveillance Modeling network that annual screening will save 2 additional lives with 82 additional biopsies and 6 overdiagnosed breast tumors for every 1000 women screened between 50 and 74 years of age. This model did not include women younger than 50 years for which the benefit of more frequent screening was thought to be greater.[13] Annual screening results in the least number of breast cancer deaths, especially in younger women. Therefore, the NCCN recommends annual screening.[14] The ACS recommends that women should have the opportunity to have annual screening at 40 years of age and, after 55 years of age, transition to biennial screening or have the opportunity to continue annual screening, stating that annual screening seems to have an additional benefit over biennial screening, especially in younger women.[9] The US Preventive Services Task Force recommends biennial screening for all patients stating the mortality benefit with fewer harms, including callbacks and benign breast biopsies.[11]

Another area lacking data and clarity is when to stop obtaining mammograms. It Is agreed on that women should continue screening mammography until at least 75 years of age. However, after 75 years of age, the decision is based on shared decision-making and, often, life expectancy. This issue becomes challenging, especially because more than 25% of breast cancer cases are diagnosed in women older than 75 years.[9] Additionally, there are limited data on screening mammography in this patient population because of the lack of randomized trials to assist in decision-making. The results of 2 observational guideline articles show a reduction in breast cancer mortality associated with mammographic detection of breast cancer in women 75 years of age and older.[15,16] There have been simulation studies showing a benefit in older women. A simulation study included women aged 70 to 74 years and showed a reduction in mortality with screening mammography in women only if they are in good health without significant medical problems. A Cancer Intervention and Surveillance Modeling Network included women up to 84 years of age and showed a benefit in screening mammography.[13] Overall, decision-making for women older than 75 years should involve examining their general health, quality of life, and life expectancy. There are many women of this age group who are in good health and more than half of women older than 75 years can be expected to live longer than 10 years.[17] The assessment of life expectancy should also be used for women younger than 75 years with significant comorbidities and short life expectancy who may not benefit from mammographic screening.

In addition to the positive benefits of mammography, there has been a focus on the adverse effects. False-positive results lead to callbacks, additional imaging, and possible biopsies that are benign, which causes increased cost and patient anxiety. The most common adverse effect is recall for additional imaging in 9.6% to 11.6% of women.[2] The 11.6% recall rate has a cancer detection rate of 5.1 per 1000 with a sensitivity of 87% and specificity of 89%.[18] Although lower recall rates may decrease benign workup and anxiety, it can be at the expense of cancer detection. Recall rates of 10% to 14% have better cancer detection rates than recall rates of less than 10%. However, recall rates greater than 14% did not continue to demonstrate the same benefit.[19] The Breast Cancer Surveillance Consortium saw a 10-year cumulative false-positive rate of 61% with annual screening and a 42% with biennial screening. Biopsies occurred in 7% of annual screenings and 5% of biennial screenings. Other studies have reported lower rates of biopsies, occurring in only 2% of screened women.[20] A woman who undergoes annual screening from 40 to 49 years of age will have a benign biopsy 0.67% each year.[21] Benign biopsies also decrease with age.[2] The US Preventative Task Force found that women who were given negative results had minimal anxiety compared with increased anxiety and breast cancer–specific distress in women who were called back for additional testing and/or biopsy. However, although anxiety is important, it is difficult to quantify. The amount of anxiety and consistent data about anxiety in the overall population has not been well evaluated. Additionally, most studies have described short-term anxiety without discussing potential long-term effects.[2,22] When women were asked if they would accept the risk of recall to detect cancer at an earlier stage, 86% agreed.[23] Patients with false-positive results add to health care costs, and those patients were less likely to resume regular screening.

There has also been controversy surrounding the overdiagnosis and overtreatment related to the management of DCIS. Particularly, are screening mammograms finding disease whose natural progression would not cause harm to patients? Sixteen publications by EUROSCREEN showed overdiagnosis to be from 0% to 10% with the inclusion of DCIS.[24] If so, are subsequent biopsies and excisions causing patient anxiety, additional procedures and associated risks as well as increased health care costs. The US Preventive Service Task Force concluded that 1 in 8 women who receive biennial screening from 50 to 75 years of age will be overdiagnosed. Using this estimate, for every woman who avoids a breast cancer death, 2 to 3 women will be treated unnecessarily.[11] The ACS commented that although there is overdiagnosis, all the estimates provided use unverifiable assumptions or biased methods, including inadequate follow-up or failure to adequately adjust for trends in incidence and lead time, which leads to overinflation of estimates.[9]

Another potential side effect of mammography is exposure to radiation. Although there have been no definitive studies of radiation exposure from mammography, the US Preventative Services Task Force had a modeling study that estimated the number of deaths from mammography radiation-induced cancer was 2 per 100,000 among women aged 40 to 49 years screened annually.[12] In contrast, another modeling study estimated that the potential mortality benefit of early breast cancer detection through annual screening starting at 40 years of age outweighed the risk of dying of mammography radiation-induced cancer by 60-fold. This model estimated radiation from annual screening of 100,000 women aged 40 to 74 years induced approximately 125 cases of breast cancer and 16 cancer deaths, while preventing 968 cancer deaths through early detection screening.[25]

Currently in medicine with increasing patient autonomy, shared decision-making has been discussed as a part of screening mammography guidelines. This shared decision-making combines physician knowledge of benefits as well as harms and includes the patients' opinions on how current evidence should guide each individual's decision. For example, some women may prefer additional screening in order to decrease their rate of breast cancer death. Other women could place more emphasis on the potential harms of screening and anxieties associated with potential unnecessary biopsies or overtreatment and opt for a less vigorous screening schedule.

The Centers for Disease Control and Prevention reports data on the percentage of women receiving yearly mammograms. **Fig. 1** shows the percentage of women in the United States undergoing mammography in the past 2 years during 1987 to 2015.

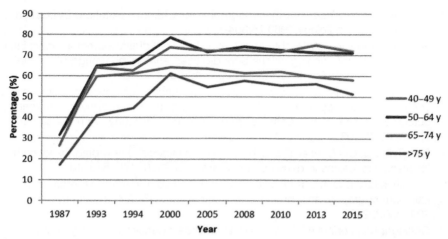

Fig. 1. Percentage of women in the United States by age. The graph displays women in each year surveyed who underwent a mammogram within the past 2 years of the year shown. (*Data from* Centers for Disease Control and Prevention. CDC health. 2016. Available at: www.cdc.gov/nchs/data/hus/2016/070.pdf.)

SUMMARY

Although the value of screening mammography is not debated, controversies exist surrounding initiation age, frequency of screening, and cessation age. The focus of screening mammography remains to prevent breast cancer deaths through early detection and treatment with the goal of increased survival. Screening mammography, however, does have associated risks and potential harms. Although one perspective is that the value of even one life outweighs anxiety caused by false positives or health care costs, this may not be the perspective of every patient. Therefore, one very important and essential component is the shared decision-making between patient and practitioner. Over time, as the population ages, this joint decision-making process will likely become more important. Additionally, as the life expectancy of the average person increases, screening after 75 years of age will warrant further investigation. Although it is clear that good performance status adds value to screening in this age group, there is still uncertainty of the cessation time. Unfortunately, randomized trials are not available to add in decision-making. If feasible, a prospective randomized trial would add to our current knowledge. However, it is essential to properly inform and educate patients so anxiety does not overshadow the value of early detection and added years of life gained by screening mammography.

REFERENCES

1. Practice bulletin no. 179 summary: breast cancer risk assessment and screening in average-risk women. Obstet Gynecol 2017;130(1):241–3.
2. Monticciolo DL, Newell MS, Hendrick RE, et al. Breast cancer screening for average-risk women: recommendations from the ACR commission on breast imaging. J Am Coll Radiol 2017;14(9):1137–43.
3. Saadatmand S, Bretveld R, Siesling S, et al. Influence of tumour stage at breast cancer detection on survival in modern times: population based study in 173,797 patients. BMJ 2015;351:h4901.

4. Egan RL. Experience with mammography in a tumor institution. Evaluation of 1,000 studies. Radiology 1960;75:894–900.

5. Garg AS, Rapelyea JA, Rechtman LR, et al. Full-field digital mammographic interpretation with prior analog versus prior digitized analog mammography: time for interpretation. AJR Am J Roentgenol 2011;196(6):1436–8.

6. Nederend J, Duijm LE, Louwman MW, et al. Impact of transition from analog screening mammography to digital screening mammography on screening outcome in The Netherlands: a population-based study. Ann Oncol 2012; 23(12):3098–103.

7. Bian T, Lin Q, Cui C, et al. Digital breast tomosynthesis: a new diagnostic method for mass-like lesions in dense breasts. Breast J 2016;22(5):535–40.

8. Agasthya GA, D'Orsi E, Kim YJ, et al. Can breast compression be reduced in digital mammography and breast tomosynthesis? AJR Am J Roentgenol 2017; 209(5):W322–32.

9. Oeffinger KC, Fontham ET, Etzioni R, et al. Breast cancer screening for women at average risk: 2015 guideline update from the American Cancer Society. JAMA 2015;314(15):1599–614.

10. Myers ER, Moorman P, Gierisch JM, et al. Benefits and harms of breast cancer screening: a systematic review. JAMA 2015;314(15):1615–34.

11. Siu AL. Screening for breast cancer: U.S. Preventive Services Task Force recommendation statement. Ann Intern Med 2016;164(4):279–96.

12. Nelson HD, Cantor A, Humphrey L, et al. U.S. Preventive Services Task Force evidence syntheses, formerly systematic evidence reviews. In: Screening for breast cancer: a systematic review to update the 2009 U.S. Preventive Services Task Force recommendation. Rockville (MD): Agency for Healthcare Research and Quality (US); 2016. p. 1–45.

13. Mandelblatt JS, Stout NK, Schechter CB, et al. Collaborative modeling of the benefits and harms associated with different U.S. breast cancer screening strategies. Ann Intern Med 2016;164(4):215–25.

14. NCCN. Breast cancer screening and diagnosis. Version 1.2016.

15. Roder D, Houssami N, Farshid G, et al. Population screening and intensity of screening are associated with reduced breast cancer mortality: evidence of efficacy of mammography screening in Australia. Breast Cancer Res Treat 2008; 108(3):409–16.

16. Jonsson H, Bordas P, Wallin H, et al. Service screening with mammography in Northern Sweden: effects on breast cancer mortality - an update. J Med Screen 2007;14(2):87–93.

17. Arias E. United States Life Tables, 2011. National vital statistics reports: from the Centers for Disease Control and Prevention, National Center for Health Statistics, National Vital Statistics System. 2015;64(11):1–63.

18. Lehman CD, Arao RF, Sprague BL, et al. National performance benchmarks for modern screening digital mammography: update from the breast cancer surveillance consortium. Radiology 2017;283(1):49–58.

19. Grabler P, Sighoko D, Wang L, et al. Recall and cancer detection rates for screening mammography: finding the sweet spot. AJR Am J Roentgenol 2017; 208(1):208–13.

20. Blanchard K, Colbert JA, Kopans DB, et al. Long-term risk of false-positive screening results and subsequent biopsy as a function of mammography use. Radiology 2006;240(2):335–42.

21. Hendrick RE, Helvie MA. United States Preventive Services Task Force screening mammography recommendations: science ignored. AJR Am J Roentgenol 2011; 196(2):W112–6.
22. Sutton S, Saidi G, Bickler G, et al. Does routine screening for breast cancer raise anxiety? Results from a three wave prospective study in England. J Epidemiol Community Health 1995;49(4):413–8.
23. Ganott MA, Sumkin JH, King JL, et al. Screening mammography: do women prefer a higher recall rate given the possibility of earlier detection of cancer? Radiology 2006;238(3):793–800.
24. Puliti D, Duffy SW, Miccinesi G, et al. Overdiagnosis in mammographic screening for breast cancer in Europe: a literature review. J Med Screen 2012;19(Suppl 1): 42–56.
25. Miglioretti DL, Lange J, van den Broek JJ, et al. Radiation-induced breast cancer incidence and mortality from digital mammography screening: a modeling study. Ann Intern Med 2016;164(4):205–14.

Breast Cancer Genetics and Indications for Prophylactic Mastectomy

Helen Krontiras, MD[a],*, Meagan Farmer, MS, CGC, MBA[b],
Julie Whatley, RN, BSN, CRNP[a]

KEYWORDS

- Risk-reducing mastectomy • Contralateral prophylactic mastectomy
- Multigene panel testing • BRCA • Genetic counseling

KEY POINTS

- The initial evaluation of patients who may be at risk for hereditary breast cancer begins with a risk assessment.
- There are 3 possible results from genetic testing: positive, negative, or uninformative.
- There are many strategies for breast cancer risk reduction, which include surveillance, risk reducing or prophylactic surgery, and chemoprevention.
- Management decisions should be individualized and may be based on genetic factors as well as personal and family history of breast and other cancers.

Since the first molecular diagnostic test for hereditary breast and ovarian cancer was introduced in 1996, there has been an explosion in the understanding and availability of genetic testing. Multigene panel testing, which uses next-generation sequencing technology to analyze several cancer predisposition genes simultaneously, has become commonplace for individuals suspected to have or be at risk for hereditary breast cancer.

As more genetic information becomes available to inform breast cancer treatment, screening, and risk-reduction approaches, clinicians must become more knowledgeable about possible genetic testing and prevention strategies, including outcomes, benefits, risks, and limitations. The aim of this article is to define and distinguish high- and moderate-risk breast cancer predisposition genes, summarize the clinical recommendations that may be considered based on the identification of pathogenic

Disclosure Statement: The authors have nothing to disclose.
[a] Division of Surgical Oncology, Department of Surgery, University of Alabama at Birmingham, Faculty Office Tower Suite 1153, 1720 2nd Avenue South, Birmingham, AL 35294-3411, USA;
[b] Department of Genetics, University of Alabama at Birmingham, Kaul Human Genetics Building, Suite 230, 720 20th Street, South Birmingham, AL 35294-0024, USA
* Corresponding author.
E-mail address: hkrontir@uabmc.edu

variants (mutations) in these genes, and indications for risk-reducing and contralateral prophylactic mastectomy.

DEFINING HIGH RISK

Initial evaluation of patients who may be at risk for hereditary breast cancer begins with a risk assessment. This assessment includes obtaining detailed information about cancer in the individual and in the family. Specifically, the types of cancer and age of onset are important to determine the potential for inherited breast cancer. Both maternal and paternal sides of the family are relevant and should be considered independently. Various guidelines establish criteria for genetic testing. The National Comprehensive Cancer Network's (NCCN) guidelines[1] are updated annually and provide evidence-based guidance for clinicians to decide which patients should undergo genetic testing (**Box 1**). Ideally, women with or at risk for hereditary breast cancer should be cared for by multidisciplinary teams including both breast and genetics specialists.

If patients meet criteria, it is recommended that they undergo pretest counseling with a complete pedigree evaluation and computational assessment of risk using available statistical models and tables. Using this information as well as the qualitative criteria from the NCCN, the clinician can provide patients with the probability of testing positive in addition to the risk of developing breast cancer. Reflecting on these data as well as the expectations and motivations for testing, patients can then make an informed decision about whether to pursue testing.

The next decision is which test to order and which family member should be tested first. Testing an affected relative is preferable and will yield the most useful information. With the widespread availability and the rapidly decreasing cost of DNA sequencing, the provider has multiple commercial tests to choose from, each with varying turnaround time, insurance coverage, and number of genes analyzed. For patients who have a personal or family history clearly suggestive of a specific hereditary breast cancer syndrome, genetic testing for genes associated with that syndrome makes sense. However, in many circumstances this is not the case. Multigene testing gives the provider the opportunity to analyze multiple genes associated with breast cancer all at one time in an efficient and cost-effective manner. This testing can be particularly helpful when there are other types of cancers in the family in addition to breast and ovarian cancer. These multigene panels often include high-risk genes or high-penetrance genes, meaning pathogenic variants in these genes cause a relatively high risk for female breast cancer, and moderate-risk genes or moderate-penetrance genes, meaning pathogenic variants in these genes cause a moderately increased risk for female breast cancer. Genes considered high risk are generally ones associated with a 50% or greater lifetime risk of breast cancer, and moderate genes are ones generally associated with a 20% to 49% lifetime risk of breast cancer. Pathogenic variants in BRCA1 and BRCA2 (50%–85% lifetime risk of breast cancer), PALB2 (33%–58%), TP53 (Li-Fraumeni Syndrome (50%–90%),[2] PTEN (Cowden syndrome/PTEN hamartoma tumor syndrome) (25%–50%), STK11 (32%–54%), and CDH1 (30%–50%) cause a relatively high lifetime risk for breast cancer.[3] Pathogenic variants in CHEK2 (20%–40% [c.1100delC]), ATM (20%), and NBN (20%–30% [c.675del5]) cause a moderately increased risk for female breast cancer. Pathogenic variants in other genes, such as MRE11A and RAD50, may cause an increased risk for breast cancer; but the exact level of risk is undetermined at this time. **Table 1** lists the lifetime risk of high-penetrance and moderate-penetrance genes and associated cancers.[4]

Box 1
Criteria for genetic risk evaluation

- Patients without a personal history of cancer
  - A close relative with any of the following:
    - A known mutation in a cancer susceptibility gene within the family
    - A first- or second-degree relative with breast cancer at or before 45 years of age
    - Two or more individuals with breast cancer on the same side of the family and at least one diagnosed at or before 50 years of age
    - Two or more breast cancer primaries in a single individual
    - An individual with ovarian cancer, fallopian cancer, or primary peritoneal cancer
    - Male breast cancer
    - Family history of 3 or more of the following (especially if diagnosed at or before 50 years of age): breast cancer, pancreatic cancer, prostate cancer (Gleason score ≥7 or metastatic), melanoma, sarcoma, adrenocortical carcinoma, brain tumors, leukemia, di use gastric cancer, colon cancer, endometrial cancer, thyroid cancer, kidney cancer, dermatologic manifestations and/or macrocephaly, or hamartomatous polyps of gastrointestinal tract

- An individual with a breast cancer diagnosis with any of the following:
  - A known mutation in a cancer susceptibility gene within the family
  - Breast cancer diagnosed at or before 50 years of age
  - Triple negative (ER−, PR−, HER2−) breast cancer diagnosed at or before 60 years of age
  - Two breast cancer primaries
  - Breast cancer at any age and more than 1 close blood relative with breast cancer diagnosed at or before 50 years of age or 1 or more close blood relatives with invasive ovarian cancer at any age
  - Two or more close blood relatives with breast cancer, prostate cancer (Gleason score ≥7 or metastatic), and/or pancreatic cancer at any age
  - Personal history of pancreatic cancer at any age
  - An individual of Ashkenazi Jewish descent with breast, ovarian, or pancreatic cancer at any age
  - Male breast cancer
  - An individual with a personal and/or family history of 3 or more of the following (especially if diagnosed at or before 50 years of age): breast cancer, pancreatic cancer, prostate cancer (Gleason score ≥7 or metastatic), melanoma, sarcoma, adrenocortical carcinoma, brain tumors, leukemia, di use gastric cancer, colon cancer, endometrial cancer, thyroid cancer, kidney cancer, dermatologic manifestations and/or macrocephaly, or hamartomatous polyps of gastrointestinal tract

Abbreviations: ER−, estrogen receptor negative; HER−, human epidermal growth factor receptor 2; PR−, progesterone receptor negative.
Data from Daly MB, Pilarski R, Berry M, et al. NCCN guidelines insights: genetic/familial high-risk assessment: breast and ovarian, version 2.2017. J Natl Compr Canc Netw 2017;15(1):9–20; and American Society of Breast Surgeons. Consensus guideline on hereditary genetic testing for patients with and without breast cancer. 2017. Available at: https://www.breastsurgeons.org/new_layout/about/statements/PDF_Statements/BRCA_Testing.pdf. Accessed December 30, 2017.

INTERPRETATION OF RESULTS

Interpretation of genetic testing results is a critical part of the process. There are 3 possible results from genetic testing: positive, negative, or uninformative. A positive result indicates that a harmful (deleterious or pathogenic) mutation was identified. Negative results are somewhat more complicated, as the results have to be interpreted in the context of the family pedigree. A true negative is when there is a known pathogenic or deleterious mutation in the family and the patients presenting for testing are negative. These individuals have a substantially lower risk of developing breast cancer than a member of the family who does carry the mutation.[5–7] Negative results

Table 1
Genes associated with hereditary breast cancer

Gene	Genes Associated with Hereditary Breast Cancer	Associated Cancers	Lifetime Breast Cancer Risk in Women with Mutation (%)
BRCA1	Hereditary breast and ovarian cancer (HBOC)	Breast cancer, ovarian/fallopian tube cancers, primary peritoneal malignancies	50–85
BRCA2	Hereditary breast and ovarian cancer (HBOC)	Breast cancer, ovarian/fallopian tube cancers, pancreatic cancers, melanomas, prostate cancer	50–85
PALB2	Familial breast cancer	Spectrum of associated cancers may be similar to those in BRCA2	40–60
TP53	Li-Fraumeni syndrome (LFS)	Multiple primary cancers, sarcomas, brain tumors, premenopausal breast cancers, leukemias, adrenocorticocarcinomas	50–90
PTEN	Cowden syndrome (CS)	Breast cancer, thyroid cancers, endometrial cancer, renal cell carcinoma, melanoma, colorectal cancer, endometrial cancers	25–50 (may be up to 85)
STK11	Peutz-Jeghers syndrome (PJS)	Breast cancer, colorectal cancer, gastric cancer, pancreatic cancer, lung cancer, ovarian and testicular cancers	45–50
CGH1	Hereditary diffuse gastric cancer (HDGC)	Diffuse gastric cancer, lobular breast cancer	39–52
CHEK2	Familial breast cancer	Breast cancer, possibly colorectal cancer	20–40 (c.1100delC)
ATM	Familial breast cancer	Breast cancer	20
NBN	Familial breast cancer	Breast cancer	20–30 (c.675del5)
MRE11A	Familial breast cancer	Breast cancer	Undetermined
RAD50	Familial breast cancer	Breast cancer	Undetermined
BRIP1	Familial breast cancer	Breast cancer	20

Data from Rainville IR, Rana HQ. Next-generation sequencing for inherited breast cancer risk: counseling through the complexity. Curr Oncol Rep 2014;16(3):371.

in an unaffected individual when there is not a known deleterious mutation in the family should be interpreted with caution, and every attempt should be made to test an affected relative if possible. Ideally, the youngest and closest in relation to the patients should be tested to clarify the pedigree. When no other relatives are available for testing, a negative result does not eliminate the risk in those patients. Another example of an uninformative result is a variant of unknown significance (VUS). A VUS is a mutation in a gene that is not yet defined to be associated with an increased risk of developing cancer or a normal change in the gene. Over time as more information is gained about the particular mutation, these may be reclassified as deleterious or benign. It is recommended that patients with VUS be managed based on their personal and family history of breast cancer.

MANAGEMENT OF INCREASED RISK

There are many strategies for breast cancer risk reduction. These strategies include surveillance, risk-reducing or prophylactic surgery, and chemoprevention. Management decisions should be individualized and may be based on genetic factors as well as personal and family history of breast and other cancers. In the individual with a known breast cancer, the risk of subsequent cancer should also be taken into consideration.

A systematic review of studies comparing prophylactic bilateral total mastectomy with observation yielded 2 contemporary studies.[8] Neither study demonstrated a survival benefit for prophylactic bilateral mastectomy. Although there has not been a randomized controlled trial to determine the efficacy of prophylactic mastectomy for women at increased risk of breast cancer, retrospective and prospective observational studies demonstrate that prophylactic bilateral mastectomy is effective and decreases the incidence of breast cancer by as much as 90% (and up to 100%) in women with genetic predisposition to breast cancer.[9–12]

Women opting for bilateral prophylactic mastectomy with either skin-sparing or nipple and skin sparing approaches can have synchronous reconstruction without impacting the preventive effects.[13–15] Subcutaneous mastectomy, however, is not recommended for prevention, as it leaves too much glandular breast tissue behind.

Contralateral prophylactic mastectomy (CPM) is a mastectomy of the other breast in the setting of unilateral breast cancer to reduce the risk of a second breast cancer. The use of contralateral mastectomy in the United States is increasing.[16] Characteristics associated with the increasing use of CPM are Caucasian race, higher socioeconomic status, private insurance, high-volume centers, younger age, increasing use of MR imaging, genetic testing, and reconstructive surgery.[17,18] Most patients undergoing CPM do so for "peace of mind."[19] Anxiety and fear of cancer or recurrence of cancer can be a contributing factor in the perception of risk. Many patients often overestimate the cancer outcome benefits of CPM. CPM does reduce the risk of contralateral breast cancer (CBC), but for most patients that risk is quite small. In fact, there has been a declining incidence of CBC in the United States among most women diagnosed with breast cancer.[20] In a study using data from the US Surveillance, Epidemiology, and End Results database, the estimated risk of CBC at 10 years for patients whose first breast cancers were estrogen receptor (ER) positive and who were diagnosed between 2001 and 2005 was less than 5% for all age groups. For women 40 years of age or older with ER-negative first cancers, the estimated 10-year risk of CBC was between 4.7% and 6.3%. For women younger than 40 years with ER-negative first cancers, it was between 6.4% and 12.6%. In a population-based case-control study,[21] the 10-year cumulative risk of CBC in noncarriers of BRCA mutations with unilateral breast cancer and no known family history of breast cancer ranged from 5% to 7% in women diagnosed with their first cancer in their 20s and 30s to approximately 4% in women diagnosed in their 50s. As expected the 10-year cumulative risk of CBC in BRCA 1 and 2 mutation carriers diagnosed with first cancer in their 20s and 30s was much higher at 24% to 31%. Interestingly, in noncarriers with a family history of bilateral breast cancer the 10-year cumulative risk of CBC for the same age group was similar to that of BRCA mutation carriers (18%–24%). Additionally, a large retrospective study from the German Consortium for Hereditary Breast and Ovarian Cancer of more than 2000 women with BRCA1 or 2 deleterious mutations demonstrated that the cumulative risk for CBC after 25 years after first breast cancer diagnosis was 47.4% and was even higher in younger women with BRCA1 mutations specifically.[22] There is a paucity of data regarding CBC risk in other hereditary breast cancer syndromes; however, one study found that the risk of a CBC primary within 5 years in women with a pathogenic PALB2 variant was estimated to be 10%.[23]

Although CPM does reduce the risk of a CBC, CPM does not change the risk of recurrence associated with the index cancer. Compared with less favorable index cancers, the CBCs that do develop are often stage I, T1, node negative, and ER positive.[24] Thus, for most patients, CBCs have very little, if any, impact on survival. However, for a small subset of patients there may be a potential survival benefit. In a retrospective analysis of 181 patients with breast cancer with deleterious BRCA mutations, CPM was associated with a 48% reduction in death from breast cancer.[25] Furthermore, the 20-year survival rate for BRCA1 and 2 carriers undergoing a CPM was 88% compared with a 66% survival rate for carriers treated with a unilateral mastectomy even after controlling for factors, such as age and treatment. In a smaller study of 105 BRCA mutation carriers with case-matched controls, the 10-year overall survival was 89% for the CPM group and 71% for the non-CPM group.[26] As these are retrospective studies, selection bias may confound the results.

When counseling patients considering risk-reducing mastectomy or CPM, it is important to inform patients about the risks, benefits, and alternatives of the operation. In addition, the patients should understand the various options for reconstruction, and a formal consultation with a plastic surgeon is encouraged. Overall health and comorbidities should also be taken into account when considering prophylactic surgery. The decision-making process for patients considering mastectomy is based on many factors, including personal choice as well as influences from clinicians, family, and friends. The NCCN's guidelines for genetic/familial high-risk assessment for breast and ovarian cancer offer recommendations for the management of risk based on genetic test results.[1] For instance, in the case that a pathogenic variant has been identified in BRCA1, BRCA2, TP53, or PTEN, the option of risk-reducing mastectomy should be discussed. However, in the case of other genes associated with breast and ovarian cancer, there is insufficient evidence regarding the benefit of risk-reducing surgery to recommend consideration of prophylactic mastectomy and management should be tailored based on family history.

As with any operation there are risks related to bleeding, infection, and anesthesia. But there are potential side effects and complications unique to mastectomy, such as seroma, skin flap necrosis, nipple necrosis, pain, phantom breast syndrome, arm mobility issues, and lymphedema. The frequency of surgical complications following a bilateral mastectomy is greater than with a unilateral mastectomy, with rates ranging from 5% to 35%.[27–29] Data from the National Surgical Quality Improvement Program confirm these findings.[30,31] Patients who had a bilateral mastectomy were 1.9 times more likely to have postoperative complications than those patients who had unilateral mastectomy. More specifically, bilateral mastectomy was also associated with longer hospital stays and increased transfusion rates. When implant reconstruction was used, there was also an increase in reoperation rates for bilateral mastectomy compared with unilateral mastectomy. However, the rate of surgical site infection and prosthesis or flap failure was less than 5%; there was no statistical difference between the two groups. In addition to potential surgical complications, patients who undergo mastectomy, whether bilateral prophylactic or CPM, may experience changes in body image, self-esteem, perception of femininity, libido, and sexual function.[32–34] Still, most patients report satisfaction with the decision to have CPM and would choose CPM again.[35]

For women who desire to delay or not pursue risk-reducing surgery, breast cancer surveillance is an acceptable option. Based on current the NCCN's guidelines, recommendations for surveillance for those at high risk for breast cancer include annual mammogram and annual breast MRI. At the authors' institution, they stagger each of these by 6 months.[36] Because of the concern for the development of interval cancers, a clinical breast examination every 6 to 12 months is also recommended.[1] Although there are some data about the efficacy of screening breast ultrasound in women who are at an increased risk or with dense breasts,[37] breast ultrasound is not recommended for routine screening but may be used in adjunct to clinical breast examinations, MRI, and mammogram.

Chemoprevention is the use of medications or drugs to reduce the risk of developing cancer. Chemoprevention is less effective than prophylactic mastectomy in the reduction of breast cancer risk. Chemoprevention for the prevention of breast cancer includes selective ER modulators (SERMs) and aromatase inhibitors. Tamoxifen is a SERM that can be considered for high-risk women who opt against or to delay mastectomy, especially if they have a pathogenic BRCA2 variant. There are limited data in the preventive benefit of tamoxifen use in women with pathogenic BRCA variants.[38] The NSABP P-1 trial demonstrated a 62% reduction in breast cancer risk with pathogenic BRCA2 variants versus no risk reduction in women with pathogenic BRCA1 variants.[38] This finding makes sense given the fact that breast cancers that arises in patients with BRCA2 mutations are often ER positive. However, this study was limited in the number of patients with deleterious mutations in BRCA 1 or 2 who developed breast cancer. There are no data regarding raloxifene (another SERM) or aromatase inhibitors and patients with BRCA mutations specifically, but there is evidence of significant reduction in breast cancer risk in women at an increased risk for breast cancer.[39,40]

SUMMARY

Genetic testing for breast cancer has become more complex in the era of next generation sequencing. Physicians charged with the management of patients at increased risk for hereditary breast cancer should individualize recommendations based on genetic factors and personal and family history of breast and other cancers while at the same time listening to and respecting the patient's motivations and desires.

REFERENCES

1. Daly MB, Pilarski R, Berry M, et al. NCCN guidelines insights: genetic/familial high-risk assessment: breast and ovarian, version 2.2017. J Natl Compr Canc Netw 2017;15(1):9–20.

2. Mai PL, Best AF, Peters JA, et al. Risks of first and subsequent cancers among TP53 mutation carriers in the National Cancer Institute Li-Fraumeni syndrome cohort. Cancer 2016;122(23):3673–81.

3. Grignol VP, Agnese DM. Breast cancer genetics for the surgeon: an update on causes and testing options. J Am Coll Surg 2016;222(5):906–14.

4. Rainville IR, Rana HQ. Next-generation sequencing for inherited breast cancer risk: counseling through the complexity. Curr Oncol Rep 2014;16(3):371.

5. Katki HA, Gail MH, Greene MH. Breast-cancer risk in BRCA-mutation-negative women from BRCA-mutation-positive families. Lancet Oncol 2007;8(12):1042–3.

6. Korde LA, Mueller CM, Loud JT, et al. No evidence of excess breast cancer risk among mutation-negative women from BRCA mutation-positive families. Breast Cancer Res Treat 2011;125(1):169–73.

7. Metcalfe KA, Finch A, Poll A, et al. Breast cancer risks in women with a family history of breast or ovarian cancer who have tested negative for a BRCA1 or BRCA2 mutation. Br J Cancer 2009;100(2):421–5.

8. Ludwig KK, Neuner J, Butler A, et al. Risk reduction and survival benefit of prophylactic surgery in BRCA mutation carriers, a systematic review. Am J Surg 2016;212(4):660–9.

9. Hartmann LC, Schaid DJ, Woods JE, et al. Efficacy of bilateral prophylactic mastectomy in women with a family history of breast cancer. N Engl J Med 1999; 340(2):77–84.

10. Hartmann LC, Sellers TA, Schaid DJ, et al. Efficacy of bilateral prophylactic mastectomy in BRCA1 and BRCA2 gene mutation carriers. J Natl Cancer Inst 2001; 93(21):1633–7.

11. Meijers-Heijboer H, van Geel B, van Putten WL, et al. Breast cancer after prophylactic bilateral mastectomy in women with a BRCA1 or BRCA2 mutation. N Engl J Med 2001;345(3):159–64.

12. Domchek SM, Friebel TM, Singer CF, et al. Association of risk-reducing surgery in BRCA1 or BRCA2 mutation carriers with cancer risk and mortality. JAMA 2010; 304(9):967–75.

13. Yao K, Liederbach E, Tang R, et al. Nipple-sparing mastectomy in BRCA1/2 mutation carriers: an interim analysis and review of the literature. Ann Surg Oncol 2015;22(2):370–6.

14. Peled AW, Irwin CS, Hwang ES, et al. Total skin-sparing mastectomy in BRCA mutation carriers. Ann Surg Oncol 2014;21(1):37–41.

15. Manning AT, Wood C, Eaton A, et al. Nipple-sparing mastectomy in patients with BRCA1/2 mutations and variants of uncertain significance. Br J Surg 2015; 102(11):1354–9.

16. Kurian AW, Lichtensztajn DY, Keegan TH, et al. Use of and mortality after bilateral mastectomy compared with other surgical treatments for breast cancer in California, 1998-2011. JAMA 2014;312(9):902–14.

17. Arrington AK, Jarosek SL, Virnig BA, et al. Patient and surgeon characteristics associated with increased use of contralateral prophylactic mastectomy in patients with breast cancer. Ann Surg Oncol 2009;16(10):2697–704.

18. Yao K, Sisco M, Bedrosian I. Contralateral prophylactic mastectomy: current perspectives. Int J Womens Health 2016;8:213–23.

19. Jagsi R, Hawley ST, Griffith KA, et al. Contralateral prophylactic mastectomy decisions in a population-based sample of patients with early-stage breast cancer. JAMA Surg 2017;152(3):274–82.

20. Nichols HB, Berrington de González A, Lacey JV Jr, et al. Declining incidence of contralateral breast cancer in the United States from 1975 to 2006. J Clin Oncol 2011;29(12):1564–9.

21. Reiner AS, John EM, Brooks JD, et al. Risk of asynchronous contralateral breast cancer in noncarriers of BRCA1 and BRCA2 mutations with a family history of breast cancer: a report from the Women's Environmental Cancer and Radiation Epidemiology Study. J Clin Oncol 2013;31(4):433–9.

22. Graeser MK, Engel C, Rhiem K, et al. Contralateral breast cancer risk in BRCA1 and BRCA2 mutation carriers. J Clin Oncol 2009;27(35):5887–92.

23. Cybulski C, Kluzniak W, Huzarski T, et al. Clinical outcomes in women with breast cancer and a PALB2 mutation: a prospective cohort analysis. Lancet Oncol 2015; 16(6):638–44.

24. Liederbach E, Piro R, Hughes K, et al. Clinicopathologic features and time interval analysis of contralateral breast cancers. Surgery 2015;158(3):676–85.

25. Metcalfe K, Gershman S, Ghadirian P, et al. Contralateral mastectomy and survival after breast cancer in carriers of BRCA1 and BRCA2 mutations: retrospective analysis. BMJ 2014;348:g226.

26. Evans DG, Ingham SL, Baildam A, et al. Contralateral mastectomy improves survival in women with BRCA1/2-associated breast cancer. Breast Cancer Res Treat 2013;140(1):135–42.

27. Craft RO, Colakoglu S, Curtis MS, et al. Patient satisfaction in unilateral and bilateral breast reconstruction [outcomes article]. Plast Reconstr Surg 2011;127(4): 1417–24.

28. Koslow S, Pharmer LA, Scott AM, et al. Long-term patient-reported satisfaction after contralateral prophylactic mastectomy and implant reconstruction. Ann Surg Oncol 2013;20(11):3422–9.

29. Eck DL, Perdikis G, Rawal B, et al. Incremental risk associated with contralateral prophylactic mastectomy and the effect on adjuvant therapy. Ann Surg Oncol 2014;21(10):3297–303.

30. Osman F, Saleh F, Jackson TD, et al. Increased postoperative complications in bilateral mastectomy patients compared to unilateral mastectomy: an analysis of the NSQIP database. Ann Surg Oncol 2013;20(10):3212–7.

31. Silva AK, Lapin B, Yao KA, et al. The effect of contralateral prophylactic mastectomy on perioperative complications in women undergoing immediate breast reconstruction: a NSQIP analysis. Ann Surg Oncol 2015;22(11):3474–80.

32. Gopie JP, Mureau MA, Seynaeve C, et al. Body image issues after bilateral prophylactic mastectomy with breast reconstruction in healthy women at risk for hereditary breast cancer. Fam Cancer 2013;12(3):479–87.

33. Brandberg Y, Sandelin K, Erikson S, et al. Psychological reactions, quality of life, and body image after bilateral prophylactic mastectomy in women at high risk for breast cancer: a prospective 1-year follow-up study. J Clin Oncol 2008;26(24): 3943–9.

34. Frost MH, Schaid DJ, Sellers TA, et al. Long-term satisfaction and psychological and social function following bilateral prophylactic mastectomy. JAMA 2000; 284(3):319–24.

35. Boughey JC, Hoskin TL, Hartmann LC, et al. Impact of reconstruction and reoperation on long-term patient-reported satisfaction after contralateral prophylactic mastectomy. Ann Surg Oncol 2015;22(2):401–8.

36. Lowry KP, Lee JM, Kong CY, et al. Annual screening strategies in BRCA1 and BRCA2 gene mutation carriers: a comparative effectiveness analysis. Cancer 2012;118(8):2021–30.

37. Brem RF, Lenihan MJ, Lieberman J, et al. Screening breast ultrasound: past, present, and future. AJR Am J Roentgenol 2015;204(2):234–40.

38. Dunn BK, Ford LG. Breast cancer prevention: results of the National Surgical Adjuvant Breast and Bowel Project (NSABP) breast cancer prevention trial (NSABP P-1: BCPT). Eur J Cancer 2000;36(Suppl 4):S49–50.

39. Vogel VG. The NSABP study of tamoxifen and raloxifene (STAR) trial. Expert Rev Anticancer Ther 2009;9(1):51–60.

40. Goss PE, Ingle JN, Ales-Martinez JE, et al. Exemestane for breast-cancer prevention in postmenopausal women. N Engl J Med 2011;364(25):2381–91.

Incorporating Biologic Factors into the American Joint Committee on Cancer Breast Cancer Staging System

Review of the Supporting Evidence

Anna Weiss, MD[a], Tari A. King, MD[b], Kelly K. Hunt, MD[c], Elizabeth A. Mittendorf, MD, PhD[a],*

KEYWORDS

- AJCC staging System • Breast cancer • Anatomic stage • Prognostic stage
- Biomarkers

KEY POINTS

- The AJCC 8th edition has defined clinical and pathologic prognostic stages incorporating biologic factors with standard tumor (T), node (N), and metastasis (M) categories.
- The prognostic staging systems facilitate more refined stratification with respect to survival outcomes than the anatomic stage.
- Given the large number of possible combinations of T, N, and M categories with grade, ER, PR, and HER2, there will be challenges incorporating the prognostic staging system into the multidisciplinary care of patients with breast cancer.

BREAST CANCER STAGING: THE FUNDAMENTALS

Historically, the American Joint Committee on Cancer (AJCC) staging system has assigned stage for patients with breast cancer based on the size of their primary tumor (T), the presence and extent of lymph node involvement (N), and the presence or absence of distant metastasis (M). The T, N, and M categories are determined and this corresponds with a specific disease stage. A clinical stage is assigned at the time of

Disclosure Statement: Dr E.A. Mittendorf is a member of the AJCC expert panel. Dr A. Weiss, T. A. King, and K.K. Hunt have nothing to disclose.
[a] Breast Surgical Oncology, Dana-Farber/Brigham and Women's Cancer Center, 450 Brookline Avenue, Suite 1470, Boston, MA 02215, USA; [b] Breast Surgical Oncology, Dana-Farber/Brigham and Women's Cancer Center, 450 Brookline Avenue, Suite 1220, Boston, MA 02215, USA; [c] Department of Breast Surgical Oncology, The University of Texas MD Anderson Cancer Center, 1400 Pressler Street, Unit 1434, Houston, TX 77030, USA
* Corresponding author.
E-mail address: emittendorf@bwh.harvard.edu

Surg Clin N Am 98 (2018) 687–702
https://doi.org/10.1016/j.suc.2018.03.005
surgical.theclinics.com
0039-6109/18/© 2018 Elsevier Inc. All rights reserved.

diagnosis with a pathologic stage assigned after surgery. The primary goal of staging is to inform prognosis. In addition, staging information has been incorporated into management guidelines and is used to help determine a treatment plan.[1] By providing a common framework, staging also facilitates communication between providers, is used to define groups of patients for inclusion on clinical trials, and can facilitate standardized data collection allowing for the evaluation of the impact of changes in clinical practice.

Since publication of the first AJCC staging manual in 1977,[2] the breast cancer staging system has undergone multiple revisions to reflect advances in diagnosis and treatment. For example, with the 6th edition published in 2002, there were significant changes related to the detection method, size, number, and location of regional lymph node metastases.[3] These changes reflected several factors to include the routine use of sentinel lymph node dissection in patients with clinically node-negative breast cancer; use of immunohistochemistry (IHC) in the pathologic evaluation of sentinel lymph nodes leading to the identification of small-volume metastatic disease; and new information regarding the clinical importance of the total number of positive axillary lymph nodes and the outcomes associated with metastases to the supraclavicular, infraclavicular, and internal mammary lymph nodes.[4]

Although previous revisions to the AJCC breast cancer staging system largely reflected improvements in imaging, surgery, and pathology leading to earlier detection and more refined determination of the anatomic extent of disease, they failed to account for biologic factors that are known to have predictive and prognostic value. Included among these are grade, estrogen (ER) and progesterone (PR) receptor status, and HER2 status, which are part of the routine pathologic assessment of breast tumors and influence management of patients with breast cancer.[5,6] Recommendations for treatment and the response to therapy are determined by these factors, therefore patient prognosis within each TNM stage varies based on these biologic features.[1,7–10] Recognizing this, the recently revised 8th edition of the AJCC breast cancer staging manual has incorporated biologic factors into newly defined clinical and pathologic prognostic stages.[11] These prognostic stages provide more refined stratification with respect to survival estimates for patients receiving appropriate systemic therapy.

EVIDENCE TO SUPPORT THE INCLUSION OF BIOLOGIC FACTORS IN BREAST CANCER STAGING

The breast cancer expert panel convened to revise the AJCC staging system, which included one author of the current article (EAM), noted that breast cancer represents a group of diseases with different molecular characteristics resulting in different patterns of dissemination, recurrence, sensitivities to available therapies, and prognoses.[11] Furthermore, it was noted that when breast cancer clinicians communicate regarding patients, they do so most often by referring to the specific biologic subtype: hormone receptor (HR)-positive/HER2-negative, HR+/HER2+, HR-/HER2+ or triple negative (HR-/HER2-). Therefore, for the 8th edition staging system to maintain relevance in clinical practice, the panel believed it important to include biologic factors. Having made that determination, the panel was challenged by the lack of level I evidence available to support the impact of biologic factors on prognosis.

Novel Staging System Incorporating Prognostic Factors

Several groups have called the classic anatomic staging system into question and proposed staging models incorporating biologic factors to provide more refined prognostic information than anatomic factors alone.[7,12–16] One such model was developed by our group at The University of Texas MD Anderson Cancer Center using a prospectively maintained database that included 3728 patients with invasive breast cancer treated with surgery as the first intervention between 1997 and 2006.[16] For all patients, the AJCC TNM stage, grade, and ER and PR status were known. Importantly, the study predated routine HER2 testing and use of trastuzumab in patients with HER2-positive disease. Univariate and multivariate analyses were performed to identify factors associated with disease-specific survival (DSS) calculated from the time of surgery to breast cancer–specific death. Candidate factors included pathologic stage; Black nuclear grade; the presence of lymphovascular invasion; ER status; PR status; combination of ER and PR; and combination of ER, PR, and HER2 status. Factors identified as independent predictors for DSS on univariate analyses were assigned points based on the hazard ratio from the multivariate analyses. Binary factors with increased risk over their reference group were assigned 1 point; ordinal factors with a hazard ratio of 1.1 to 3 were assigned 1 point; and factors with a hazard ratio of 3.1 to 6 were assigned 2 points (**Table 1**). A staging score was calculated by summing scores for the individual DSS predictors. Using definitive pathologic stage as the backbone, models were then created by varying combinations of those prognostic factors. There were six models generated: (1) pathologic stage alone; (2) pathologic stage and grade; (3) pathologic stage, grade, and lymphovascular invasion; (4) pathologic stage, grade, and ER; (5) pathologic stage, grade, and combination of ER and PR; and (6) pathologic stage, grade, and combination of ER, PR, and HER2. The predictive abilities of the model staging systems were calculated by Harrell concordance index (C-index),[17] which measures the concordance of predicted and observed outcomes and can range from 0 (perfect discordance) to 1 (perfect concordance), and Akalke Information Criterion (AIC), which measures model fit.[18] A model with a lower AIC value is more accurate. Using C-index and AIC, the best models were determined to be pathologic stage + grade + ER (C-index = 0.80, AIC = 1931.9), and pathologic stage + grade + ER/PR combination (C-index = 0.80, AIC = 1927.3) (**Fig. 1**). In contrast, for pathologic stage alone, the C-index was 0.68 and AIC was 2038.4. These data showed that a staging model that included biologic factors facilitated better survival discrimination than a staging system using anatomic factors alone. This model was internally validated using bootstrapping technique, and externally validated using a dataset of 26,711 patients from Surveillance, Epidemiology, and End Results (C-index of 0.80).[16]

Bioscore

The initial effort undertaken at MD Anderson to develop a staging model incorporating biologic factors was limited by the fact that the time period studied predated routine HER2 testing and use of trastuzumab in the treatment of patients with HER2-positive disease. Analyses were therefore repeated in a subsequent cohort of 3327 patients with invasive breast cancer treated with surgery as a first intervention at MD Anderson between 2007 and 2013.[13] This second study included 306 patients with HER2-positive breast cancer that were treated with trastuzumab. For this analysis, two sets of models were created: one using pathologic stage as the backbone, and one using T and N categories as separate factors (TN). Multivariate analyses were again performed and points assigned to prognostic factors based on hazards ratios. When models were evaluated, the two models that incorporated grade, ER, and HER2 performed best. The pathologic

Table 1
Points assigned for prognostic factors in initial MD Anderson staging system

Factor	Points Assigned
Pathologic stage	
I	0
IIA	1
IIB	1
IIIA	2
Grade	
I	0
II	0
III	1
ER status	
Positive	0
Negative	1
ER and PR status	
ER+/PR+	0
ER+/PR−	0
ER−/PR−	1
ER−/PR+	2
HR and HER2	
HR+/HER2−	0
HR+/HER2+	0
HR−/HER2+	0
HR−/HER2−	1
Lymphovascular invasion	
Absent	0
Present	1

HR designated as positive if either ER or PR were positive.

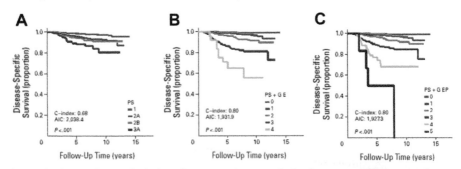

Fig. 1. Kaplan-Meier survival plots demonstrating association between different staging systems and disease-specific survival in patients with breast cancer. (*A*) PS. (*B*) PS plus G and E status. (*C*) PS plus G, E, and P status. E, estrogen receptor; G, nuclear grade; P, progesterone receptor; PS, pathologic state. *P* value indicates log-rank test for comparison. (*From* Yi M, Mittendorf EA, Cormier JN, et al. Novel staging system for predicting disease-specific survival in patients with breast cancer treated with surgery as the first intervention: time to modify the current American Joint Committee on Cancer Staging System. J Clin Oncol 2011;29:4658; with permission.)

stage + grade + ER + HER2 model had a C-index of 0.813 and AIC of 993.9 (**Fig. 2A**). The T + N + grade + ER + HER2 model had a C-index of 0.811 and AIC of 988.8 (**Fig. 2B**). Both of these were superior to the AJCC pathologic stage alone, which had a C-index of 0.74 and AIC of 1041.5 (**Fig. 2C**). Based on these data, the Bioscore, which incorporates pathologic stage and biologic factors to stratify patients with respect to DSS, was proposed (**Table 2**). An individual patient's Bioscore ranges from 0 (ie, a T1, N0 [pathologic stage I], grade 1, ER+, HER2+ breast cancer) to 7 (ie, a T3, N3 [pathologic stage IIIC], grade 3, ER-, HER2- breast cancer) depending on the points assigned for the pathologic stage and each of the biologic factors. The increased discriminatory capacity of the Bioscore was shown by variation in the 5-year DSS from 33.3% to 100% by Bioscore versus 79.5% to 99.1% for the AJCC pathologic stage (**Table 3**). The Bioscore model was subsequently validated using data from 67,944 patients with breast cancer treated between 2005 and 2010 identified in the California Cancer Registry, a large population-based database.[13]

Although the Bioscore incorporates the pathologic stage as determined by T, N, and M categories, it does not strictly maintain the traditional pathologic stage. Specifically, the Bioscore translates the pathologic stage to a point score then adds additional points to reflect the biologic characteristics. This was a concern of the AJCC expert panel when the Bioscore was considered for inclusion in the 8th edition revisions of the breast cancer staging system. Maintenance of a TNM anatomic stage within the 8th edition was believed to be important for several reasons, primarily because in low- and middle-income countries, resources are not always available to evaluate for molecular markers.[11] In addition, expensive therapies, to include those targeting HER2 for patients with HER2-positive breast cancer, may not be available. It is anticipated therefore that the TNM anatomic stage will continue to be used in evaluating patients with breast cancer and making treatment decisions in these countries. The anatomic stage will also remain a common terminology for clinicians regardless of the country where they practice. Finally, the anatomic stage will remain a link to the past allowing for comparison of studies and patient populations.[11]

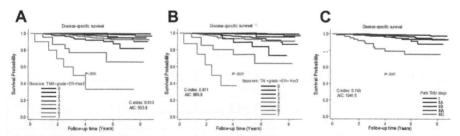

Fig. 2. Kaplan-Meier survival plots demonstrating association between revised biology-based staging systems and disease-specific survival in patients with breast cancer. (*A*) Bioscore using pathologic stage (TNM) as backbone with the additional biologic factors grade, ER, and HER2 status incorporated. (*B*) Tumor and node (TN) categories as backbone with the additional biologic factors grade, ER, and HER2 status incorporated. (*C*) Anatomic pathologic stage (TNM). *P* value indicates log-rank test for comparison. (*Modified from* Mittendorf EA, Chavez-MacGregor M, Vila J, et al. Bioscore: a staging system for breast cancer patients that reflects the prognostic significance of underlying tumor biology. Ann Surg Oncol 2017;24:3506; with permission.)

Table 2
Points assigned for prognostic factors to calculate the Bioscore

Factor	Points Assigned
Pathologic stage	
I (A and B)	0
IIA	1
IIB	2
IIIA	3
IIIC	4
Grade	
I	0
II	0
III	1
ER status	
Positive	0
Negative	1
HER2 status	
Positive	0
Negative	1

Risk Score

To address the concern regarding maintaining an anatomic stage, our group at MD Anderson subsequently developed a risk score that is used to modify a patient's TNM stage to provide refined prognostic information based on biologic features. The risk score was initially developed in the cohort of patients treated at MD Anderson from 2007 to 2013 with surgery as an initial intervention. A Cox proportional hazards model was used to identify factors independently associated with outcome.[19] Taking the results of the multivariable model into account, a point-based risk score system (range, 0–3 points) was created (**Table 4**). To calculate the risk score, one point was assigned for each one of the following tumor characteristics: HR-negative status,

Table 3
Five-year DSS based on AJCC pathologic stage versus Bioscore

Pathologic Stage	DSS (%)	95% CI	Bioscore	DSS (%)	95% CI
I (A and B)	99.1	98.5–99.5	0	100	—
IIA	98.0	96.5–98.8	1	99.4	98.8–99.8
IIB	95.6	92.3–97.5	2	99.2	98.0–99.7
IIIA	95.4	89.7–98.0	3	97.2	95.2–98.4
IIIC	79.5	65.6–88.2	4	94.2	90.1–96.7
			5	92.0	84.5–96.0
			6	77.3	53.6–89.9
			7	33.3	6.3–64.6

Abbreviation: CI, confidence interval.
Modified from Mittendorf EA, Chavez-MacGregor M, Vila J, et al. Bioscore: a staging system for breast cancer patients that reflects the prognostic significance of underlying tumor biology. Ann Surg Oncol 2017;24:3506; with permission.

Table 4
Points assigned to calculate the risk score

Factor	0 Points	1 Point
Grade	1 or 2	3
ER status	Positive	Negative
HER2 status	Positive	Negative

HER2-negative status, and grade 3. Thus, a patient with an invasive ductal carcinoma grade 1, HR-positive, HER2-positive breast cancer has a risk score of 0; one with a grade 3 HR-negative, HER2-positive tumor is assigned a risk score of 2; and a patient with a grade 3 triple negative breast cancer has a risk score of 3. Univariate survival analyses according to stage (I, IIA, IIB, IIIA, and IIIC) and risk score were performed for DSS and overall survival (OS) using the Kaplan-Meier method. The log-rank test was used to compare differences among groups. The distribution of AJCC pathologic stage with risk score modification is shown in **Table 5**. Within each pathologic stage, the risk score stratified patients with respect to 5-year DSS and OS. The ability of the risk score to stratify patients within an AJCC pathologic stage was more pronounced in patients with higher pathologic stage.

A subsequent analysis performed in a cohort of 43,938 patients with stage I-IV breast cancer treated between 2005 and 2008 identified in the California Cancer Registry further supported use of the risk score.[7] In this study, patients were placed into four breast cancer subtypes: (1) HR+/HER2-, (2) HR+/HER2+, (3) HR-/HER2+, and (4) HR-/HER2-. A Cox proportional hazards model was used and grade, ER, and HER2 were again identified as the most important prognostic factors in addition to pathologic stage. Applying the same risk score, it was again shown that survival

Table 5
Survival outcomes by risk score

Stage	Risk Score	n	5-y DSS	95% CI	5-y OS	95% CI
I (IA and IB)	0	36	100	—	97	80.4–99.6
	1	1177	99.4	98.7–99.8	96.7	95.4–97.6
	2	278	98.8	96.4–99.6	94.6	91.1–96.8
	3	119	96.6	91.1–98.7	93.8	87.5–97.0
IIA	0	31	100	—	96.8	79.2–99.5
	1	637	99.4	97.5–99.8	97.1	94.7–98.5
	2	236	97.5	93.2–99.1	94.1	88.7–97.0
	3	98	91	81.8–95.7	88.2	78.5–93.8
IIB	0	11	100	—	100	—
	1	309	96.9	92.6–98.8	94.6	89.6–97.2
	2	107	92.9	83.6–97.0	89.3	80.1–94.4
	3	40	91.5	75.6–97.2	91.5	75.6–97.2
IIIA	0	3	100	—	100	—
	1	135	98.3	88.4–99.8	91.7	82.8–96.1
	2	51	92.4	77.8–97.6	90.5	76.2–96.4
	3	7	68.6	21.3–91.2	68.6	21.3–91.2
IIIC	0	0	—	—	—	—
	1	39	92.2	72.1–98.0	84.4	63.7–93.9
	2	16	80.8	51.4–93.4	80.8	51.4–93.4
	3	10	33.3	6.3–64.6	33.3	6.3–64.6

outcomes (breast cancer–specific survival and OS) vary by the risk score within a pathologic stage group (**Fig. 3**). One benefit of the risk score is that it is consistent intuitively with how clinicians think about breast cancer subtype impacting prognosis within a stage group.

National Cancer Database

A group led by Dr David Winchester, another member of the AJCC breast cancer expert panel, used the National Cancer Data Base (NCDB) to evaluate the prognostic significance of biologic factors in breast cancer. The analysis included 238,265 patients with invasive breast cancer treated from 2010 to 2011 with a complete set of variables that included the AJCC 7th edition stage group, tumor grade, ER, PR, and HER2 status.[11] Median follow-up for the cohort was 37.6 months. Survival calculations were performed for each prognostic subgroup based on the possible combinations of stage group with biologic variables. These analyses showed that patients with triple negative tumors, regardless of grade, had decreased survival comparable with patients with at least one stage higher disease as determined by the 7th edition TNM stage. Conversely, subgroups with tumors expressing both ER and PR had improved survival compared with others with the same 7th edition TNM stage grouping. These findings were consistent with the observations made with implementation of the risk score. These combinations of T, N, and M category with grade, ER, PR, and HER2 status could then be assigned one of nine stage groups (0, IA, IB, IIA, IIB, IIIA, IIIB, IIIC, IV) to maintain consistency with previous breast cancer staging groups.

THE 8TH EDITION AMERICAN JOINT COMMITTEE ON CANCER PROGNOSTIC STAGE

The AJCC breast cancer expert panel used the NCDB analyses to establish a prognostic stage that was incorporated into the 8th edition of the staging manual published in October 2016 with the intent to begin use by cancer registrars in January 2018.[11] When using the NCDB data, the panel cited the fact that the NCDB captures patients

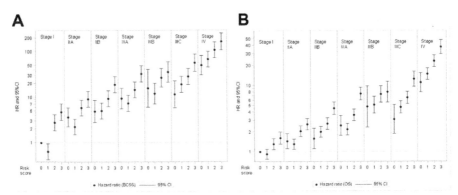

Fig. 3. HR among patients with breast cancer for (*A*) breast cancer specific survival and (*B*) overall survival according to stage and risk score. Risk score was assigned according to a point system: 1 point if estrogen receptor negative, 1 point if HER2 negative, and 1 point for grade 3 disease. Reference group was stage 1 risk 0. Bars represent 95% CI. Adjusted for age, receipt of radiation therapy, receipt of chemotherapy, and surgery type (breast conservation/mastectomy/none). CI, confidence interval; HR, hazard ratio. (*From* Chavez-MacGregor M, Mittendorf EA, Clarke CA, et al. Incorporating tumor characteristics to the American Joint Committee on Cancer breast cancer staging system. Oncologist 2017;22:1297; with permission.)

treated at approximately 1500 Commission on Cancer accredited facilities, representing more than 70% of newly diagnosed cancers. In addition, most women in the NCDB were treated with appropriate systemic therapy to include endocrine therapy, HER2-targeted therapy, and chemotherapy.[11] Finally, the NCDB analysis maintained consistency with previous staging editions by using the T, N, and M categories (ie, the anatomic stage) as the backbone and by grouping combinations of T, N, M, grade, ER, PR, and HER2 into the widely recognized nine breast cancer stages (0, IA, IB, IIA, IIB, IIIA, IIIB, IIIC, IV).

To determine a patient's prognostic stage, the T category, N category, M category, grade, ER status, PR status, and HER2 status must be known. With respect to determining grade, the Nottingham combined histologic grade is recommended. Using this system, grade is determined by assessing the morphologic features of tubule formation, nuclear pleomorphism, and mitotic count.[20,21] ER and PR status are to be determined using IHC with staining of 1% or more of cells being considered positive.[5] HER2 status is determined either by IHC staining for protein expression or by in situ hybridization (either fluorescent or chromogenic) to assess gene copy number. Using IHC, a score of 3+ is considered positive; using in situ hybridization, a HER2/CEP17 ratio greater than or equal to 2.0 or HER2 copy number greater than or equal to six regardless of ratio is considered positive.[6] Once all of the variables are known, the published 8th edition AJCC staging manual provides tables that allow for determination of the prognostic stage. For example, for a patient with a T2 N1 M0 tumor that is grade 1, HER2-, ER+, and PR-, the prognostic stage is IIIA. If that patient's T2 N1 M0 tumor is grade 3, HER2-, ER+, and PR-, the stage is IIIB. If T2 N1 M0, grade 3, HER2-, ER-, and PR-, it is stage IIIC. In total, there are 152 possible combinations of T, N, M, grade, HER2, ER, and PR included in this original prognostic stage.

The expert panel revising the AJCC staging system also discussed incorporation of multigene panels into the staging system. Most of these panels test for levels of expression of a large number of genes in the tumor at the RNA level. Several multigene panels are in use because of studies showing their value in providing more specific prognostic information and in defining sensitivity to systemic therapy, especially chemotherapy. Among these panels are Oncotype Dx,[22–24] Mammaprint,[25,26] Endo-Predict,[27] PAM50,[28–30] and Breast Cancer Index.[31,32] At the time the 8th edition staging system was submitted for publication in August 2016, it was believed that the only multigene panel for which there was level one evidence was Oncotype Dx based on the first publication of results from the TAILORx study.[24] Oncotype Dx is a genomic test that assesses 21 genes, and based on the result of a mathematical formula of the weighted expression of each gene, reports a recurrence score. Studies using Oncotype DX in archived tissues collected from National Surgical Adjuvant Breast and Bowel Project trials have demonstrated that the recurrence score has prognostic and predictive value in patients with node negative, HR+ breast cancer.[22,23] The TAILORx study, which was designed as a prospective validation of the Oncotype Dx recurrence score, enrolled patients with HR+, HER2-, node negative breast cancer with a primary tumor between 1.1 and 5.0 cm (or 0.6–1.0 cm if intermediate or high grade). Patients with an Oncotype Dx recurrence score less than 11 were thought to be at very low risk, therefore they were assigned to receive endocrine therapy alone without chemotherapy. The trial enrolled 10,253 patients including 1626 with a recurrence score less than 11. At 5 years, the invasive disease-free survival rate for these patients was 93.8%, the rate of freedom from local regional or distant recurrence of breast cancer was 98.7%, the rate of freedom from distant recurrence was 99.3%, and the OS rate was 98.0%.[24] These data confirmed a low-risk population that did well with endocrine therapy alone and prompted the AJCC expert panel to incorporate the Oncotype Dx recurrence score into the 8th edition prognostic stage. Specifically, for patients with T1-T2 N0 M0, ER+, HER2-breast cancer with a recurrence score less than 11, the prognostic stage is IA.[11]

Validation of the 8th Edition of the American Joint Committee on Cancer Prognostic Stage

Following publication of the 8th edition AJCC prognostic stage in October 2016, our group sought to validate this staging system using a single institution cohort from MD Anderson and the large California Cancer Registry population database.[33] The MD Anderson cohort included 3327 patients with stage I-IIIC breast cancer treated between 2007 and 2013. A critical observation was that in 451 (13.6%) patients, a prognostic stage could not be assigned because of the presence of N1mi disease in patients with tumors larger than T1 (n = 96) or because of uncategorized combinations of T and N categories with grade, ER, PR, and HER2 status (n = 355). For those in whom a prognostic stage could be determined, compared with the AJCC anatomic stage, 29.5% of patients were upstaged and 28.1% were downstaged. DSS was calculated using the Kaplan-Meier method for all patients in whom both an anatomic and prognostic stage could be determined. Median follow-up was 5 years. The prognostic staging system (C-index = 0.8357 and AIC = 816.8) provided more accurate stratification with respect to DSS than the anatomic stage (C-index = 0.737 and AIC = 1039.8) (Fig. 4A, B).

In the cohort of 54,727 patients with breast cancer with stage I-IV disease identified in the California Cancer Registry, median follow-up of 7 years, a prognostic stage could not be determined in 3745 (6.8%) because of the presence of N1mi disease in patients with tumors larger than T1 (n = 1181) or uncategorized combinations of T and N stage with biologic factors (n = 2654). In patients in whom a prognostic stage

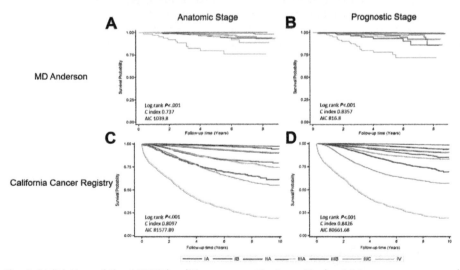

Fig. 4. Validation of the AJCC 8th edition prognostic stage. Kaplan-Meier curves were used to determine disease-specific survival for a cohort of patients treated with surgery as an initial intervention at the MD Anderson Cancer Center according to anatomic and prognostic stages (A, B) and for a cohort from the California Cancer Registry (C, D). (*Modified from* Weiss A, Chavez-MacGregor M, Lichtensztajn DY, et al. Validation Study of the American Joint Committee on Cancer eighth edition prognostic stage compared with the anatomic stage in breast cancer. JAMA Oncol 2018;4(2):206; with permission.)

could be assigned, this upstaged 30.9% and downstaged 20.6%. When the prognostic stage was used to stratify patients with respect to DSS, it again outperformed the anatomic stage with a C-index of 0.8426 versus 0.8097 and an AIC of 80661.68 versus 81,577.89 (**Fig. 4**C, D). Although this work confirmed that the prognostic stage incorporating biologic variables did stratify patients with respect to survival outcomes, there was concern regarding the number of patients for whom a prognostic stage could not be determined.

REVISIONS TO THE 8TH EDITION PROGNOSTIC STAGE

In light of the findings from our group and others that a percentage of patients could not be assigned a prognostic stage, the expert panel has revised the 8th edition AJCC breast cancer staging manual. Important revisions addressed (1) staging for patients with pN1mi disease and T2 or T3 tumors, (2) uncategorized combinations of T and N stage and biologic factors, and (3) additional data available regarding the use of multigene molecular profiling. The revised version is available online (https://cancerstaging.org/references-tools/deskreferences/Pages/Breast-Cancer-Staging.aspx).

Staging for Patients with pN1mi Disease

It is uncommon that patients with tumors larger than 2 cm have micrometastases in their sentinel lymph nodes in the absence of macrometastases. In the study performed to validate the 8th edition AJCC staging system, this occurred in 2.9% of patients in the MD Anderson cohort and 2.1% of patients in the California Cancer Registry cohort.[33] It was acknowledged, however, by the AJCC expert panel that clarification regarding how to stage these patients was required. Therefore, in the revised 8th edition breast cancer staging manual, a note was added to the anatomic stage tables indicating that T2, T3, and T4 tumors with nodal micrometastases (N1mi) are staged using the N1 category based on expert consensus. Therefore, a patient with pT2N1mi disease is staged the same as a patient with pT2N1 disease, anatomic stage IIB. The anatomic stage IB designation is reserved for patients with T0N1mi or T1N1mi disease. Future revisions to the AJCC breast cancer staging system should further evaluate the pN1mi designation. Specifically, additional analyses of available data should be performed to determine whether outcomes for patients with T2-T4N1mi disease more closely resemble those of patients with T2-T2N0 or T2-T4N1 disease. In a previous study from our group we evaluated the significance of the anatomic stage IB designation, so the impact of pN1mi disease in patients with T1 tumors. The study included a cohort of 3474 patients treated at MD Anderson and 4590 patients treated on the American College of Surgeons Oncology Group Z0010 trial showed no significant differences between patients with stage IA and stage IB disease with respect to 5-year or 10-year recurrence-free survival, DSS, or OS.[34] These data indicated that for patients with T1 tumors, those with pN1mi disease had outcomes similar to those with pN0 disease. In that study, grade and ER status significantly stratified stage I patients with respect to these survival end points providing additional evidence regarding the importance of biologic factors in informing prognosis.

Uncategorized Combinations of T and N Stage and Biologic Factors

The identification of uncategorized combinations of T and N stage and biologic factors was the primary impetus behind the AJCC expert panel providing a revision so quickly after initial publication of the 8th edition staging system. To revise the prognostic stage, two analyses were performed resulting in a clinical prognostic stage that is to be determined for all patients with breast cancer and a pathologic prognostic stage that is to be determined for patients that undergo surgery as the first intervention.[35] These analyses used an expanded dataset from the NCDB that included 334,243 patients diagnosed with invasive breast cancer between 2010 and 2012 (initial analysis included patients diagnosed 2010–2011). Median follow-up was 41.7 months. The first analysis, used to define the clinical prognostic stage, included all patients. The second analysis, used to define the pathologic prognostic stage, included 305,519 patients from that cohort who had surgery as their initial intervention. In both analyses, T, N, and M categories were again combined with grade, ER, PR, and HER2 to define prognostic stage groups. The 3-year OS was calculated for each prognostic stage group and compared with the 7th edition staging for each patient. If the calculated survival of a prognostic stage group was higher or lower than the 95% confidence interval of the 7th edition stage, then the subgroup was either downstaged or upstaged as appropriate. Similar to the first iteration of the prognostic stage, based on the survival analyses, the combinations of T, N, M, grade, ER, PR, and HER2 were assigned to the established stage groups: stage 0 for ductal carcinoma in situ, stage IV for metastatic disease, and seven intervening stage groups (IA, IB, IIA, IIB, IIIA, IIIB, IIIC). As had been established with the initial publication of the 8th edition Prognostic Stage, patients with pT1 or pT2, N0, M0 tumors that are ER positive and HER2 negative with an Oncotype DX score less than 11 are assigned to pathologic prognostic stage group IA. The clinical prognostic stage does not include a category to reflect Oncotype DX testing.

Multigene Molecular Profiling

At the time the 8th edition AJCC breast cancer staging system was written and sent to press (August 2016), the only available level 1 evidence evaluating use of multigene panels was from the TAILORx study, which demonstrated an excellent prognosis for patients with pT1 or pT2, N0, M0 tumors that are ER positive, HER2 negative, and have an Oncotype DX recurrence score less than 11.[24] Shortly thereafter, data from the MINDACT trial was reported. These data showed that patients with ER-positive, HER2-negative tumors with a Mammaprint low genomic risk of recurrence might be spared chemotherapy, even in the setting of being identified as high clinical risk using the Adjuvant! OnLine system.[36] In preparing the revision to the 8th edition AJCC breast cancer staging system, the MINDACT data were discussed extensively by the expert panel. Ultimately it was determined that Mammaprint would not be incorporated into the Pathologic Prognostic Stage table for several reasons to include the fact that the clinical risk of recurrence that was used in the MINDACT trial cannot be determined currently because it was based on survival estimates from Adjuvant! OnLine, which as of July 2017 when the revision was written was not available. The system is being updated and it is unknown when the Web site will become available again for use. In addition, the panel noted that the Mammaprint result does not predict benefit of chemotherapy. The panel emphasized that it was not endorsing use of a specific multigene panel assay and that clinicians should make decisions regarding use of such assays based on evidence available at the time of treatment and the anticipated value of the results of the assay in informing treatment decisions.[35] It is anticipated that additional data will become available evaluating different assays and comparing assays.[37] As more is learned regarding which molecular profiles provide the best prognostic and predictive information, those data will be incorporated into future revisions of the AJCC breast cancer staging system.

ADDITIONAL CONSIDERATIONS

One important caveat to use of the newly defined Pathologic Prognostic Stage is that it is limited to patients that undergo surgery as the initial intervention. For patients receiving neoadjuvant therapy, following surgery they are to be assigned T and N categories of clinical (ycT and ycN) or pathologic (ypT and ypN) post-therapy tumor and node status. Response to therapy (complete, partial, no response) is also to be recorded. This is unchanged from the 7th edition AJCC staging system. The 2010 to 2012 NCDB data did include 44,189 patients who received neoadjuvant therapy to include cytotoxic chemotherapy and endocrine therapy, but because of the complexity of incorporating degree of response to therapy and the resulting increase in the number of variables generated, and small numbers of patients, the expert panel determined that meaningful stage assignments for these patients could not be generated at this time.[35] It is noted that in current clinical practice, most patients with HER2-positive or triple negative breast cancer receive neoadjuvant systemic therapy. Therefore, there is concern that the Pathologic Prognostic Stage system will be predominately used in patients with HR-positive disease. A recent publication from the Early Breast Cancer Trialists' Collaborative Group demonstrated a steady rate of recurrence for patients with ER-positive breast cancer through 20 years.[38] The analysis included 88 trials with 62,923 patients that had ER-positive breast cancer and were disease-free at the completion of endocrine therapy at 5 years. The risk of distant recurrence correlated with T and N status. For patients with T1N0 disease, the risk of distant recurrence at 20 years was 13% versus 20% for those with T1N1 (one to three positive nodes) disease or 34% for those with T1N2 (four to nine positive nodes) disease. For patients with T2 tumors, the risk of distant recurrence was 19%, 26%, and 41%, respectively, for patients with N0 disease, one to three positive nodes, or four to nine positive nodes. In addition, the absolute risk of distant recurrence varied by tumor grade. This suggests that the 41.7-month median follow-up in the NCDB cohort used to determine the 8th edition Clinical and Pathologic Prognostic Stages may be too short to provide optimal stratification of patients with ER-positive disease.

Another important consideration for implementation of the 8th edition Clinical and Pathologic Prognostic Stages is the complexity. It is unlikely that a busy clinician will use the available tables that include the numerous combinations of T, N, M, grade, ER, PR, and HER2. Similarly, cancer registrars will be challenged by the time required to stage patients using this system. For the Prognostic Stages to be used, it is critical that staging be incorporated into electronic medical record platforms. In addition, it is anticipated that clinicians and registrars will use online tools or applications for smart phones that are now available.

SUMMARY

Biologic factors are critical in determining treatment plans and prognosis for patients with breast cancer. Although this has long been recognized, available level 1 data have been limited thereby making it challenging to incorporate such factors in previous editions of the AJCC staging system. The expert panel convened to generate the 8th edition of the AJCC breast cancer staging system prioritized incorporation of biologic factors based on the best available evidence. As reviewed here, this evidence confirms that patients with breast cancer are better stratified for survival outcomes based on the combination of anatomic extent of disease and biologic factors to include grade, ER, PR, and HER2 status. This initial effort to incorporate such factors was deemed as critical to maintain relevance of the staging system. It is anticipated that subsequent revisions required because of the availability of clinical and scientific data will be made more frequently than the historical 6- to 8-year cycle of staging revisions.[35] In addition, it is likely that more advanced staging models will be required as the complexity of survival predictions increases. At the current time, however, it is encouraged that patients be staged as appropriate according to the 8th edition anatomic stage, clinical prognostic stage, and pathologic prognostic stage to acquire the data necessary to inform future revisions.

REFERENCES

1. Clinical Practice Guidelines in Oncology: Breast, National Comprehensive Cancer Network (NCCN), 2017. Available at: https://www.nccn.org/professionals/physician_gls/default.aspx. Accessed April 27, 2018.
2. Bears OH, Car DT, Ruben P, editors. Manual for staging of cancer. 1st edition. Philadelphia: Lippincott; 1977.
3. Greene FL, Page DL, Fleming ID, et al. AJCC cancer staging handbook. New York: Springer; 2002.
4. Singletary SE, Connolly JL. Breast cancer staging: working with the sixth edition of the AJCC cancer staging manual. CA Cancer J Clin 2006;56:37–47.
5. Hammond ME, Hayes DF, Dowsett M, et al. American Society of Clinical Oncology/College of American Pathologists guideline recommendations for immunohistochemical testing of estrogen and progesterone receptors in breast cancer. J Clin Oncol 2010;28:2784–95.
6. Wolff AC, Hammond ME, Hicks DG, et al. Recommendations for human epidermal growth factor receptor 2 testing in breast cancer: American Society of Clinical Oncology/College of American Pathologists clinical practice guideline update. J Clin Oncol 2013;31:3997–4013.
7. Chavez-MacGregor M, Mittendorf EA, Clarke CA, et al. Incorporating tumor characteristics to the American Joint Committee on Cancer breast cancer staging system. Oncologist 2017;22:1292–300.
8. Coates AS, Winer EP, Goldhirsch A, et al. -Tailoring therapies-improving the management of early breast cancer: St Gallen International Expert Consensus on the primary therapy of early breast cancer 2015. Ann Oncol 2015;26:1533–46.
9. Harris LN, Ismaila N, McShane LM, et al. Use of biomarkers to guide decisions on adjuvant systemic therapy for women with early-stage invasive breast cancer: American Society of Clinical Oncology clinical practice guideline. J Clin Oncol 2016;34:1134–50.
10. Van Poznak C, Somerfield MR, Bast RC, et al. Use of biomarkers to guide decisions on systemic therapy for women with metastatic breast cancer: American Society of Clinical Oncology Clinical practice guideline. J Clin Oncol 2015;33:2695–704.
11. Hortobagyi GN, Connolly JL, Edge SB, et al. Breast. AJCC cancer staging manual. 8th edition. New York: Springer International Publishing; 2016.
12. Bagaria SP, Ray PS, Sim MS, et al. Personalizing breast cancer staging by the inclusion of ER, PR, and HER2. JAMA Surg 2014;149:125–9.
13. Mittendorf EA, Chavez-MacGregor M, Vila J, et al. Bioscore: a staging system for breast cancer patients that reflects the prognostic significance of underlying tumor biology. Ann Surg Oncol 2017;24:3502–9.
14. Park YH, Lee SJ, Cho EY, et al. Clinical relevance of TNM staging system according to breast cancer subtypes. Ann Oncol 2011;22:1554–60.
15. Veronesi U, Zurrida S, Viale G, et al. Rethinking TNM: a breast cancer classification to guide to treatment and facilitate research. Breast J 2009;15:291–5.

16. Yi M, Mittendorf EA, Cormier JN, et al. Novel staging system for predicting disease-specific survival in patients with breast cancer treated with surgery as the first intervention: time to modify the current American Joint Committee on Cancer staging system. J Clin Oncol 2011;29:4654–61.
17. Harrell FE Jr, Califf RM, Pryor DB, et al. Evaluating the yield of medical tests. JAMA 1982;247:2543–6.
18. Akaike H. New look at statistical-model identification. IEEE Trans Automat Contr 1974;19:716–23.
19. Mittendorf EA, Vila J, Chavez-MacGregor M, et al. Evaluation of a risk score based on biologic factors to enhance prognostic stratification by the American Joint Committee on Cancer (AJCC) staging system. Cancer Res 2017;77(4 Suppl) [abstract: P6-09-17].
20. Bloom HJ, Richardson WW. Histological grading and prognosis in breast cancer; a study of 1409 cases of which 359 have been followed for 15 years. Br J Cancer 1957;11:359–77.
21. Elston CW, Ellis IO. Pathological prognostic factors in breast cancer. I. The value of histological grade in breast cancer: experience from a large study with long-term follow-up. Histopathology 1991;19:403–10.
22. Paik S, Shak S, Tang G, et al. A multigene assay to predict recurrence of tamoxifen-treated, node-negative breast cancer. N Engl J Med 2004;351: 2817–26.
23. Paik S, Tang G, Shak S, et al. Gene expression and benefit of chemotherapy in women with node-negative, estrogen receptor-positive breast cancer. J Clin Oncol 2006;24:3726–34.
24. Sparano JA, Gray RJ, Makower DF, et al. Prospective validation of a 21-gene expression assay in breast cancer. N Engl J Med 2015;373:2005–14.
25. van't Veer LJ, Paik S, Hayes DF. Gene expression profiling of breast cancer: a new tumor marker. J Clin Oncol 2005;23:1631–5.
26. Buyse M, Loi S, van't Veer L, et al. Validation and clinical utility of a 70-gene prognostic signature for women with node-negative breast cancer. J Natl Cancer Inst 2006;98:1183–92.
27. Fitzal F, Filipits M, Rudas M, et al. The genomic expression test EndoPredict is a prognostic tool for identifying risk of local recurrence in postmenopausal endocrine receptor-positive, her2neu-negative breast cancer patients randomised within the prospective ABCSG 8 trial. Br J Cancer 2015;112:1405–10.
28. Bastien RR, Rodriguez-Lescure A, Ebbert MT, et al. PAM50 breast cancer subtyping by RT-qPCR and concordance with standard clinical molecular markers. BMC Med Genomics 2012;5(44):10.
29. Wallden B, Storhoff J, Nielsen T, et al. Development and verification of the PAM50-based Prosigna breast cancer gene signature assay. BMC Med Genomics 2015; 8(54):10.
30. Dowsett M, Sestak I, Lopez-Knowles E, et al. Comparison of PAM50 risk of recurrence score with oncotype DX and IHC4 for predicting risk of distant recurrence after endocrine therapy. J Clin Oncol 2013;31:2783–90.
31. Sestak I, Zhang Y, Schroeder BE, et al. Cross-stratification and differential risk by breast cancer index and recurrence score in women with hormone receptor-positive lymph node-negative early-stage breast cancer. Clin Cancer Res 2016; 22:5043–8.
32. Sgroi DC, Sestak I, Cuzick J, et al. Prediction of late distant recurrence in patients with oestrogen-receptor-positive breast cancer: a prospective comparison of the

breast-cancer index (BCI) assay, 21-gene recurrence score, and IHC4 in the TransATAC study population. Lancet Oncol 2013;14:1067–76.

33. Weiss A, Chavez-MacGregor M, Lichtensztajn DY, et al. Validation study of the American Joint Committee on Cancer eighth edition prognostic stage compared with the anatomic stage in breast cancer. JAMA Oncol 2018;4(2):203–9.

34. Mittendorf EA, Ballman KV, McCall LM, et al. Evaluation of the stage IB designation of the American Joint Committee on Cancer staging system in breast cancer. J Clin Oncol 2015;33:1119–27.

35. Available at: https://cancerstaging.org/references-tool)/deskreferences/Pages/Breast-Cancer-Staging.aspx. Accessed December 12, 2017.

36. Cardoso F, van't Veer LJ, Bogaerts J, et al. 70-gene signature as an aid to treatment decisions in early-stage breast cancer. N Engl J Med 2016;375:717–29.

37. Bartlett JM, Bayani J, Marshall A, et al. Comparing breast cancer multiparameter tests in the OPTIMA prelim trial: no test is more equal than the others. J Natl Cancer Inst 2016;108(9) [pii:djw050].

38. Pan H, Gray R, Braybrooke J, et al. 20-year risks of breast-cancer recurrence after stopping endocrine therapy at 5 Years. N Engl J Med 2017;377:1836–46.

Impact of Advancing Technology on Diagnosis and Treatment of Breast Cancer

Heather I. Greenwood, MD[a,1,*], Katerina Dodelzon, MD[b,1], Janine T. Katzen, MD[b,1]

KEYWORDS

- Tomosynthesis • Breast MRI • Abbreviated protocol MRI
- Diffusion-weighted imaging • Radioactive seed localization • MAGSEED
- SAVI SCOUT

KEY POINTS

- Three-dimensional imaging of the breast (digital breast tomosynthesis) minimizes the effects of overlapping fibroglandular tissue seen with standard mammography, improving lesion detection, characterization, and localization.
- Digital breast tomosynthesis has demonstrated improved diagnostic accuracy compared with full-field digital mammography alone, with consistently reported decreased recall rates and increased cancer detection rates.
- Fast abbreviated breast MRI reduces time and costs associated with full diagnostic protocol breast MRI while maintaining diagnostic accuracy in the evaluation for breast cancer.
- Diffusion-weighted imaging is a functional MRI technique that has shown promise in breast cancer screening, lesion detection/characterization, and the evaluation of treatment response.
- Recent years have introduced several new localization techniques which increase patient satisfaction and decrease operating room delays compared with traditional needle/wire localization.

TOMOSYNTHESIS

Breast screening with mammography is widely recognized as the most effective method of detecting early breast cancer[1] and has consistently demonstrated a 20% to 40% decrease in mortality among screened women.[2,3] In fact, a 2014 study by

Disclosure Statement: The authors have nothing to disclose.
[a] Department of Radiology, University of California San Francisco, UCSF Medical Center at Mount Zion, 1600 Divisadero Street Room C-250, San Francisco, CA 94115, USA;
[b] Department of Radiology, Weill Cornell Medical Center, New York-Presbyterian, 425 East 61st Street, 9th Floor, New York, NY 10065, USA
[1] All authors contributed equally to this work.
* Corresponding author.
E-mail address: Heather.greenwood@ucsf.edu

Surg Clin N Am 98 (2018) 703–724
https://doi.org/10.1016/j.suc.2018.03.006
0039-6109/18/© 2018 Elsevier Inc. All rights reserved.

surgical.theclinics.com

Webb and colleagues[4] demonstrated that 71% of breast cancer deaths are seen in unscreened women. Despite advances in treatment, stage at diagnosis is the greatest predictor of breast cancer survival and, therefore, early detection leads to improved breast cancer survival.[5]

However, the sensitivity of mammography is far from perfect ranging from 70% to 85%[6] with overlapping dense fibroglandular tissue presenting the greatest impediment to detection. This limitation is due to the inherent nature of mammography, which captures a 2-dimensional (2D) image of a 3-dimensional structure (the breast) with resultant superimposition of fibroglandular tissue, which can obscure underlying malignancy.

Improvement in sensitivity was seen with the switch from screen film mammography to full-field digital mammography (FFDM), in particular in women younger than 50 and those with dense breasts[7,8]; however, it remains suboptimal, in particular with increasing breast densities. In addition to obscuring malignancy, the superimposition of normal fibroglandular tissue can also mimic mammographic appearance of cancer and thus increase the number of false positive recall rates. Digital breast tomosynthesis (DBT) was developed to address both of these deficiencies of FFDM.

Technique

First described by Niklason and colleagues[9] in 1997 and receiving approval from the US Food and Drug Administration (FDA) in 2011, DBT is a technique that enables 3-dimensional visualization of the breast. Unlike standard mammography, which uses a single x-ray beam exposure produced at a fixed angle to the stationary breast and detector, DBT acquires multiple low dose images as the x-ray tube moves in an arc that varies between 15° and 60° (depending on the manufacturer) above the breast and detector (**Fig. 1**). Also depending on the manufacturer, the detector may rotate

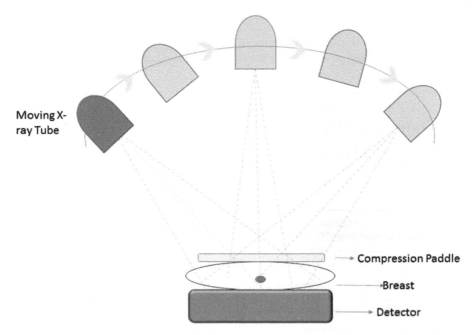

Moving X-ray Tube

Compression Paddle

Breast

Detector

Fig. 1. Schematic of tomosynthesis. The x-ray tube moves in an arch producing low radiation exposures of the breast.

during the acquisition or remain stationary as with standard mammography. Obtained images can then be reconstructed parallel to the detector producing a 3-dimensional image of the entire breast composed of a stack of multiple 2D "slices" in focus that are separated from each other by a fixed increment.[9–11] Not an isotropic imaging modality like computed tomography or MRI, DBT cannot be reconstructed in any direction with the same resolution; therefore, two standard views (craniocaudal and mediolateral oblique) of the breast are obtained just like with standard mammography. Although studies do demonstrate the added benefit of a single view DBT to standard mammography, two-view DBT added to standard mammography provided double the gain of diagnostic accuracy over mammography with single view DBT.[12]

The reconstructed DBT images can be then read by the radiologist either as a dynamic movie format (cine mode) or scrolled through manually by the reader at their chosen speed concentrating on an area of interest. Because the images are reconstructed sequentially from skin surface to skin surface, that is, from the medial skin surface to the lateral skin surface in the case of a mediolateral oblique view, and are separated by a fixed interval, usually 1 mm, DBT allows for lesion localization. To aid in localization, the reconstructed DBT images are accompanied by a scroll bar, indicating the slice location within the breast (**Fig. 2**).

Screening Performance Outcomes of Tomosynthesis

Its ability to decrease the Impact of overlapping tissue allots DBT the dual benefit of increasing the diagnostic accuracy of mammography while decreasing false-positive recall rates. One of the landmark studies on the diagnostic performance of DBT was the Oslo Tomosynthesis Trial, which prospectively compared women screened with mammography alone versus mammography with two-view DBT. A total of 12,631 women who elected to participate in the trial underwent screening with both mammography and DBT and the investigators found that addition of DBT yielded a 27% increase in cancer detection rate and 15% decrease in recall rates.[13] Most

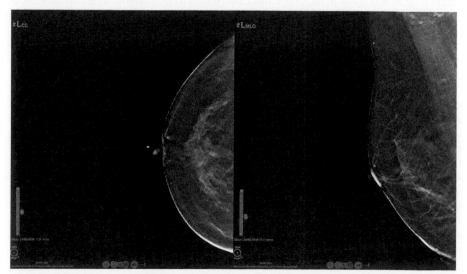

Fig. 2. Routine craniocaudal and mediolateral oblique tomosynthesis views. A scroll bar accompanies the images indicating slice position within the breast and relative orientation compared with head versus feet and medial versus lateral breast, respectively.

notably, the increased cancer detection rate was seen across all densities and was particularly significant for invasive cancers (increase invasive cancer yield of 40%). These findings were similarly replicated in the United States and other European populations with multiple studies[14-17] including a multicenter study by Rafferty and colleagues[14] in 2013 which demonstrated superior diagnostic accuracy of digital mammography with DBT compared with that of digital mammography alone. McDonald and colleagues[18] found that decreased recall rate and increased cancer detection rate is most pronounced in younger patients and those with baseline screening examination. They reported a 22% decrease in recall rates for baseline screened patients compared with a 14.5% decrease for previously screened patients and increase in cancer detection in the baseline subgroup of 40.5% versus increase in previously screened group of 17.4% over FFDM alone. The investigators confirmed that the improvement in diagnostic accuracy with the use of DBT is in fact sustainable over consecutive years of screening across all breast densities and ages,[18] validating that the preliminary clinical investigations of DBT, which yielded an increased cancer detection rate are not just a "prevalence" detection bias.

The incremental increase in cancer detection rate of DBT to digital mammography seems to be predominately represented by lesions presenting as architectural distortion, which account for approximately 73% of lesions seen on DBT only.[19,20] Although architectural distortion is only the third most common presentation of breast cancer, it represents up to 45% of cases of missed breast cancer.[21] Ray and colleagues[19] in a small series further characterized all lesions occult on digital mammography and seen on DBT only. Although these reflected only 7% of lesions recommended for biopsy, more than one-half of these were found to be malignant (53%) and remainder represented high-risk lesions, underscoring the importance of tissue sampling for all such lesions[19] (**Fig. 3**).

Diagnostic Performance of Tomosynthesis

In addition to improved conspicuity, DBT has been shown to outperform FFDM in lesion characterization. In fact, DBT has been found to be superior in lesion classification according to level of malignancy suspicion with equivalent if not superior mass margin characterization, as compared with conventional supplemental views. Consequently, DBT allows for either a downgrade of a lesion at the time of screening or obviates the need of additional mammographic views at diagnostic workup, at which time only targeted ultrasound evaluation can be obtained[22-26] (**Fig. 4**).

Lesion triangulation and localization is an added performance feature of DBT. As described, DBT images are accompanied by a scroll bar that depicts the slice number and location relative to superior versus inferior (on a craniocaudal view), or medial versus lateral (on a mediolateral oblique view) portions of the breast. This feature allows the reader to localize a lesion to a particular quadrant, which is especially useful for those lesions seen only on one tomosynthesis view—not an infrequent occurrence. Identifying the correct quadrant decreases the number of additional mammographic views, which would otherwise be attempted to visualize the lesion in two-views, as well as focuses the targeted area to be scanned by ultrasound examination. Those findings, which are within the skin, also become readily apparent on tomosynthesis, seen within a handful of the initial slices at each edge of the stack, eliminating the need of tangential views and allowing for definitive characterization.

DBT is superior to FFDM in the estimation of the extent of malignancy, which has implications for surgical planning. Luparia and colleagues[27] compared preoperative lesions on MRI, DBT, ultrasound examination, and FFDM and found that, although MRI remained most accurate in estimating true lesion size as compared with final pathologic

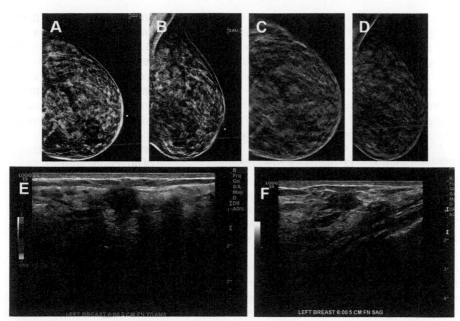

Fig. 3. A 51-year-old asymptomatic woman presented for screening. (*A, B*) full-field digital mammography craniocaudal (CC) and mediolateral oblique (MLO) views demonstrate no abnormality (*C, D*). Tomosynthesis CC and MLO views obtained as part of routine screening demonstrate a 1.4-cm architectural distortion in the lower inner left breast middle to posterior depth. (*E, F*) Targeted sonographic images demonstrate and irregular hypoechoic poorly circumscribed mass with antiparallel orientation measuring 1.1 cm, which correlates with the architectural distortion seen on tomosynthesis. The patient underwent ultrasound-guided core biopsy yielding moderately differentiated invasive ductal carcinoma.

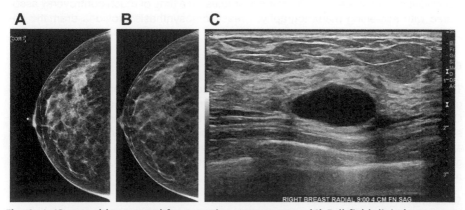

Fig. 4. A 42-year-old presented for screening mammogram. (*A*) Full-field digital mammography craniocaudal view demonstrates a mass in the outer breast with obscured margins. (*B*) Tomosynthesis images demonstrate an oval isodense well circumscribed mass—the margins are readily characterized; therefore, the patient was recalled for only targeted ultrasound examination, rather than additional mammographic views. (*C*) Ultrasound examination demonstrated a benign 1.8-cm simple cyst in the area of mammographic concern.

specimens, DBT approached MRI level of accuracy with correlation of pathologic tumor size of R = 0.89 and R = 0.92, respectively. Multifocality and multicentricity have also been shown to be more frequently identified with the addition of DBT, in particular in the setting of invasive lobular pathology.[28] Although preoperative MRI remains the most sensitive method for detecting additional ipsilateral and contralateral disease in the setting of known index malignancy, the addition of second look DBT to the conventional second look ultrasound examination has been demonstrated in one series to increase additional lesion detection from 52% to 75%, thus, decreasing the need for often uncomfortable and expensive MRI-guided needle biopsy.[29]

Radiation Dose and Synthetic 2D Mammogram

Despite its advantages, one of the main concerns with DBT is the increased radiation dose to patients. Because the female breast is radiosensitive, the Mammography Quality Standard Act dictate a breast dose restriction of 3 mG per acquisition.[30] Although DBT uses low-dose exposures, there are multiple exposures per view, as discussed, ranging from 10 to 50; therefore, early studies using DBT demonstrate a dose ratio (dose of DBT/dose of FFDM) of 0.68 to 1.17 and the combination of DBT with FFDM yields dose ratios of 1.5 to 2.2 times that of FFDM alone.[31] A proposed solution to dose reduction has been the use of a synthetic 2D mammogram that is reconstructed from images acquired during DBT, and requires no additional radiation exposure. Replacement of FFDM with 2D views results in reduction of the dose of FFDM with DBT by one-half, thus, resulting in radiation exposure levels comparable with that of FFDM. Approved by the FDA, synthetic 2D mammograms have consistently demonstrated equivalent diagnostic accuracy to FFDM in recent studies[32–34] (**Fig. 5**).

Summary

Studies have demonstrated that DBT is superior to standard mammography both in the screening and diagnostic setting, with improved cancer detection, decreased recall rate, and improved lesion characterization. The increased radiation dose associated with the combination of DBT to FFDM will likely be resolved with the replacement of FFDM with synthetic 2D mammograms, which have been showing equivalent performance to FFDM in initial studies. At a time of much controversy associated with screening mammography, breast tomosynthesis provides dramatic improvements, ushering in a new era in screening.

BREAST MRI

There are several imaging modalities available to radiologists for the detection and diagnosis of breast cancer, including mammography, ultrasound, and breast MRI. Of all these modalities, MRI has been shown to have the greatest sensitivity for screening for breast cancer[35,36] (**Fig. 6**). Advancing technology in MRI, such as fast abbreviated protocol breast MRI and diffusion-weighted imaging (DWI), have shown great promise as future applications in breast cancer screening, extent of disease, and response to neoadjuvant therapy.

Screening

Women of average risk are screened for breast cancer with mammography. However, in women with the greatest risk for developing breast cancer, additional screening with MRI in addition to mammography is recommended. These women include those with a lifetime risk of greater than 20% of developing breast cancer, BRCA1 or BRCA2 mutation, a first-degree relative with a BRCA1 or BRCA2 mutation but who are themselves

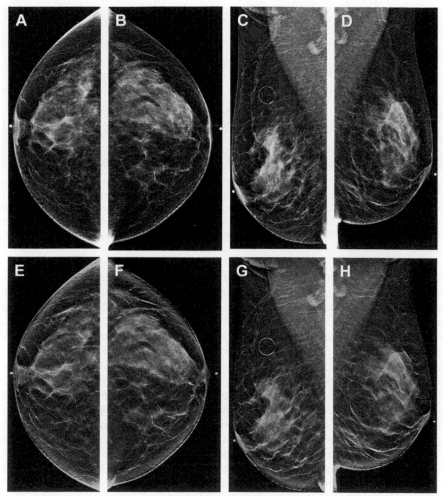

Fig. 5. A 45-year-old asymptomatic woman presenting for screening. (*A–D*) Full-field digital mammography mammogram. (*E–H*) Concurrent synthetic 2-dimensional mammogram reconstructed from the tomosynthesis data.

untested, a history of chest wall radiation between the ages of 10 and 30 years, and patients with Li-Fraumeni syndrome, Cowden syndrome, or Bannayan-Riley-Ruvalcaba syndrome, or a patient with a first-degree relative with one of these syndromes.[35,37] Numerous prospective studies have shown that, in women at risk for familial breast cancer, MRI has increased breast cancer detection rates compared with mammography.[38–43] There is currently insufficient evidence to recommend for or against screening MRI in patients at intermediate risk, those with a lifetime breast cancer risk of 15% to 20%, personal history of breast cancer, prior biopsy revealing high-risk pathology (atypical ductal hyperplasia, atypical lobular hyperplasia, lobular carcinoma in situ), or heterogeneously or extremely dense breasts on mammography.[35]

It is known that women with a personal history of breast cancer have a statistically significant increased risk of future breast cancer.[44–47] However, according to the American Cancer Society guidelines, and endorsed by the Society of Breast Imaging,

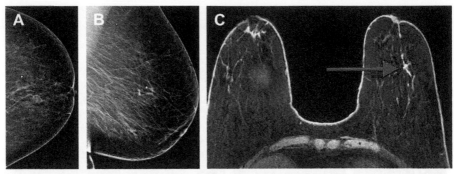

Fig. 6. A 69-year-old woman with intermittent clear and bloody nipple discharge (*A*, *B*). Craniocaudal (CC) and mediolateral oblique mammograms show no abnormality (*C*). Axial fat-saturated postcontrast image shows suspicious nonmass enhancement with a clumped internal enhancement pattern and a linear distribution (*arrow*). Subsequent MRI-guided breast biopsy intermediate grade ductal carcinoma in situ, which was mammographically occult.

patients with a personal history of breast cancer fall into the insufficient evidence group for supplementary screening with breast MRI, because there is a lack of data validating the use of breast MRI in this group given that most prior studies have evaluated MRI in patients at genetic/familial risk. However, several recent studies have examined the outcomes of screening MRI in patients with a personal history of breast cancer. These studies (with numbers of participants ranging from 141 to 915) demonstrated an MRI cancer detection rate of 9.9 to 28.8 per 1000 examinations.[48–54] The largest study by Lehman and colleagues[54] compared 915 women who underwent breast MRI for a personal history of breast cancer with 606 women who underwent breast MRI owing to a genetic or family risk for breast cancer. They found no difference in sensitivity and cancer detection rate between the 2 groups (P>.99). Interestingly, there was a lower false-positive rate in patients with a personal history of breast cancer compared with those with genetic/familial risk (12.3% vs 21.6%; P<.001). This study, and several prior studies,[49–52] suggest that MRI should be used in conjunction with mammography in women with personal history of breast cancer.[54]

Women at less than 15% risk for developing breast cancer are not currently recommended to undergo screening breast MRI.[35,37] A recent prospective observational study by Kuhl and colleagues[55] evaluated the usefulness of breast MRI as a supplemental breast cancer screening tool in women at average risk for breast cancer. A total of 3861 screening MRI studies were performed in 2120 asymptomatic women at average risk for breast cancer (lifetime risk of <15%). Breast cancer was diagnosed in 61 of the participants—41 invasive cancers and 20 cases of ductal carcinoma in situ (DCIS). The supplemental cancer detection rate for breast MRI was 15.5 per 1000 cases. The cancers detected with MRI had a medial size of 8 mm and 93.4% were node negative; 4 women had node-positive cancer, and none had distant metastases. None of the participants developed an interval cancer. The specificity of breast MRI was 97.1%. This study suggests that screening women of average risk with breast MRI is useful.

Fast Abbreviated MRI

Given its high sensitivity and ability to detect clinically, mammographically, and sonographically occult breast cancers[36,42,56–58] the use of breast MRI has increased over the past decade.[36,40,43,59] However, the specificity of breast MRI is moderate, and breast

MRI is limited owing to the high cost, long examination time, long interpretation time, and lower availability compared with mammography and ultrasound examination.[60] Exact full diagnostic protocol breast MRIs vary across institutions, but traditionally consist of the following sequences: T2 fat-suppressed, precontrast T1 non–fat-suppressed, precontrast T1 fat-suppressed, and then several postcontrast T1 fat-suppressed images. This examination takes approximately 40 minutes to perform, varying with the amount of sequences obtained. Over recent years an abbreviated breast MRI protocol (AP) has been developed to address the limitations of FDP breast MRI. AP MRI usually consists of a single precontrast and single postcontrast series, along with the images derived from them by standard reconstruction tools (subtraction and a maximum intensity projection image). Some protocols also include a T2-weighted sequence (**Fig. 7**).

The concept behind AP breast MRI, is based on tumor angiogenesis and neovascularity. Cancers tend to exhibit fast initial enhancement and thus are best seen on the early arterial phase/initial postcontrast sequence. Background parenchymal enhancement tends to increase as time progresses, so cancers tend to stand out most from the normal fibroglandular tissue enhancement at the early postcontrast time point.[60]

Multiple studies have shown that an AP breast MRI can shorten both acquisition and reading time, while maintaining diagnostic accuracy.[61–66] One of the first prospective observation reader study on abbreviated breast MRI by Kuhl and colleagues[61] included 606 MRI studles in 443 women (mean age of 54 years) referred for breast MRI owing to a personal or family history of breast cancer or dense breasts. All of the women had a normal or benign finding on screening mammography. They compared an FDP with AP MRI and found that AP MRI had an equivalent diagnostic accuracy compared with FDP, with a sensitivity and negative predictive value of 100%, specificity of 94.3%, and positive predictive value of 24.4%. There was an additional cancer yield of 18.2 per 1000 from MRI screening with 11 total breast cancers, the majority of which (64%) were invasive and all of the cancers detected at an early stage (T1N0). Interpretation of only the maximum intensity projection image missed 1 cancer, with the negative predictive value remaining high at 99.8%.[61]

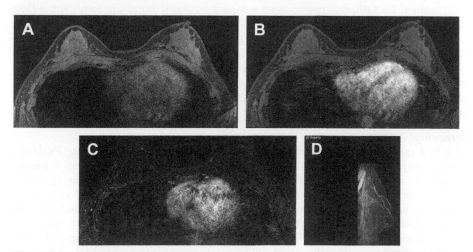

Fig. 7. A 49-year-old woman with a BRCA2 mutation with a negative fast abbreviated breast MRI protocol. (*A*) T1-weighted fat-saturated precontrast sequence. (*B*) Single T1-weighted fat-saturated postcontrast image. (*C*) Axial postcontrast subtraction image. (*D*) Sagittal reconstructed maximum intensity projection image.

Overall, studies have shown both a decreased acquisition time and also a decreased interpretation time for AP breast MRI, compared with FDP. The average acquisition time for FDP among these studies was 24 minutes (range, 16–40 minutes), and the average time for abbreviated protocol was 9 minutes (range, 3–15 minutes), saving approximately 15 minutes (range, 6–30 minutes).[67] Reduced interpretation times have varied from study to study. Kuhl[60] found an average interpretation time for the AP breast MRI of 28 seconds, and for a single maximum intensity projection image of 2.8 seconds. All but 1 of the 6 studies showed decreased interpretation time for AP compared with FDP.[61–66]

The literature to date has shown that AP breast MRI protocols are able to maintain the diagnostic accuracy obtained in traditional full diagnostic protocols, while decreasing the acquisition time and interpretation time and therefore cost of screening MRI. AP breast MRI has shown great promise to be the potential standard breast cancer imaging tool in the future.

Diffusion-Weighted Imaging

DWI is a functional MRI technique that is not currently a part of routine clinical breast MRI protocols. It is a short, 120- to 180-second technique that has shown potential in breast cancer imaging.[68] It has the benefit of not requiring intravenous gadolinium, and takes less time and is of lower cost than a full protocol traditional contrast-enhanced MRI. DWI is a microstructurally sensitive technique based on random thermal motion (Brownian motion) of water molecules.[69] It quantifies the random motion of water in biologic tissue. The diffusion of water molecules is inversely proportional to tissue cellularity and cell membrane integrity. Signal intensity on DWI is typically higher in an area with restricted diffusion, such as a cancer. However, molecules with long T2 relaxation times may also produce high signal intensity on DW images, an effect called T2 shine through. This T2 shine through effect may be eliminated by calculating apparent diffusion coefficients (ADCs) from DW images. Thus, it is important to look at both the DWI and the ADC map. Cancers tend to have high cellularity and, therefore, restrict the diffusion of free water, and consequently show restricted diffusion and low ADC values. On MRI, this phenomena appears as bright signal intensity on the DWI sequences and relatively dark signal on ADC maps[70] (**Fig. 8**).

Promising applications of DWI include a noncontrast breast MRI screening technique, lesion detection and characterization, and the evaluation of neoadjuvant treatment response. Multiple studies have looked at the application of DWI in differentiating benign from malignant lesions in the breast. Malignant breast lesions have been shown to show restricted diffusion on DWI, with significantly lower ADC values than normal breast/benign breast lesions.[71–74]

Screening

DWI is a promising noncontrast technology for breast cancer screening. Partridge and colleagues[73] investigated the performance of DWI for differentiating mammographically and clinically occult malignant (n = 27) from benign lesions (n = 91). They found that the 27 carcinomas in their series exhibited significantly lower ADC compared with 91 benign lesions (*P*<.001).[73] Kuroki-Suzuki and colleagues[75] studied the capability of using DWI with short T1 inversion recovery imaging to detect for breast cancer. DWI and short T1 inversion recovery together were able to detect 68 of 70 malignancies (sensitivity of 97%).[75] A recent study by McDonald and colleagues[76] evaluated the performance of DWI in detecting mammographically occult breast cancer in women with dense breasts. They found that the mammographically occult malignancies (18 invasive, 8 DCIS) had higher signal intensity on DWI than

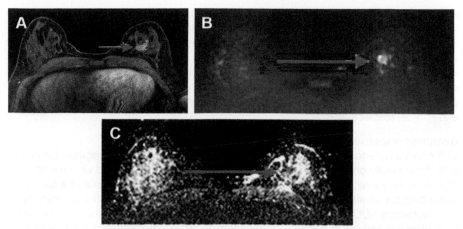

Fig. 8. A 37-year-old woman with a new diagnosis of invasive ductal carcinoma (IDC) with MRI for extent of disease (*A*). Postcontrast T1-weighted fat-suppressed sequence demonstrates an irregular spiculated mass in the inner left breast compatible with known IDC (*arrow*) (*B*). Diffusion-weighted high B value MRI shows corresponding high signal (*arrow*) (*C*). Apparent diffusion coefficient map shows corresponding low signal compatible with restricted diffusion in the tumor (*arrow*).

Ipsilateral normal tissue, and the ADCs of the lesions were lower than the ADCs of ipsilateral normal tissue (*P*<.0001).[76]

However, there remain some challenges in using DWI as a screening tool, because DWI does not detect all lesions that are identified on dynamic contrast enhanced-MRI. Tozaki and Fukama[77] found that although DWI was able to detect all the cases of invasive carcinoma and mass forming DCIS, it missed 8 of 28 cases of DCIS that presented as nonmass enhancement. Yabuuchi and colleagues[78] conducted a retrospective reader study looking at the detectability of nonpalpable breast cancers in asymptomatic women by mammogram, DCE-MRI, and unenhanced MRI using DWI and T2-weighted images. They found that the sensitivity for nonpalpable breast cancers using a combination of DW images and T2-weighted images was 69% and specificity was 86%, compared with mammography alone (sensitivity of 40%). However, the sensitivity of DW images and T2-weighted images was less than that for standard DCE-MRI, which was 86% in their study.[78]

Lesion detection and characterization

Not only has DWI shown potential in discriminating benign from malignant breast lesions, it has also shown potential in malignancy characterization. Some studies have found a lower ADC value in high-grade cancers than in intermediate- and low-grade cancers and DCIS.[79,80] Studies have also looked at the relationship between ADC values and hormone receptor status. Martincich and colleagues examined the correlation between ADC and histopathological and immunohistochemical breast tumor characteristics in 190 patients with 192 cancers undergoing breast MRI for local staging. They found that median ADC values were significantly higher in estrogen receptor (ER)-negative tumors than ER-positive tumors, and that HER2-enriched tumors had the highest median ADC value.[81] Youk and colleagues[82] studied 269 patients with 271 invasive cancers. They found that mean ADC value for triple negative breast cancer was higher than mean ADC values for ER-positive and HER2-positive breast cancers. In addition, studies have shown a higher ADC values for DCIS compared with invasive breast carcinomas.[83,84] More specifically, DWI has also demonstrated the ability to differentiate low-grade and high-grade DCIS, which could have a significant clinical impact. Rahbar and colleagues[83] evaluated 74 cases of DCIS in 69 women undergoing DWI. They found that not only did DCIS demonstrate lower ADC values compared with normal tissue, but non–high-grade DCIS had greater DWI intensity compared with high-grade DCIS.[83] Iima and colleagues[84] found lower mean ADC values for high and intermediate grade DCIS compared with low grade DCIS ($P<.01$ and $P = .3$, respectively).

Treatment response

DWI may be able to detect treatment response earlier and more accurately than DCE-MRI. Traditionally on imaging, treatment response has been assessed via tumor size on DCE-MRI. However, DWI is a technique sensitive to the microstructure of a tumor. As tumor cells die after successful treatment, there is less restriction to diffusion and, therefore, increased ADC. Some studies have shown that changes in diffusion occur earlier than changes in size in patients undergoing neoadjuvant treatment for breast cancer.[84,85] Sharma and colleagues[86] evaluated ADC values of breast tumors before and after multiple cycles of chemotherapy, and found that the mean ADC values of tumors were significantly lower those that of normal breast tissue of controls as well as disease-free contralateral breast tissue of patients. After the first cycle of chemotherapy, the ADC was significantly higher than pretherapy and showed further increase after the second and third cycles.[85,86] Woodhams and colleagues[87] compared contrast-enhanced breast MRI with DWI in assessing treatment response following neoadjuvant chemotherapy for breast carcinomas. They found a sensitivity of DWI for residual breast cancer after neoadjuvant chemotherapy were 97% and 93% ,respectively, with specificities of 89% and 56%, and accuracies of 96% and 89%, respectively.[87]

In conclusion, of all breast imaging modalities, MRI has the highest sensitivity for the detection of breast cancer. Traditional limitations of breast MRI include accessibility, time, and cost. These limitations are being overcome by new MRI techniques such as fast abbreviated MRI and DWI, which have shown great promise in screening, lesion evaluation/characterization, and the evaluation of treatment response.

NEW TECHNIQUES FOR LOCALIZATION

With advances in breast cancer treatment, breast conservation therapy plus radiation therapy has become a viable and desirable alternative to modified radical mastectomy. Studies have demonstrated no significant difference in survival rates between patients with early stage breast cancer (stages I and II) undergoing breast conservation therapy versus mastectomy.[45,88]

Many early stage breast cancers are not palpable and thus must be localized before surgery. Historically, this localization was performed by placing a wire or needle/wire combination into the region of concern using mammographic, ultrasound, or MRI guidance. Some of the disadvantages of this technique include patient discomfort, wire displacement, wire transection/retained fragments, and surgical delays because the wire needs to be placed on the day of surgery.[89] The rate of positive margins for wire localizations ranges from 20% to 70%.[89]

Recent years have produced several alternatives to this method that allow for localization up to 30 days before surgery. This results in decreased delays on the day of surgery, as well as increased patient convenience and comfort. One disadvantage of these newer techniques is that they cannot be placed under MRI guidance. To date only wire localizations can be performed under MRI guidance. Herein we review some of the newer, nonwire localization techniques.

Radioactive Seed Localization

Radioactive I-125 seeds were initially used for interstitial radiation treatment for prostate cancer. These I-125 seeds emit low-dose radiation (0.08–0.4 mCi) that can be detected with a gamma probe through the skin at the time of surgery.[90–92] This dose of radiation is very low and the only precaution the Nuclear Regulatory Commission recommends is that breastfeeding women not feed from that breast until the seed is removed.[92]

The seeds consist of radioactive I-125 fully imbedded within a titanium capsule. The radioactive seed is placed into an 18-G needle and occluded with a wax tip. It is enclosed in lead before the procedure to minimize radiation exposure. The tip of the deployment device is placed at the target with sonographic or mammographic guidance and deployed via a plunger mechanism by advancing a preloaded stylet similar to the way a localizing clip is placed (**Fig. 9**A–C). The seed is visible on both mammographic and ultrasound imaging. Typically, a postprocedure mammogram is obtained to demonstrate positioning of the seed relative to the target (**Fig. 9**D).

The half-life of the I-125 seed is 60 days; however, the current recommendation is that it be placed up to 5 to 7 days before surgery. At the time of surgery, a gamma probe is used to localize the radioactive seed. I-125 emits 27 keV of gamma radiation as opposed to the 140 keV emitted by technetium 99 used for sentinel lymph node mapping. Thus, the two energies can easily be distinguished at the time of surgery.[90]

After the removal of the surgical specimen, the gamma probe is again used to ensure that activity is now detected in the specimen outside of the patient. A specimen radiograph is also obtained, both to document excision of the targeted lesion as well as the radioactive seed (**Fig. 9**E).

Stringent tracking of the seed is necessary secondary to the associated radioactivity. It requires a multidisciplinary approach involving radiology, surgery, pathology, and nuclear medicine with the oversight of a radiation safety officer. This is one of the major drawbacks of the technique.

Radioactive seed localization has multiple advantages over wire localizations. There are significant cost savings relative to wire localization.[93,94] Bloomquist and

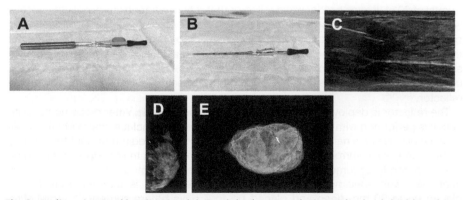

Fig. 9. Radioactive seed localization (*A*). Seed deployment device with a lead shield in place. A "stopper" is present to prevent unintentional deployment of the seed. (*B*) Radioactive seed deployment device with removal of lead shield and stopper. (*C*) Ultrasound image of tip of deployment device within the mass. (*D*) Mammogram after seed placement. (*E*) Specimen radiograph showing the presence of the localizing clip and radioactive seed.

colleagues[95] demonstrated that patients have reported less pain, greater convenience, and increased overall satisfaction with radioactive seed localization versus wire localizations. In addition, several studies have demonstrated improved to equivalent margin status compared with wire localization.[93–99] In these studies positive margin rates range from 12% to 27% with radioactive seed localization versus 13% to 46% with wire localizations. Reexcision rates range from 8% to 21% with radioactive seed localization versus 12% to 25% with wire localizations. Da Silva and colleagues[100] demonstrated decreased reexcision rates when bracketing with RS (22%) versus wire localizations (53%). Decreased operating room delays, decreased vasovagal reactions, and minimal seed migration are additional benefits.[93,96,99,101] For all of these reasons, radioactive seed localization is now frequently being performed across the country.

Magseed

Magseed (Endomag, Austin, TX) received clearance from the FDA in April 2016. It is a magnetic metallic marker, similar in size to an I-125 radioactive seed (5 mm). As with radioactive seeds, the Magseed is preloaded within a sterile 18-G needle occluded with a wax tip. It is deployed in a near identical method to a radioactive seed with an 18-G needle that comes in varying lengths.

A major benefit of the Magseed is that there is no associated radiation, sparing the necessary regulatory oversight that is associated with radioactive seed localization. It can be placed under mammographic or ultrasound guidance and is meant to stay in place for up to 30 days. Similar to radioactive seed localization, a postprocedure mammogram confirms appropriate positioning and a specimen radiograph is obtained to confirm Magseed retrieval (**Fig. 10**).

At the time of surgery, a Sentimag probe is used to detect the Magseed. The detector allows for multidirectional sensing and can detect at up to 30 mm depth. The detector allows for estimating the distance to the target. Bracketing may be performed as long as the seeds are placed greater than 20 mm from one another.[102]

SAVI SCOUT

The SAVI SCOUT radar localization system (Cianna Medical, Aliso Viejo, CA) is another alternative to wire localizations. The SAVI SCOUT system received FDA approval in August of 2014. It uses a radar wave reflector that is activated with infrared light to assist with localization. The 1.2-cm radar wave-reflective device (reflector) is percutaneously placed under imaging guidance (ultrasound or mammogram; **Fig. 11**A–C). The detector then emits radar waves and infrared light into the breast tissue. The reflector sends a signal to the detector displayed on a console with audible cues, which increase in cadence and visual numeric real-time distance measured in millimeters from the reflector.[103,104]

The reflector is deployed through a preloaded 16-G needle. After placement, verification is performed with the detector handpiece to ensure that a signal is identified. At the time of surgery, a handpiece is placed on the skin and used throughout the surgery to target the tissue surrounding the reflector. Once removed, the handpiece is used on the specimen to document that the reflector has been resected. This is subsequently confirmed with specimen radiography. Recommendation is that the reflector be placed up to 30 mm deep and placed up to 7 days before surgery.[103] Bracketing may be performed with the 2 reflectors placed at least 20 mm from one another. Mango and colleagues[105] demonstrated clear margins in a total of 8 bracketed cases. The reexcision rates from initial publications with SAVI SCOUT range from 0% to 18.5%.[103–106]

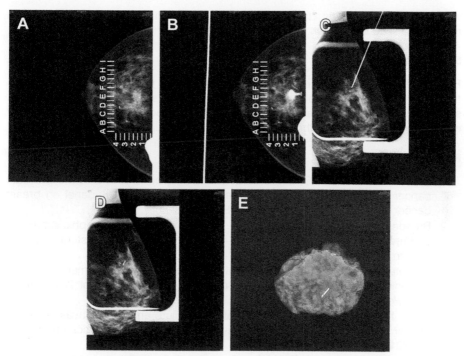

Fig. 10. MAGSEED (*A*). Alphanumeric grid at site of targeted localization. (*B*) Placement of MAGSEED at site. (*C*) Predeployment image (in opposing view) with needle tip adjacent to target. (*D*) Postdeployment image with seed adjacent to targeted localizing clip. (*E*) Specimen radiograph documenting excision of MAGSEED as well as targeted localizing clip. Another clip adjacent localizing clip happened to be excised as well.

Disadvantages of the technique include the possibility of nondetection after placement (2.0%–2.5%) and that it cannot be placed at greater than 45 mm depth.[103–106] Cox and colleagues[104] describe older halogen lights in the operating room interfering with the detection of the device in two cases. A major advantage of this technique is the avoidance of the previously described potential complications associated with

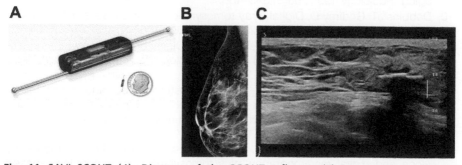

Fig. 11. SAVI SCOUT (*A*). Diagram of the SCOUT reflector. (*B*) Mammogram with the SCOUT reflector in place next to localizing clip. (*C*) Ultrasound image of the SCOUT reflector in place. IR, infrared. (*Courtesy of* [*A, B*] Cianna Medical; and [*C*] Cianna Medical, Aliso Viejo, CA.)

wire localization as well as a lack of extensive multidisciplinary oversight required with radioactive seed localization.[103]

SUMMARY

Recent years have introduced several new techniques that provide alternatives to traditional needle and needle/wire localization. Benefits include improved patient satisfaction as well as decrease costs and operating room delays. Each have their own advantages, providing the surgeon with several options.

REFERENCES

1. Marmot MG, Altman DG, Cameron DA, et al. The benefits and harms of breast cancer screening: an independent review. Independent UK panel on breast cancer screening. Lancet 2012;380(9855):1778–86.
2. Broeders M, Moss S, Nystrom L, et al. The impact of mammographic screening on breast cancer mortality in Europe: a review of observational studies. J Med Screen 2012;19(1):14–25.
3. Coldman A, Phillips N, Wilson C, et al. Pan-Canadian study of mammography screening and mortality from breast cancer. J Natl Cancer Inst 2015;107(1). https://doi.org/10.1093/jnci/dju404.
4. Webb ML, Cady B, Michaelson JS, et al. A failure analysis of invasive breast cancer: most deaths from disease occur in women not regularly screened. Cancer 2014;120(18):2839–46.
5. Saadatmand S, Bretveld R, Siesling S, et al. Influence of tumour stage at breast cancer detection on survival in modern times: population based study in 173, 797 patients. BMJ 2015;351. https://doi.org/10.1136/bmj.h4901.
6. Mushlin AI, Kouides RW, Shapiro DE. Estimating the accuracy of screening mammography: a meta-analysis. Am J Prev Med 1998;14(2):143–53.
7. Pisano ED, Gastonis C, Hendrick E, et al. Diagnostic performance of digital versus film mammography for breast cancer screening. N Engl J Med 2005; 353(17):1773–83.
8. Skaane P. Studies comparing screen-film mammography and full-field digital mammography in breast cancer screening: updated review. Acta Radiol 2009;50(1):3–14.
9. Niklason LT, Christian BT, Niklason LE, et al. Digital tomosynthesis in breast imaging. Radiology 1997;205(3):399–406.
10. Dobbins JT, Godfrey D. Digital x-ray tomosynthesis: current state of the art and clinical potential. Phys Med Biol 2003;48(19):R65–106.
11. Roth RG, Maidment ADA, Weinstein SP, et al. Digital breast tomosynthesis: lessons learned from early clinical implementation. Radiographics 2014;34(4): E89–102.
12. Rafferty EA, Park JM, Philpotts LE, et al. Diagnostic accuracy and recall rates for digital mammography and digital mammography combined with one-view and two-view tomosynthesis: results of an enriched reader study. AJR Am J Roentgenol 2014;202(2):273–81.
13. Skaane P, Bandos AI, Gullien R, et al. Comparison of digital mammography alone and digital mammography plus tomosynthesis in a population-based screening program. Radiology 2013;267(1):47–56.
14. Rafferty EA, Park JM, Philpotts LE, et al. Assessing radiologist performance using combined digital mammography and breast tomosynthesis compared with

digital mammography alone: results of a multicenter, multireader trial. Radiology 2013;266(1):104–13.

15. Gur D, Abrams GS, Chough DM, et al. Digital breast tomosynthesis: observer performance study. AJR Am J Roentgenol 2009;193(2):586–91.

16. Wallis MG, Moa M, Zanca F, et al. -view and single-view tomosynthesis versus full-field digital mammography: high-resolution x-ray imaging observer study. Radiology 2012;262(3):788–96.

17. Gennaro G, Toledano A, di Maggio C, et al. Digital breast tomosynthesis versus digital mammography: a clinical performance study. Eur Radiol 2010;20(7): 1545–53.

18. McDonald SA, McCarthy AM, Akhtar AL, et al. Baseline screening mammography: performance of full-field digital mammography versus digital breast tomosynthesis. AJR Am J Roentgenol 2015;205(5):1143–8.

19. Ray KM, Turner E, Sickles EA, et al. Suspicious findings at digital breast tomosynthesis occult to conventional digital mammography: imaging features and pathology findings. Breast J 2015;21(5):538–42.

20. Partyka L, Laurenco AP, Mainiero MB. Detection of mammographically occult architectural distortion on digital breast tomosynthesis screening: initial experience. AJR Am J Roentgenol 2014;203(1):216–22.

21. Knutzen AM, Gisvold JJ. Likelihood of malignant disease for various categories of mammographically detected, nonpalpable breast lesions. Mayo Clin Proc 1993;68(5):454–60.

22. Hakim CM, Chough DM, Ganott MA, et al. Digital breast tomosynthesis in the diagnostic environment: a subjective side-by-side review. AJR Am J Roentgenol 2010;195:172–6.

23. Brandt KR, Craig DA, Hoskins TL, et al. Can digital breast tomosynthesis replace conventional diagnostic mammography views for screening recalls without calcifications? A comparison study in a simulated clinical setting. AJR Am J Roentgenol 2013;200(2):291–8.

24. Noroozian M, Hadjiiski L, Rahnama-Moghadam S, et al. Digital breast tomosynthesis is comparable to mammographic spot views for mass characterization. Radiology 2012;262(1):61–8.

25. Zuley ML, Bandos AI, Ganott MA, et al. Digital breast tomosynthesis versus supplemental diagnostic mammographic views for evaluation of noncalcified breast lesions. Radiology 2013;266(1):89–95.

26. Chan HP, Helvie MA, Hadjiiski L, et al. Characterization of breast masses in digital breast tomosynthesis and digital mammograms: an observer performance study. Acad Radiol 2017;24(11):1372–9.

27. Luparia A, Mariscotti G, Durando M, et al. Accuracy of tumour size assessment in the preoperative staging of breast cancer: comparison of digital mammography, tomosynthesis, ultrasound and MRI. Radiol Med 2013;118(7):1119–36.

28. Mariscotti G, Durando M, Houssami N, et al. Digital breast tomosynthesis as an adjunct to digital mammography for detecting and characterizing invasive lobular cancers: a multi-reader study. Clin Radiol 2016;71(9):889–95.

29. Clauser P, Corbonar LA, Pancot M. Additional findings at preoperative breast MRI: the value of second-look digital breast tomosynthesis. Eur Radiol 2015; 25(10):2830–9.

30. Destouet JM, Bassett LW, Yaffe MJ, et al. The ACR's mammography accreditation program: ten years of experience since MQSA. J Am Coll Radiol 2005;2(7): 585–94.

31. Svah TM, Houssami N, Sechopoulos I, et al. Review of radiation dose estimates in digital breast tomosynthesis relative to two-view full-field digital mammography. Breast 2015;24(2):93–9.

32. Gur D, Zuley ML, Anello MI, et al. Dose reduction in digital breast tomosynthesis (DBT)screening using synthetically reconstructed projection images: an observer performance study. Acad Radiol 2012;19(2):166–71.

33. Houssami N, Skaane P. Overview of the evidence on digital breast tomosynthesis in breast cancer detection. Breast 2013;22(2):101–8.

34. Skaane P, Bandos AI, Eben EB, et al. Two view digital breast tomosynthesis screening with synthetically reconstructed projection images: comparison with digital breast tomosynthesis with full field digital mammographic images. Radiology 2014;271(3):655–63.

35. Lee CH, Dershaw DD, Kopans D, et al. Breast cancer screening with imaging: recommendations from the Society of Breast Imaging and the ACR on the use of mammography, breast MRI, breast ultrasound, and other technologies for the detection of clinically occult breast cancer. J Am Coll Radiol 2010;7(1):18–27.

36. Berg WA, Zhang Z, Lehrer D, et al. Detection of breast cancer with addition of annual screening ultrasound or a single screening MRI to mammography in women with elevated breast cancer risk. JAMA 2010;307(13):1394–404.

37. American College of Radiology. ACR practice parameter for the performance of contrast-enhanced magnetic resonance imaging (MRI) of the breast. 2013. Available at: https://www.acr.org/~/media/2a0eb28eb59041e2825179afb72ef624.pdf. Accessed November 30, 2015.

38. Warner E, Plewes D, Hill K, et al. Surveillance for BRCA1 and BRCA2 mutation carriers with magnetic resonance imaging, ultrasound mammography and clinical breast examination. JAMA 2004;292(11):1317–25.

39. Sardanelli F, Podo F, D'Agnolo G, et al. Multicenter comparative multimodality survey of women at genetic-familial high risk for breast cancer (HIBCRIT study): preliminary results. Radiology 2007;242(3):1317–25.

40. Kriege M, Brekelmans C, Boetes C, et al. Efficacy of MRI and mammography for breast-cancer screening in women with familial or genetic predisposition. N Engl J Med 2004;351(5):427–37.

41. Leach M, Boggis C, Dixon A, et al. Screening with magnetic resonance imaging and mammography of a UK population at high familial risk of breast cancer: a prospective multicenter cohort study. Lancet 2005;365(9473):1769–78.

42. Kuhl C, Schrading S, Leutner C, et al. Mammography, breast ultrasound, and magnetic resonance imaging for surveillance of women at high familial risk for breast cancer. J Clin Oncol 2005;23(33):8469–76.

43. Lehman C, Blume J, Weatherall P, et al. Screening women at high risk for breast cancer with mammography and magnetic resonance imaging. Cancer 2005; 103(9):1898–905.

44. Early Breast Cancer Trialists' Collaborative Group (EBCTCG), Darby S, McGale P, Correa C, et al. Effect of radiotherapy after breast-conserving surgery on 10-year recurrence and 15-year breast cancer death: meta-analysis of individual patient data for 10,801 women in 17 randomised trials. Lancet 2011; 378(9804):1707–16.

45. Poggie M, Danforth D, Sciuto L, et al. Eighteen-year results in the treatment of early breast carcinoma with mastectomy versus breast conservation therapy: the National Cancer Institute Randomized Trial. Cancer 2003;98(4):697–702.

46. Veronesi U, Cascinelli N, Mariani L, et al. Twenty-year follow-up of a randomized study comparing breast-conserving surgery with radical mastectomy for early breast cancer. N Engl J Med 2002;347(16):1227–32.
47. Clarke M, Collins R, Darby S, et al. Effects of radiotherapy and of differences in the extent of surgery for early breast cancer on local recurrence and 15-year survival: an overview of the randomized trials. Lancet 2011;378(9804): 1707–16.
48. Elmore L, Margenthaler JA. Breast MRI surveillance in women with prior curative-intent therapy for breast cancer. J Surg Res 2010;163(1):58–62.
49. Brennan S, Liberman L, Dershaw D, et al. Breast MRI screening of women with a personal history of breast cancer. AJR Am J Roentgenol 2010;195(2):510–6.
50. Schacht D, Yamaguchi K, Lai J, et al. Importance of a personal history of breast cancer as a risk factor for the development of subsequent breast cancer as a risk factor for the development of subsequent breast cancer: results from screening breast MRI. AJR Am J Roentgenol 2014;202(2):289–92.
51. Gweon HM, Cho N, Han W, et al. Breast MR imaging screening in women with a history of breast conservation therapy. Radiology 2014;272(2):366–73.
52. Giess C, Poole P, Chikarmane S, et al. Screening breast MRI in patients previously treated for breast cancer: diagnostic yield for cancer and abnormal interpretation rate. Acad Radiol 2015;22(11):1331–7.
53. Weinstock C, Campassi C, Goloubeva O, et al. Breast magnetic resonance imaging (MRI) surveillance in breast cancer survivors. Springerplus 2015;4:459.
54. Lehman CD, Lee JM, DeMartini WB, et al. Screening MRI in women with a personal history of breast cancer. J Natl Cancer Inst 2016;108(3) [pii:djv349].
55. Kuhl C, Strobel K, Bieling H, et al. Supplemental breast MR imaging screening of women with average risk of breast cancer. Radiology 2017; 283(2):361–70.
56. Sardanelli F, Podo F, Santoro F, et al. Multicenter surveillance of women at high genetic breast cancer risk using mammography, ultrasonography, and contrast-enhanced magnetic resonance imaging (the high breast cancer risk Italian 1 study): final results. Invest Radiol 2011;46(2):94–105.
57. Lehman C, Isaacs C, Schnall M, et al. Cancer yield of mammography, MR, and US in high-risk women: prospective multi-institution breast cancer screening study. Radiology 2007;244(2):381–8.
58. Lehman C. Clinical Indications: what is the evidence? Eur J Radiol 2012;81(S1): s82–4.
59. Kuhl CK, Schrading S, Leutner C, et al. Mammography, breast ultrasound, and magnetic resonance imaging for surveillance of women at high familial risk for breast cancer. J Clin Oncol 2015;20(33):1769–78.
60. Kuhl C. The current status of breast MR imaging. Part I. Choice of technique, image interpretation, diagnostic accuracy, and transfer to clinical practice. Radiology 2007;244(2):356–78.
61. Kuhl CK, Schrading S, Strobel K, et al. Abbreviated breast magnetic resonance imaging (MRI): first postcontrast subtracted images and maximum-intensity projection—a novel approach to breast cancer screening with MRI. J Clin Oncol 2014;32(22):2304–10.
62. Mango VL, Morris EA, David Dershaw D, et al. Abbreviated protocol for breast MRI: are multiple sequences needed for cancer detection? Eur J Radiol 2015; 84(1):65–70, 19.
63. Grimm LJ, Soo MS, Yoon S, et al. Abbreviated screening protocol for breast MRI: a feasibility study. Acad Radiol 2015;22(9):1157–62.

64. Harvey SC, Di Carlo PA, Lee B, et al. An abbreviated protocol for high risk screening breast MRI saves time and resources. J Am Coll Radiol 2016;13(4): 374–80.
65. Heacock L, Melsaether AN, Heller SL, et al. Evaluation of a known breast cancer using an abbreviated breast MRI protocol: correlation of imaging characteristics and pathology with lesion detection and conspicuity. Eur J Radiol 2016;85(4): 815–23.
66. Moschetta M, Telegrafo M, Rella L, et al. Abbreviated combined MR protocol: a new faster strategy for characterizing breast lesions. Clin Breast Cancer 2016; 16(3):207–11.
67. Chor C, Mercado C. Abbreviated MRI protocols: wave of the future of breast cancer screening. AJR Am J Roentgenol 2017;208(2):284–9.
68. Partridge S, McDonald E. Diffusion weighted magnetic resonance imaging of the breast: protocol optimization, interpretation, and clinical applications. Magn Reson Imaging Clin N Am 2013;1(3):601–24.
69. Neil JJ. Diffusion imaging concepts for clinicians. J Magn Reson Imaging 2008; 27(1):1–7.
70. Partridge S, DeMartini W, Kurland B, et al. Quantitative diffusion-weighted imaging as an adjunct to conventional breast MRI for improved positive predictive value. AJR Am J Roentgenol 2009;193(6):1716–22.
71. Partridge S. Future applications and innovations of clinical breast magnetic resonance imaging. Top Magn Reson Imaging 2008;19(3):171–6.
72. Koh D, Collins D. Diffusion-weighted MRI in the body: applications and challenges in oncology. AJR Am J Roentgenol 2007;188(6):1622–35.
73. Woodhams R, Matsunaga K, Iwabuch K, et al. Diffusion-weighted imaging of malignant breast tumors: the usefulness of apparent diffusion coefficient (ADC) value and ADC map for the detection of malignant breast tumors and evaluation of cancer extension. J Comput Assist Tomogr 2005;29(5):644–9.
74. Patridge S, Demartini W, Kurland B, et al. Differential diagnosis of mammographically and clinically occult breast lesions on diffusion-weighted MRI. J Magn Reson Imaging 2010;31(3):562–70.
75. Kuroki-Suzuki S, Kuroki Y, Nasu K, et al. Detecting breast cancer with non-contrast MR imaging: combining diffusion-weighted imaging and STIR imaging. Magn Reson Med Sci 2007;6(1):21–7.
76. McDonald E, Hammersley J, Chou S, et al. Performance of DWI as a rapid unenhanced technique for detecting mammographically occult breast cancer in elevated-risk women with dense breasts. AJR Am J Roentgenol 2016;207(1): 205–16.
77. Tozaki E, Fukuma E. 1H MR spectroscopy and diffusion-weighted imaging of the breast: are they useful tools for characterizing breast lesions before biopsy? AJR Am J Roentgenol 2009;193(3):840–9.
78. Yabuuchi H, Matsuo Y, Sunami S, et al. Detection of non-palpable breast cancer in asymptomatic women by using unenhanced diffusion-weighted and T2-weighted MR imaging: comparison with mammography and dynamic contrast-enhanced MR imaging. Eur Radiol 2011;21(1):11–7.
79. Constantini M, Belli P, Rinalid P, et al. Diffusion weighted imaging in breast cancer: relationship between apparent diffusion coefficient and tumour aggressiveness. Clin Radiol 2010;65(12):1005–12.
80. Razek A, Gaballa G, Denewer A, et al. Invasive ductal carcinoma: correlation of apparently diffusion coefficient value with pathological prognostic factors. NMR Biomed 2010;23(6):619–23.

81. Martincich LM, Deantoni V, Bertollo I, et al. Correlations between diffusion-weighted imaging and breast cancer biomarkers. Eur Radiol 2012;22(7):1519–28.
82. Youk J, Son E, Chung J, et al. Triple-negative invasive breast cancer on dynamic contrast-enhanced and diffusion-weighted MR imaging comparison with other breast cancer subtypes. Eur Radiol 2012;8(22):1724–34.
83. Rahbar H, Partridge S, Eby P, et al. Characterization of ductal carcinoma in situ on diffusion weighted breast MRI. Eur Radiol 2011;21(9):2011–9.
84. Iima M, Le Bihan D, Okumura R, et al. Apparent diffusion coefficient as an MR imaging biomarker of low-risk ductal carcinoma in situ: a pilot study. Radiology 2011;269(2):364–74.
85. Pickles M, Gibbs P, Lowry M, et al. Diffusion changes precede size reduction in neoadjuvant treatment of breast cancer. Magn Reson Imaging 2006;24(7):843–7.
86. Sharma U, Danishad K, Seenu V, et al. Longitudinal study of the assessment by MRI and diffusion-weighted imaging of tumor response in patients with locally advanced breast cancer undergoing neoadjuvant chemotherapy. NMR Biomed 2009;22(1):104–13.
87. Woodhams R, Kakita S, Hata H, et al. Identification of residual breast carcinoma following neoadjuvant chemotherapy: diffusion-weighted imaging—comparison with contrast-enhanced MR imaging and pathologic findings. Radiology 2010;254(2):357–66.
88. Ye J, Yan W, Christos P, et al. Equivalent survival with mastectomy or breast-conserving surgery plus radiation in young women aged <40 years with early-stage breast cancer: a national registry-based stage-by-stage comparison. Clin Breast Cancer 2015;15:390–7.
89. Besic N, Zgajnar J, Hocevar M, et al. Breast biopsy with wire localization: factors influencing complete excision of nonpalpable carcinoma. Eur Radiol 2002;12(11):2684–9.
90. Jakub J, Gray R, Degnim A, et al. Current status of radioactive seed for localization of non palpable breast lesions. Am J Surg 2010;199(4):522–8.
91. Best Medical International. Radioactive seeds. Available at: http://www.teambest.com/products/BMI_Catalog_RadioactiveSeeds_Oct2014.pdf. Accessed October 5, 2017.
92. Nuclear Regulatory Commission. Advisory Committee on the Medical Use of Isotopes. Available at: https://www.nrc.gov/docs/ML1514/ML15149A508.pdf. Accessed October 5, 2017.
93. Zhang Y, Seely J, Cordeiro E, et al. Radioactive seed localization versus wire-guided localization for nonpalpable breast cancer: a cost and operating room efficiency analysis. Ann Surg Oncol 2017;24(12):3567–73.
94. Sharek D, Zuley ML, Zhang JY, et al. Radioactive seed localization versus wire localization for lumpectomies: a comparison of outcomes. AJR Am J Roentgenol 2015;204(4):872–7.
95. Bloomquist E, Ajkay N, Patil S, et al. A randomized prospective comparison of patient-assessed satisfaction and clinical outcomes with radioactive seed localization versus wire localization. Breast J 2016;22(2):151–7.
96. Sung J, King V, Thornton C, et al. Safety and efficacy of radioactive seed localization with I-125 prior to lumpectomy and/or excisional biopsy. Eur J Radiol 2013;82(9):1453–7.
97. Dryden M, Dogan B, Fox P, et al. Imaging factors that influence surgical margins after preoperative I radioactive seed localization of breast lesions: comparison with wire localization. AJR Am J Roentgenol 2016;206(5):1–7.

98. Langhans L, Tvedskov T, Klausen T, et al. Radioactive seed localization or wire-guided localization of nonpalpable invasive and in situ breast cancer: a randomized, multicenter, open-label trial. Ann Surg 2017;266(1):29–35.

99. Hughes J, Mason M, Gray R, et al. A multi-site validation trial of radioactive seed localization as an alternative to wire localization. Breast J 2008;14(2):153–7.

100. Da Silva M, Porembka J, Mokdad A, et al. Bracketed radioactive seed localization vs bracketed wire-localization in breast surgery. Breast J 2018;24(2):161–6.

101. Alderliesten T, Loo C, Pengel K, et al. Radioactive seed localization of breast lesions: an adequate localization method without seed migration. Breast J 2011; 17(6):594–601.

102. Endomag. Lesion localization. Available at: http://us.endomag.com/lesion-localisation. Accessed September 21, 2017.

103. Cox C, Garcia-Henriquez N, Glancy M, et al. Pilot study of a new nonradioactive surgical guidance technology for locating nonpalpable breast lesions. Ann Surg Oncol 2016;23(6):1824–30.

104. Cox C, Russell S, Prowler V, et al. A prospective, single arm, multi-site, clinical evaluation of a nonradioactive surgical guidance technology for the location of nonpalpable breast lesions during excision. Ann Surg Oncol 2016;23(10): 3168–74.

105. Mango V, Wynn R, Feldman S, et al. Beyond wires and seeds: reflector-guided breast lesion localization and excision. Radiology 2017;284(2):365–71.

106. Mango V, Ha R, Gomberawalla A, et al. Evaluation of the SAVI SCOUT surgical guidance system for localization and excision of nonpalpable breast lesions: a feasibility study. AJR Am J Roentgenol 2016;15:W1–4.

Ductal Carcinoma In Situ

FangMeng Fu, MD[a], Richard C. Gilmore, MD[b], Lisa K. Jacobs, MD[b],*

KEYWORDS

- Ductal carcinoma in situ • Incidence • Mortality • Radiation therapy
- Hormonal therapy • Breast cancer

KEY POINTS

- Ductal carcinoma in situ has been stable in incidence over the past decade and has an excellent prognosis within a multidisciplinary treatment approach.
- Breast conservation therapy is a safe and effective surgical treatment for most Ductal carcinoma in situ patients at the current time.
- Adjuvant whole breast radiation therapy is recommended to reduce the risk of local recurrence in ductal carcinoma in situ undergoing breast conservation therapy.
- Accelerated partial breast irradiation is a promising alternative for some selected patients to decreased toxicity and improve cosmetic results.

EPIDEMIOLOGY AND ETIOLOGY

Ductal carcinoma in situ (DCIS) of the breast is characterized by abnormal ductal epithelial cells that have not yet invaded through the myoepithelial cells overlying the ductal basement membrane and, thus, is by definition noninvasive. The incidence of DCIS has increased dramatically over the last few decades, thought to be largely attributable to the widespread adoption and use of population-based mammographic screening for breast cancer in the United States.[1] Before 1982, the incidence of DCIS was relatively stable at approximately 12 per 100,000, comprising less than 1% to 2% of diagnosed breast cancer.[2] With the increased use of mammographic screening between 1982 and 1991, its incidence reached approximately 30 per 100,000. After 1991, the age-standardized incidence of DCIS continued to increase to 50 per 100,000 women in 1999, and then stabilized.[1] In the United States, DCIS accounts for 20% of all newly diagnosed breast cancers and about 1 in 33 women will be diagnosed with breast carcinoma in situ in their lifetime.[3] In 2015, there were an estimated 60,000 diagnosed cases of breast carcinoma in situ, representing 25% of all breast cancer diagnoses, with most of them (83%) being DCIS.[4]

The authors have nothing to disclose.
[a] Fujian Medical University Union Hospital, 29 Xinquan Rd, DongJieKou SangQuan, Gulou Qu, Fuzhou Shi, Fujian Sheng 350001, China; [b] Johns Hopkins Hospital, The Johns Hopkins University School of Medicine, 1800 Orleans Street, Baltimore, MD 21287, USA
* Corresponding author. Johns Hopkins Medicine, 601 North Caroline Street, Baltimore, MD 21287.
E-mail address: Ljacob14@jhmi.edu

Surg Clin N Am 98 (2018) 725–745
https://doi.org/10.1016/j.suc.2018.03.007
0039-6109/18/© 2018 Elsevier Inc. All rights reserved.

The incidence of DCIS varies according to both age and ethnicity. Because mammographic screening for women younger than 40 years of age is not routinely recommended, DCIS is rarely identified in young women.[5] In women over 40 years of age, DCIS incidence tends to increase rapidly with increasing age and peaks in the 70 to 79 years of age range.[4] With regard to ethnicity, the incidence of DCIS is nearly equal for non-Hispanic white and black women, lower for Asian/Pacific Islander and Hispanic women, and lowest for American Indian and Alaska Native women.[4]

The long-term prognosis of DCIS is excellent, with mortality rates at 10 years being less than 5%. Recently, a large retrospective study using Surveillance, Epidemiology, and End Results (SEER) data investigated the 10- and 20-year breast cancer-specific survival in 956 patients after a diagnosis of DCIS.[6] They found a 20-year cause-specific DCIS mortality rate of 3.3% (95% confidence interval [CI], 3.0%-3.6%), which decreased to 1.7% when contralateral recurrence was excluded. The breast cancer-specific survival of DCIS was associated with age at diagnosis, ethnicity, tumor size, tumor grade, and estrogen receptor (ER) status. Among patients who received breast conservation therapy (BCT)/lumpectomy and whole breast radiation therapy (WBRT), there was an associated reduction in risk of ipsilateral invasive recurrence at 10 years (2.5% vs 4.9%; adjusted hazard ratio [HR], 0.47; 95% CI, 0.42–0.53), but not of breast cancer-specific survival at 10 years (0.8% vs 0.9%; HR, 0.86; 95% CI, 0.67–1.10).[6] This study has been criticized for its absence of central pathology review to exclude occult invasive breast cancer, its retrospective nature with inherent selection bias, and its survival statistical methods.[7–9] Despite these limitations, the study clearly demonstrates the excellent prognosis of DCIS when treated appropriately.

DCIS is generally considered as the nonobligate precursor lesion of invasive ductal carcinoma (IDC), but its own etiology is poorly understood compared with IDC. Epidemiologic studies indicate that both DCIS and IDC share similar environmental risk factors, which include reproductive risk factors, such as age at menarche, parity, age at first birth, and age at menopause, as well as nonreproductive risk factors, such as family history, alcohol intake, and hormone replacement therapy.[10–18] Interestingly, the association of body mass index (BMI) with DCIS remains unclear. Longnecker and colleagues[11] found that increasing BMI was inversely related to the risk of DCIS (excluding 11 lobular carcinoma in situ cases), but was unrelated to the risk of developing IDC. Conversely, Reinier and colleagues[19] demonstrated that BMI was associated with an increased risk of IDC in postmenopausal women, but was not related to DCIS regardless of menopausal status. Similarly, a much larger study found that BMI was positively associated with the risk of invasive breast cancer but not DCIS (relative risks [RR] per 5 kg/m^2 = 1.20 and 1.01, respectively; P for heterogeneity = .002).[17] Further study is needed to more clearly define the association between BMI and DCIS.

Germline mutations in BRCA1 and BRCA2 are associated with a significantly increased risk of both invasive breast cancer and DCIS. It is reported that about 3.2% of patients with DCIS have mutations in one of these two genes.[20] Patients with DCIS with a family history of ovarian cancer or a first-degree relative with breast cancer are much more likely to be BRCA mutation carriers.[20,21] Most BRCA1-associated DCIS cases have triple negative receptor status, whereas most BRCA2-associated DCIS cases are ER and/or progesterone receptor (PR) positive, similar to invasive breast cancer.[22]

Outside of BRCA mutations, few studies have attempted to search the low-risk common loci predisposing a patient to DCIS in comparison with invasive breast cancer. One study of 873 women with DCIS and 4959 women with IDC reported that locus rs1982073 on TGFB1 was associated with a per-allele relative risk of 0.93 (95% CI, 0.84–1.03) for DCIS and 1.03 (95% CI, 0.98–1.09) for IDC (P = .05).[17] Campa and colleagues[23] genotyped 39 single nucleotide polymorphisms from the subjects recruited in the National Cancer Institute's Breast and Prostate Cancer Cohort Consortium. In this study, CDKN2BAS-rs1011970 showed a positive association with breast cancer in situ, but no association with invasive breast cancer with subsequent subgroup analyses indicating this variant was also associated with DCIS, albeit less significantly (odds ratio, 1.25; 95% CI, 1.09–1.42; $P<.01$). More recently, Petridis and colleagues[24] pooled data from 38 studies comprising 5067 cases of DCIS, 24,584 cases of IDC, and 37,467 cancer-free controls, all of which were genotyped and found to contain 76 known breast cancer predisposition single nucleotide polymorphisms, with no differences in association with IDC and DCIS.[24]

Although several investigators focus on differences in etiology between DCIS and IDC, both DCIS and IDC have similar risk factors whether environmental or genetic, supporting the hypothesis that DCIS and IDC are different phases, but in fact, a continuum of the same disease.

MULTIDISCIPLINARY MANAGEMENT OF DUCTAL CARCINOMA IN SITU
Breast Surgery for Ductal Carcinoma In Situ

The goal of surgery for DCIS is to eliminate the potential progression to IDC. Therefore, its management has traditionally been similar to those approaches used to manage early IDC. The surgical procedures available for DCIS include either mastectomy or BCT/lumpectomy.

Before the 1990s, DCIS was always regarded as early invasive breast cancer and mastectomy was the historical surgical treatment for DCIS without considering the intrinsic biology of the disease.[25] Long-term follow-up after mastectomy demonstrated that both local control and long-term survival were excellent.[26–28] Recently, a study-level metaanalysis including 8 retrospective studies (8 mastectomy studies including 936 patients with DCIS) manifested a 10-year local recurrence rate of 2.6%.[29] Yet, successful treatment of IDC with BCT has raised the question of less extensive surgical treatment for DCIS. For many patients with DCIS, mastectomy is a more than adequate treatment from an oncologic perspective and distinctly affects the patient's long-term quality of life.[30–32] For this reason, mastectomy for the treatment of DCIS has decreased rapidly in favor of BCT, especially for small localized DCIS. SEER data demonstrate that mastectomy for treatment of DCIS was used in only 28.3% of patients (including 4.5% bilateral mastectomy) in 2010 compared with 43% in 1992.[33] However, mastectomy remains the preferred surgical management for cases in which DCIS is extensive or multifocal, in which case it is difficult to achieve negative surgical margins or satisfactory cosmesis with BCT, or in those who have additional risk factors for breast cancer, such as carriers of a BRCA gene mutation, or who have contraindications to WBRT, including pregnancy, concurrent collagen vascular disease, or a prior history of WBRT.[34]

The rate of BCT for DCIS has been increasing over the last 2 decades and is now undertaken in approximately two-thirds of patients, most often in combination with WBRT.[33,35] It is critical that BCT is optimized to reduce the risk of local recurrence, while maintaining its benefits of cosmesis and improved quality of life. Thus, obtaining negative margins of resection is crucial for DCIS treated with BCT. Prospective randomized trials with long-term follow-up (>10 years) have shown ipsilateral breast recurrence rates for women with DCIS treated with BCT followed by WBRT to be 8% to 15%.[36–38] In these trials, microscopically clear margins were defined as no ink on tumor, with ipsilateral breast recurrence rates being higher than those of IDC treated with BCT. Other retrospective studies from single institutions have indicated that a negative margin up to or more than 1 cm conferred better protection against or even eliminated ipsilateral breast recurrence.[39–41] Nevertheless, wider margins are more likely to compromise cosmesis and the patients' body image. More recently, a multidisciplinary consensus panel reviewed 20 studies including 7883 patients and completed a metaanalysis of margin width and ipsilateral breast recurrence for DCIS.[42] The consensus panel recommended 2-mm margins as the standard for DCIS treated with BCT, which they concluded was associated with lower rates of ipsilateral breast recurrence, improved cosmetic outcomes, and decreased health care costs.[43] Despite some limitations, this standard has been adopted as a guideline by the Society of Surgical Oncology, American Society of Radiation Oncology, and American Society of Clinical Oncology.[43]

Apart from simple mastectomy and BCT as the major surgical treatment options for DCIS, it is important to note the increasing application of contralateral prophylactic mastectomy (CPM) in DCIS. Current guidelines only recommend CPM for BRCA gene mutation carriers and do not support its use in routine clinical practice. However, as shown in a retrospective assessment of trends in the local management of DCIS in the United States using the National Cancer Database, CPM has been increasing over time, particularly among women under 50 years of age.[44] Apart from age and BRCA receptor status, white race, higher educational level, family history, and private insurance type are other predictors for CPM.[45] Notably, there have been several studies using a variety of approaches definitively demonstrating negligible to no overall survival advantage obtained from CPM.[46–48] Other studies showing improvement in breast cancer–specific or overall mortality after CPM have been criticized for potential selection bias.[49–51] Moreover, there is a much lower surgeon comfort level reported when performing CPM on patients with average genetic risk compared with those with a positive BRCA mutation (38% vs 95%).[52] The most common reasons reported for surgeon discomfort with CPM were concern for overtreatment, an unfavorable risk/benefit ratio, and inadequate patient understanding of the anticipated risks and benefits of CPM.[53] Methods proposed to reduce the CPM rate include more effective surgeon–patient communication and allowing enough time and opportunity for the patient to process the risks and benefits of CPM.[45,53]

AXILLARY EVALUATION

Axillary evaluation for DCIS diagnosed on preoperative biopsy is controversial. By definition, DCIS is a preinvasive lesion and lacks the ability to metastasize; however, when DCIS is diagnosed on core needle biopsy there is an approximately 25% rate of upgrade to invasive carcinoma at the time of surgical excision owing to sampling limitations of biopsy and pathologic analysis.[54,55] Preoperative variables that significantly increase understaging include a finer biopsy needle (14-G), greater size tumor (>20 mm), high-grade lesion, palpable lesion, and mammographic features (such as Breast Imaging Reporting and Data Systems score of IV or V and the presence of a mammographic mass).[54] Those DCIS cases harboring an invasive component will increase the risk of axillary lymph node involvement. The reported rate of positive SLN for patients with DCIS varies between 2.1% and 15% in previous studies, of which a large majority were classified as micrometastases and isolated tumor cells.[56–59]

According to American Society of Clinical Oncology and National Comprehensive Cancer Network guidelines, sentinel lymph node biopsy (SLNB) is recommended in patients with DCIS undergoing mastectomy because SLNB cannot be performed at a subsequent surgery; however, it is not routinely recommended in patients undergoing BCT. If an invasive component is found on histologic analysis of the specimen after the first complete resection of tumor, a SNLB is done as a second surgery.[60,61] SLNB may also be considered when physical examination or imaging shows a mass lesion highly suggestive of invasive cancer or when the area of DCIS by imaging is large (>5 cm).[60] Even though SLNB is a low-risk procedure, it places patients at risk for long- and short-term complications, such as permanent lymphedema, infection, and seroma, as well as neurologic and sensory deficits, including paresthesias, pain, and impaired shoulder range of motion.[62–64]

Compliance with national guidelines regarding axillary evaluation in DCIS remains varied. As demonstrated from National Cancer Database and SEER data over the past 2 decades, axillary evaluation in DCIS increased significantly with performance of SLNB, whereas the use of axillary lymph node dissection decreased dramatically.[33,65,66] The rate of SLNB in DCIS has been increasing consistently since the 1990s, reaching 19% for BCT and 63.5% for mastectomy in 2012 and 2013.[65,67]

The clinical benefit of SLNB on patients with DCIS undergoing BCT needs to be balanced against the risk of complications from the procedure. In our opinion, SLNB should not be performed routinely in DCIS cases diagnosed on core biopsy treated with BCT, unless (1) the tumor is in a location that may preclude future node sampling owing to lymphatic disruption during the procedure, (2) DCIS was diagnosed as a mass on imaging or clinical examination, or (3) there is a large volume of DCIS (>5 cm). This strategy will reduce the risk of complications and maximize the benefit of therapeutic intervention.

RADIATION THERAPY FOR DUCTAL CARCINOMA IN SITU

Adjuvant WBRT is recommended to reduce the risk of local recurrence in patients with DCIS undergoing BCT. This recommendation was initially based on data from adjuvant WBRT after IDC. In the late 1980s and the 1990s, there were 4 randomized controlled trials evaluating WBRT for IDC in combination with DCIS after BCT: the NSABP B-17 trial, EORTC 10853 trial, UK/ANZ DCIS trial, and SweDCIS trial (**Table 1**.)[38,68–71] WBRT was associated with a significant absolute decrease in ipsilateral breast tumor recurrence of more than 10% for patients with DCIS treated with BCT plus WBRT compared with those who received BCT alone. Although WBRT was associated with a decrease in ipsilateral breast recurrence (both invasive and in situ), no differences were observed in overall survival. It is important to note that the UK/ANZ DCIS trial was a 2 × 2 design evaluating the effects of WBRT and tamoxifen on ipsilateral breast recurrence. In this study, tamoxifen decreased recurrent ipsilateral DCIS (HR, 0.70; 95% CI, 0.51–0.86) and contralateral tumors (HR, 0.44; 95% CI, 0.25–0.77), but had no effect on ipsilateral invasive disease (HR, 0.95; 95% CI, 0.66–1.38). These results highlight the importance of WBRT in DCIS undergoing BCT and also suggest a role for tamoxifen primarily for new contralateral disease. A recent metaanalysis including these 4 randomized controlled trials confirmed a statistically significant benefit from the addition of WBRT on all ipsilateral breast events (HR, 0.49; 95% CI, 0.41–0.58; $P<.00001$), both for ipsilateral invasive recurrence (HR, 0.50; 95% CI, 0.32–0.76; $P = .001$) and ipsilateral DCIS recurrence (HR, 0.61; 95% CI, 0.39–0.95; $P = .03$).[72] All of the subgroups, analyzed by surgical excision, age, tumor size, and histology, benefited from the addition of radiotherapy. These 4 randomized controlled phase III trials established the effect of adjuvant WBRT on local recurrence of DCIS after BCT.

The randomized trials found in **Table 1** were carried out in the 1970s and 1980s. More recently, there have been several clinical papers focusing on risk-adapted WBRT for patients with DCIS undergoing BCT in an attempt to identify potential low-risk DCIS that would derive no benefit from adjuvant WBRT. A SEER

Table 1
Randomized controlled trials on evaluating radiation after breast-conserving surgery for ductal carcinoma in situ

Trial	Patients	Follow-up (mo)	Margin Status	Whole Breast Irradiation	Hormonal Therapy	Ipsilateral Breast Tumor Recurrence Rate
NSABP B-17	813	207	Negative	50 Gy/25fx 9% Boost	No	35% vs 19.8%
Swe DCIS	1046	204	11.5% positive 8.8% missing	50 Gy/25fx 54 Gy/2 series	<4% tamoxifen	32% vs 20%
EORTC 10853	1010	188	21% close/ involved 4.4% missing	50 Gy/25fx 5% Boost	No known	31% vs 18%
UK/ANZ	1694	152	Negative	50 Gy/25fx No boost	Tamoxifen	19.4% vs 7.1%

population-based retrospective study by Sagara and colleagues[73] used a prognostic score for each patient based on age, tumor grade, and size to assess the benefit of adjuvant WBRT on 32,144 patients with DCIS treated with BCS. Their conclusion was that high-risk patients, defined as those with higher nuclear grade, younger age, and larger tumor size, derive breast cancer-specific and overall survival benefit from WBRT and that a patient prognostic score is associated with the magnitude of survival benefit, a finding not consistent with prior prospective randomized trials.[73] Nevertheless, these findings indicate that some "low-risk" DCIS may be exempted from WBRT after BCT.

To further identify a population of patients with low-risk DCIS in whom adjuvant WBRT could be safely omitted, prospective trials have been done as summarized in **Table 2**. The ipsilateral breast recurrence rate of "low-risk" DCIS with smaller size, larger margin width, and lower grade was decreased by adjuvant WBRT by more than 10% in Dana Farber Cancer Institute and Eastern Cooperative Oncology Group-ACRIN E5194 studies.[74,75] Adjuvant WBRT also significantly reduce the ipsilateral breast recurrence of "low-risk" DCIS in the RTOG 9804 Trial.[76] Based on these results, there is insufficient high-quality evidence demonstrating that a certain subgroup of patients with "low-risk" DCIS would fail to benefit from the addition of WBRT after BCT. Thus, further prospective randomized studies are needed to define a subset of patients with "low-risk" DCIS for whom the risks of WBRT after BCT outweigh the benefits.

The prognosis of patients with breast cancer (including DCIS) undergoing accelerated partial breast irradiation (APBI) has been studied in 4 randomized controlled trials.[77–80] The results indicate that APBI achieves the same effect on local recurrence and provides superior results regarding toxicity and cosmesis as compared with WBRT. Additional retrospective studies evaluating the efficacy of APBI on DCIS after BCT have shown low ipsilateral breast recurrence ranging from 1.4% to 5.2% with follow-up periods of 40 months to 5 years.[81–84] Given these findings, the American Brachytherapy Society consensus statement concluded that APBI is recommended for DCIS in appropriately selected women including those age 50 years and older; with DCIS 3 cm or less, negative margins, and no lymphovascular invasion; and who are lymph node negative. These results suggest that APBI may be a promising alternative to WBRT for DCIS but further prospective randomized studies are needed. Currently, a large NSABP multicenter randomized controlled trial evaluating APBI and WBRT has completed patient accrual.

Table 2

Prospective trials on the omission of radiotherapy in low-risk ductal carcinoma in situ treated with breast-conserving surgery

Trials	Design	Patients	Follow-up (y)	Risk Categorization	Radiotherapy/ET	Ipsilateral Breast Tumor Recurrence (y)
Dana Farber	Phase II, single-arm, prospective	143	11	Size ≤2.5 cm, Margin ≥1 cm Low/intermediate grade	No radiotherapy No ET	15.6% (10)
ECOG-ACRIN E−5194	Prospective, not randomized	665	12.3	Margin ≥3 mm Cohort 1: low/intermediate grade, size ≤2.5 cm Cohort 2: high grade, size ≤1 cm	No radiotherapy 30% tamoxifen	14.4%/24.6% (12)
RTOG 9804	Prospective, randomized	585	7.17	Size ≤2.5 cm, margin ≥3 mm Low/intermediate grade	Radiotherapy/observation 60% tamoxifen (optional)	0.9%/6.7% (7)

Abbreviation: ET, endocrine therapy.

HORMONAL THERAPY

DCIS is a local disease, so the need to treat it systemically with hormonal therapy is controversial. The NSABP B-24 and UK/ANZ clinical trials have addressed the role of tamoxifen in the management of DCIS.[38,68] Two prospective trials, detailed in **Table 2**, showed a significant reduction in risk of all new breast cancer events as well as ipsilateral and contralateral invasive recurrence in patients treated with tamoxifen; furthermore, the risk of ipsilateral DCIS was significantly decreased with the use of tamoxifen in the UK/ANZ trial (**Table 3**). However, after a follow-up period of more than 12 years, neither overall survival nor breast cancer-specific survival was significantly different between the tamoxifen and control groups. Nonetheless, based on these findings of reduced local recurrence, the National Comprehensive Cancer Network guidelines recommend consideration of 5 years of tamoxifen for premenopausal women with DCIS undergoing BCT, particularly if ER positive.[85]

It is important to note that the NSABP B-24 and UK/ANZ trials have been criticized for multiple reasons. First, neither study enrolled patients with DCIS based on hormonal receptor status. A retrospective evaluation of ER status in a patient subgroup of the NSABP B-24 trial showed that patients with ER-positive DCIS treated with tamoxifen had a significant decrease in subsequent breast cancer occurrence (HR, 0.49; $P<.001$) and overall survival (HR, 0.60; $P = .003$) at 10 years, which remained significant in multivariable analysis (overall HR, 0.64; $P = .003$); however, no significant benefit was observed in ER-negative DCIS.[86] A similar finding was reported by Lo et al,[87] who found that, among patients with DCIS in the post-NSABP B24 era, hormonal therapy was associated with improved event-free survival irrespective of ER status, and reduced ipsilateral breast recurrence in patients who were ER positive and ER unknown. Randomized trials are needed to confirm which patients benefit from tamoxifen based on the hormonal status of DCIS. Second, it was reported that 11% to 31% of patients with DCIS did not complete 5 years of tamoxifen.[88] Adherence to medical therapy is known to influence clinical outcomes, even in a clinical trial setting. The 2 studies found that the tamoxifen initiation and persistence rates were quite low, between 37% and 58%.[89-91] More recently, tamoxifen acceptance and adherence among patients with DCIS was evaluated in a multidisciplinary setting. Adherence rate was relative high (72%) and was related to acceptance of radiotherapy, the presence of medical insurance, and by recommendation from a medical oncologist.[92] Finally, the side effects of tamoxifen should be taken into consideration. As a selective ER modulator, tamoxifen is an estrogen agonist on bone, endometrium, and the coagulation cascade, as well as a potent antagonist in the breast. The adverse events of long-term tamoxifen medication reported in the NSABP B-24 and IBIS-1 trials were hot flashes, vaginal secretion, deep venous thrombosis, and endometrial carcinoma (0.45 per 1000 person-years vs 1.53 per 1000 person-years) compared with placebo.[86,93] Therefore, the recommendation for adjuvant tamoxifen in patients with DCIS should be based on the risk/benefit, including the hormonal receptor status.

In postmenopausal women with hormone receptor-positive invasive breast cancer, adjuvant treatment with aromatase inhibitors has proven more effective than tamoxifen in decreasing recurrence and mortality.[94] Two recently published randomized trials, NSABP B-35 and IBIS II DCIS, compared anastrozole with tamoxifen in postmenopausal women with hormone receptor-positive DCIS and invasive breast cancer (see **Table 3**).[95,96] In the NSABP B-35 trial, anastrozole significantly decreased the 10-year breast cancer event rate compared with the tamoxifen group (6.9% vs 10.9%), corresponding with a HR of 0.73 ($P = .02$) with anastrozole. This finding translated into an estimated absolute difference of 4% for the 10-year breast cancer-free

Table 3
Prospective clinical trials evaluating hormonal therapy for DCIS treated with LRT or lumpectomy

Trials	Patients	Treatment	Follow-up (mo)	All New Breast Events (%)	Ipsilateral DCIS (%)	Ipsilateral Invasive (%)	Contralateral (%)	OS and BCSS
NSABP B24	1799	LRT ± TAM	163	16.6 vs 13.2	7.6 vs 6.7	9.0 vs 6.6	8.1 vs 4.9	NS
UK/ANZ	1576	Lumpectomy ± RT ± TAM	152	24.6 vs 18.1	12.1 vs 8.6	6.9 vs 6.8	4.2 vs 1.9	NS
IBIS-II	2958	Lumpectomy + TAM/ANA	86	5 vs 5	2 vs 1	1 vs 1	2 vs <2	NS
NSABP B35	3077	LRT + TAM/ANA	108	7.9 vs 5.8	2.1 vs 1.9	1.4 vs 1.1	3.9 vs 2.5	NS

Abbreviations: ANA, anastrozole; BCSS, breast cancer specific survival; DCIS, ductal carcinoma in situ; LRT, lumpectomy followed by radiotherapy; NS, not significant; OS, overall survival; TAM, tamoxifen.

interval (89.1% for the tamoxifen group and 93.1% for the anastrozole group); in subgroup analysis, the trend was only seen in women younger than 60 years treated with anastrozole.[95] Additionally, anastrozole also decreased contralateral breast cancer events.[95] The IBIS-II DCIS trial failed to show a statistically significant difference in overall recurrence (ipsilateral and contralateral) or mortality between anastrozole and tamoxifen.[96] The rate of adverse events of anastrozole was the same as tamoxifen, but the type of side effects varied. The vasomotor and gynecologic symptoms, and thromboembolic events were more common in the tamoxifen group, whereas the risk of fracture and musculoskeletal symptoms was greater in the anastrozole group.[95,96] Although there is lack of evidence of survival benefit, anastrozole as an alternative hormonal therapy to tamoxifen allows for treatment selection based on side effect profile and younger age (≤60 years) for postmenopausal women with hormone receptor-positive DCIS.

ANTI-HUMAN EPIDERMAL GROWTH FACTOR RECEPTOR 2 THERAPY

Amplification or overexpression of the oncogene human epidermal growth factor receptor 2 (HER2) accounts for about 15% to 20% of invasive breast cancer for which HER2-targeted treatment has been proven to significantly improve the survival of this subgroup of breast cancer.[97,98] It has been reported that 20% to 44% of DCIS is HER2 positive, which is more frequent than that found in invasive breast cancer.[99–102] Furthermore, studies have shown that HER2 positivity in patients with DCIS is associated with poor prognostic features, including young age, high nuclear grade, comedotype architecture, and negative ER/PR hormone receptor status; however, the significance of HER2 expression on prognosis in patients with DCIS remains controversial.[102–104] Holmes and colleagues[105] reported that HER2 positivity in DCIS was significantly correlated with time to tumor recurrence in patients with DCIS treated with BCT alone. This result was similar to another study by Borgquist and colleagues,[100] but contradictory to a study by Noh and associates.[102] These differences may partly originate from the variation in use of adjuvant therapy in the studies and their end points. The findings of a large retrospective trial from Italy showed that HER2 overexpression remarkably increased the ipsilateral breast recurrence rate of DCIS but not IDC; moreover, they found that WBRT reduced local failure rates in HER2-positive DCIS, indicating that adjuvant WBRT might counteract the negative effect of HER-2 overexpression in DCIS.[106] This finding was confirmed by another large retrospective study based on the UK/ANZ DCIS trial, which found that HER2-positive DCIS was associated with an increased risk of local recurrence of DCIS but not IDC and that HER2-positive status was an independent predictor of radiation response.[107]

Few trials have investigated the benefit of anti-HER2 treatment in HER2-positive DCIS. A small phase II trial assessed the efficacy of 4 weeks of neoadjuvant lapatinib on 20 patients with HER2-positive DCIS and found that neoadjuvant targeted therapy decreased tumor size by inhibiting HER2 pathway signaling.[108] Kuerer and colleagues[109] observed that a single dose of neoadjuvant targeted therapy with trastuzumab for 12 patients with HER2-positive DCIS did not result in significant, clinically overt, histologic, antiproliferative, or apoptotic change, but does result in the ability to augment antibody-dependent cell-mediated cytotoxicity in all treated specimens. Currently, a prospective randomized phase III clinical trial is ongoing and aims to determine if trastuzumab in addition to radiation would reduce in-breast tumor recurrence in patients with HER2-positive DCIS treated with BCT.[110] This clinical trial may demonstrated the significance of HER2 overexpression in DCIS progression and the efficacy of anti-HER2 therapy in the treatment of DCIS.

PREDICTIVE TOOLS FOR RISK ASSESSMENT

As discussed, it is known that DCIS represents a spectrum of heterogeneous disease and the natural history of screening detected DCIS is unclear. Some forms of DCIS remain indolent, without becoming invasive or symptomatic covering the whole life span of a patient, whereas other forms have a higher risk of progression to lethal invasive cancer.[4,111] Although recent large prospective randomized clinical trials have shown that WBRT and hormonal therapy do reduce the risk of ipsilateral and/or contralateral breast cancer for patients with DCIS after BCT, there is no evidence of a survival benefit from adjuvant therapy; even for some indolent low risk DCIS, surgery may be omitted. Thus, for clinicians, the treatment of DCIS is no longer a one-size-fits-all approach. It is a challenge in the clinical management of DCIS to tailor treatment in light of individual risk to avoid overtreatment of low-risk lesions or undertreatment of DCIS with a higher risk of recurring or progressing to invasive disease. In light of this, there have been attempts to look for biomarkers or construct robust medical models to distinguish harmless from potentially hazardous disease, which may be helpful to optimize treatment of patients with DCIS.

Silverstein and colleagues[112] first introduced the Van Nuys Prognostic Index (VNPI) to predict the risk of local recurrence and aid decision making with regard to BCT with WBRT versus simple mastectomy for DCIS.[113] It was initially made up of tumor size, margin width, and pathologic classification (nuclear grade and comedo necrosis) then subsequently incorporated patient age into the algorithm.[114] The model creates a score of 1 to 3 (low risk to high risk) for each variable and the total VNPI score is the sum of the score of the 4 predictors that varies from 4 to 12. Depending on the final VNPI score a specific treatment is recommended: lumpectomy only (low risk; scores of 4–6), lumpectomy plus WBRT (moderate risk; scores of 7–9), and mastectomy (high risk; scores of 10–12).[115] The VNPI was validated by some relatively small retrospective studies, but failed in other studies.[116–120] Moreover, an Early Breast Cancer Trialists' Collaborative Group metaanalysis including 4 large prospective randomized trials of DCIS treated with BCT followed by WBRT showed that WBRT was effective in reducing ipsilateral recurrence irrespective of nuclear grade, comedonecrosis, or pathologic tumor size.[121] A survey of 52.8% of breast units in the UK was performed addressing the clinical application of this model.[122] It revealed that the VNPI was only routinely used in 12 units (15.8%) and never used in 36 units (47.4%), indicating that the VNPI was not frequently used in the decision making for WBRT after BCT. VNPI still has yet to be accepted worldwide owing to its inability to be validated by large prospective multicenter studies.

To improve on the predictive accuracy of VNPI, other predictive nomograms have attempted to incorporate more pathologic and clinical variables. The Memorial Sloan Kettering Cancer Center (MSKCC) developed a nomogram model that included 10 clinical and pathologic variables for the prediction of the 5- and 10-year risk of ipsilateral breast recurrence based on 1681 consecutive women with DCIS undergoing BCT.[123] The nomogram creates a composite score between 0 and 500, with each factor weighted based on its impact on rates of ipsilateral breast recurrence; key factors in this model include receipt of WBRT and receipt of hormonal therapy.[123] The efficacy of this nomogram has been validated by some external groups, but failed to be confirmed in other DCIS cohorts.[124–127] The inconsistency among different studies may be due to variations in study methods, sample sizes, and enrolled DCIS populations. The MSKCC nomogram has been criticized for its failure to evaluate prognosis for patients receiving BCT alone compared with adjuvant WBRT; moreover, its ability to accurately predict the rate of recurrence has been questioned.[127] In addition to these problems, the nomogram does not include molecular predictors such as ER, HER2, and Ki-67 status, and probably underestimates the true heterogeneity of DCIS lesions and the effect of innate biological trends on specific risk of invasive recurrence.[128]

Derived from the Oncotype DX 21-gene assay, the Oncotype DX DCIS score is based on expression of a panel of 7 genes including 5 proliferation genes (Ki67, STK15, Survivin, CCNB1, and MYBL2) plus PR and GSTM1, in addition to 5 reference genes. It provides data on local recurrence risk and invasive local recurrence risk in patients with DCIS and identifies those who may most benefit from WBRT.[129] It was first verified in a subset of patients enrolled in the Eastern Cooperative Oncology Group E5194 study and classified DCIS into low-, intermediate-, and high-risk groups with 10-year ipsilateral breast recurrence rates of 10.6%, 26.7%, and 25.9%, respectively ($P \leq .006$).[129] The Oncotype DX DCIS was validated in another larger respective DCIS cohort treated by BCT alone and was found to be an independent predictor for 10-year ipsilateral breast recurrence, which was 12.7%, 22%, and 28% in low-, intermediate-, and high-risk groups, respectively.[130] These studies demonstrate that multigene assays may play a promising role in risk stratification for DCIS and guide clinical management for these patients; however, there is much debate and argument about the adoption of this multigene array. First, the DCIS score was validated on low-risk patients with DCIS in the Eastern Cooperative Oncology Group cohort with specifically nonpalpable low- or intermediate-grade DCIS (≤ 2.5 cm) or high-grade DCIS (≤ 1 cm in size), with excision margin widths of at least 3 mm.[131,132] Second, even the low-risk group identified by this assay had a risk of ipsilateral breast recurrence of more than 10% in 10 years, which is high enough to be unacceptable for many physicians to withhold WBRT in this cohort.[34] Finally, the cost effectiveness and availability of this assay in areas outside the United States are of concern.[133]

Recently, the concordance of the VNPI, the MSKCC Nomogram, and the Oncotype Dx DCIS scores on prediction of DCIS recurrence risk was studied. Matlock and colleagues[134] found that the consistency and inconsistency rate among these 3 predictive tools are 29.7% and 10.8%, respectively. Concordance between all 3 models was seen only in low-risk patients.[134] Additionally, Leonard and colleagues[135] failed to verify the concordance in estimating the ipsilateral breast recurrence rate among breast radiation oncologists, VNPI, MSKCC Nomogram, and Oncotype Dx DCIS scores. In an attempt to overcome defects of these predictive tools, Altintas and colleagues[136] integrated gene expression panel information (ER, PR, HER1-4, Ki67, and c-myc) and the clinicopathologic parameters of VNPI excluding nuclear grade with the hope of developing a new predictive model with greater accuracy, efficacy, reproducibility, and clinical usefulness. The clinical usefulness of this tool remains controversial given that it has not been validated in independent patient populations. Nonetheless it has been informative as a new predictive risk pattern composed of gene expression profiles and clinicopathologic parameters for DCIS.

Apart from developing new local recurrence estimation tools for guidance in adjuvant therapy, a great deal of effort now has been devoted to detecting low-risk patients with DCIS in whom surgery may be avoided. The Surgery versus Active Monitoring for Low-Risk DCIS (LORIS) trial is a phase III, randomized, noninferiority trial of surgery versus active monitoring in low-risk patients with DCIS, which was initiated in the UK in 2014.[137] Low-risk patients with DCIS eligible for the trial include women aged 46 years or older with screening- detected calcifications and non–high-grade DCIS diagnosed by core needle biopsy. The aim of this trial is to enroll 932 patients to standard local treatment or active surveillance without receiving any antiestrogen treatment. Its primary outcome is invasive breast cancer-free survival at the 5- and 10-year follow-up. Similar studies are ongoing and include the LORD trial in Europe, the COMET trial in the United States, and the Australian LARRIKIN trial.[138–140] The deescalation of treatment for DCIS is contextualized on the basis of continual improvements in outcomes of breast cancer. In the future, the results of these prospective randomized trials will hopefully provide definitive data regarding the safety and efficacy of active surveillance in the low-risk DCIS cohort.

SUMMARY

DCIS has been stable in incidence over the past decade and has an excellent prognosis within a multidisciplinary treatment approach. BCT is a safe and effective surgical treatment for most patients with DCIS at the current time. Adjuvant WBRT is recommended to reduce the risk of local recurrence in DCIS undergoing BCT and APBI is a promising alternative for some selected patients to decreased toxicity and improve cosmetic results. The use of adjuvant hormonal therapy for DCIS treated with BCT can reduce local recurrence, but should be based on the risk/benefit ratio of the treatment as well as the hormone receptor status of the tumor. Future directions in the management of DCIS include developing predictive tools for guidance in the use of adjuvant therapy as well as selecting low-risk patients with DCIS in whom surgery may be safely omitted.

REFERENCES

1. Verdial FC, Etzioni R, Duggan C, et al. Demographic changes in breast cancer incidence, stage at diagnosis and age associated with population-based mammographic screening. J Surg Oncol 2017;115:517–22.
2. Swallow CJ, Van Zee KJ, Sacchini V, et al. Ductal carcinoma in situ of the breast: progress and controversy. Curr Probl Surg 1996;33:553–600.
3. Siegel RL, Miller KD, Jemal A. Cancer statistics. CA Cancer J Clin 2016;66:7–30.
4. Ward EM, DeSantis CE, Lin CC, et al. Cancer statistics: breast cancer in situ. CA Cancer J Clin 2015;65:481–95.
5. Smith RA, Saslow D, Sawyer KA, et al. American Cancer Society guidelines for breast cancer screening: update 2003. CA Cancer J Clin 2003;53:141–69.
6. Narod SA, Iqbal J, Giannakeas V, et al. Breast cancer mortality after a diagnosis of ductal carcinoma in situ. JAMA Oncol 2015;1:888–96.
7. Recht A, Rakovitch E, Solin LJ. Treatment and long-term risks for patients with a diagnosis of ductal carcinoma in situ. JAMA Oncol 2016;2:396.
8. Van Zee KJ, Barrio AV, Tchou J, Society of Surgical Oncology Breast Disease Site Work Group. Treatment and long-term risks for patients with a diagnosis of ductal carcinoma in situ. JAMA Oncol 2016;2:397–8.
9. Keiding N, Opdahl S, Holmberg L. Treatment recommendations for patients with a diagnosis of ductal carcinoma in situ. JAMA Oncol 2016;2:398.
10. Brinton LA, Hoover R, Fraumeni JF Jr. Epidemiology of minimal breast cancer. JAMA 1983;249:483–7.
11. Longnecker MP, Bernstein L, Paganini-Hill A, et al. Risk factors for in situ breast cancer. Cancer Epidemiol Biomarkers Prev 1996;5:961–5.
12. Kerlikowske K, Barclay J, Grady D, et al. Comparison of risk factors for ductal carcinoma in situ and invasive breast cancer. J Natl Cancer Inst 1997;89(1):76–82.
13. Trentham-Dietz A, Newcomb PA, Storer BE, et al. Risk factors for carcinoma in situ of the breast. Cancer Epidemiol Biomarkers Prev 2000;9:697–703.
14. Lambe M, Hsieh CC, Tsaih SW, et al. Parity, age at first birth and the risk of carcinoma in situ of the breast. Int J Cancer 1998;77:330–2.

15. Wohlfahrt J, Rank F, Kroman N, et al. A comparison of reproductive risk factors for CIS lesions and invasive breast cancer. Int J Cancer 2004;108:750–3.

16. Ma H, Henderson KD, Sullivan-Halley J, et al. Pregnancy-related factors and the risk of breast carcinoma in situ and invasive breast cancer among postmenopausal women in the California Teachers Study cohort. Breast Cancer Res 2010;12:R35.

17. Reeves GK, Pirie K, Green J, et al. Comparison of the effects of genetic and environmental risk factors on in situ and invasive ductal breast cancer. Int J Cancer 2012;131:930–7.

18. O'Brien KM, Sun J, Sandler DP, et al. Risk factors for young-onset invasive and in situ breast cancer. Cancer Causes Control 2015;26:1771–8.

19. Reinier KS, Vacek PM, Geller BM. Risk factors for breast carcinoma in situ versus invasive breast cancer in a prospective study of pre- and postmenopausal women. Breast Cancer Res Treat 2007;103:343–8.

20. Claus EB, Petruzella S, Matloff E, et al. Prevalence of BRCA1 and BRCA2 mutations in women diagnosed with ductal carcinoma in situ. JAMA 2005;293:964–9.

21. Bayraktar S, Elsayegh N, Gutierrez Barrera AM, et al. Predictive factors for BRCA1/BRCA2 mutations in women with ductal carcinoma in situ. Cancer 2012;118:1515–22.

22. Yang RL, Mick R, Lee K, et al. DCIS in BRCA1 and BRCA2 mutation carriers: prevalence, phenotype, and expression of oncodrivers C-MET and HER3. J Transl Med 2015;13:335.

23. Campa D, Barrdahl M, Mia M, et al. Genetic risk variants associated with in situ breast cancer. Breast Cancer Res 2015;17:82.

24. Petridis C, Brook MN, Shah V, et al. Genetic predisposition to ductal carcinoma in situ of the breast. Breast Cancer Res 2016;18:22.

25. Rosner D, Bedwani RN, Vana J, et al. Noninvasive breast carcinoma: results of a national survey by the American College of Surgeons. Ann Surg 1980;192:139–47.

26. Ashikari R, Huvos AG, Snyder RE. Prospective study of non-infiltrating carcinoma of the breast. Cancer 1977;39:435–9.

27. Sunshine JA, Moseley HS, Fletcher WS, et al. Breast carcinoma in situ. A retrospective review of 112 cases with a minimum 10 year follow-up. Am J Surg 1985;150:44–51.

28. Kinne DW, Petrek JA, Osborne MP, et al. Breast carcinoma in situ. Arch Surg 1989;124:33–6.

29. Stuart KE, Houssami N, Taylor R, et al. Long-term outcomes of ductal carcinoma in situ of the breast: a systematic review, meta-analysis and meta-regression analysis. BMC Cancer 2015;15:890.

30. Engel J, Kerr J, Schlesinger-Raab A, et al. Quality of life following breast-conserving therapy or mastectomy: results of a 5-year prospective study. Breast J 2004;10:223–31.

31. He ZY, Tong Q, Wu SG, et al. A comparison of quality of life and satisfaction of women with early-stage breast cancer treated with breast conserving therapy vs. mastectomy in southern China. Support Care Cancer 2012;20:2441–9.

32. Aerts L, Christiaens MR, Enzlin P, et al. Sexual functioning in women after mastectomy versus breast conserving therapy for early-stage breast cancer: a prospective controlled study. Breast 2014;23:629–36.

33. Worni M, Akushevich I, Greenup R, et al. Trends in treatment patterns and outcomes for ductal carcinoma in situ. J Natl Cancer Inst 2015;107:djv263.

34. Pang JM, Gorringe KL, Fox SB. Ductal carcinoma in situ - update on risk assessment and management. Histopathology 2016;68:96–109.

35. Shiyanbola OO, Sprague BL, Hampton JM, et al. Emerging trends in surgical and adjuvant radiation therapies among women diagnosed with ductal carcinoma in situ. Cancer 2016;122:2810–8.

36. Fisher B, Land S, Mamounas E, et al. Prevention of invasive breast cancer in women with ductal carcinoma in situ: an update of the National Surgical Adjuvant Breast and Bowel Project experience. Semin Oncol 2001;28:400–18.

37. EORTC Breast Cancer Cooperative Group, EORTC Radiotherapy Group, Bijker N, Meijnen P, Peterse JL, et al. Breast-conserving treatment with or without radiotherapy in ductal carcinoma-in-situ: ten-year results of European Organisation for Research and Treatment of Cancer randomized phase III trial 10853–a study by the EORTC Breast Cancer Cooperative Group and EORTC Radiotherapy Group. J Clin Oncol 2006;24:3381–7.

38. Cuzick J, Sestak I, Pinder SE, et al. Effect of tamoxifen and radiotherapy in women with locally excised ductal carcinoma in situ: long-term results from the UK/ANZ DCIS trial. Lancet Oncol 2011;12:21–9.

39. Fisher ER, Costantino J, Fisher B, et al. Pathologic findings from the National Surgical Adjuvant Breast Project (NSABP) Protocol B-17. Intraductal carcinoma (ductal carcinoma in situ). The national surgical adjuvant breast and bowel project collaborating investigators. Cancer 1995;75:1310–9.

40. Holland PA, Gandhi A, Knox WF, et al. The importance of complete excision in the prevention of local recurrence of ductal carcinoma in situ. Br J Cancer 1998;77:110–4.

41. Silverstein MJ, Lagios MD, Groshen S, et al. The influence of margin width on local control of ductal carcinoma in situ of the breast. N Engl J Med 1999;340:1455–61.

42. Morrow M, Van Zee KJ, Solin LJ, et al. Society of surgical oncology-American society for radiation oncology-American society of clinical oncology consensus guideline on margins for breast-conserving surgery with whole-breast irradiation in ductal carcinoma in situ. Pract Radiat Oncol 2016;6:287–95.

43. Morrow M, Van Zee KJ, Solin LJ, et al. Society of surgical oncology-American society for radiation oncology-American society of clinical oncology consensus guideline on margins for breast-conserving surgery with whole-breast irradiation in ductal carcinoma In Situ. J Clin Oncol 2016;34:4040–6.

44. Rutter CE, Park HS, Killelea BK, et al. Growing use of mastectomy for ductal carcinoma-In situ of the breast among young women in the United States. Ann Surg Oncol 2015;22:2378–86.

45. Jagsi R, Hawley ST, Griffith KA, et al. Contralateral prophylactic mastectomy decisions in a population-based sample of patients with early-stage breast cancer. JAMA Surg 2017;152:274–82.

46. Portschy PR, Kuntz KM, Tuttle TM. Survival outcomes after contralateral prophylactic mastectomy: a decision analysis. J Natl Cancer Inst 2014;106(8) [pii: dju160].

47. Davies KR, Brewster AM, Bedrosian I, et al. Outcomes of contralateral prophylactic mastectomy in relation to familial history: a decision analysis (BRCR-D-16-00033). Breast Cancer Res 2016;18:93.

48. Wong SM, Freedman RA, Sagara Y, et al. Growing use of contralateral prophylactic mastectomy despite no improvement in long-term survival for invasive breast cancer. Ann Surg 2017;265:581–9.

49. Yao K, Winchester DJ, Czechura T, et al. Contralateral prophylactic mastectomy and survival: report from the National Cancer Data Base, 1998-2002. Breast Cancer Res Treat 2013;142:465–76.

50. Kruper L, Kauffmann RM, Smith DD, et al. Survival analysis of contralateral prophylactic mastectomy: a question of selection bias. Ann Surg Oncol 2014;21:3448–56.
51. Jatoi I, Parsons HM. Contralateral prophylactic mastectomy and its association with reduced mortality: evidence for selection bias. Breast Cancer Res Treat 2014;148:389–96.
52. Bellavance E, Peppercorn J, Kronsberg S, et al. Surgeons' perspectives of contralateral prophylactic mastectomy. Ann Surg Oncol 2016;23:2779–87.
53. Benson JR, Winters ZE. Contralateral prophylactic mastectomy. Br J Surg 2016; 103:1249–50.
54. Brennan ME, Turner RM, Ciatto S, et al. Ductal carcinoma in situ at core-needle biopsy: meta-analysis of underestimation and predictors of invasive breast cancer. Radiology 2011;260:119–28.
55. Nicholson S, Hanby A, Clements K, et al. Variations in the management of the axilla in screen-detected ductal carcinoma in situ: evidence from the UK NHS breast screening programme audit of screen detected DCIS. Eur J Surg Oncol 2015;41:86–93.
56. van Roozendaal LM, Goorts B, Klinkert M, et al. Sentinel lymph node biopsy can be omitted in DCIS patients treated with breast conserving therapy. Breast Cancer Res Treat 2016;156:517–25.
57. Heymans C, van Bastelaar J, Visschers RGJ, et al. Sentinel node procedure obsolete in lumpectomy for ductal carcinoma in situ. Clin Breast Cancer 2017; 17:e87–93.
58. Tunon-de-Lara C, Chauvet MP, Baranzelli MC, et al. The role of sentinel lymph node biopsy and factors associated with invasion in extensive DCIS of the breast treated by mastectomy: the Cinnamome Prospective Multicenter Study. Ann Surg Oncol 2015;22:3853–60.
59. Prendeville S, Ryan C, Feeley L, et al. Sentinel lymph node biopsy is not warranted following a core needle biopsy diagnosis of ductal carcinoma in situ (DCIS) of the breast. Breast 2015;24:197–200.
60. Lyman GH, Temin S, Edge SB, et al. Sentinel lymph node biopsy for patients with early-stage breast cancer: American Society of Clinical Oncology clinical practice guideline update. J Clin Oncol 2014;32:1365–83.
61. National Comprehensive Cancer Network (NCCN). NCCN clinical practice guidelines in oncology: breast cancer. Version 3.2015. Available at: www.nccn.org. Accessed October 14, 2015.
62. Leissig A, Fallowfield LJ, Langridge CI, et al. Post-operative arm morbidity and quality of life. Results of the ALMANAC randomised trial comparing sentinel node biopsy with standard axillary treatment in the management of patients with early breast cancer. Breast Cancer Res Treat 2006;95:279–93.
63. Lucci A, McCall LM, Beitsch PD, et al. Surgical complications associated with sentinel lymph node dissection (SLND) plus axillary lymph node dissection compared with SLND alone in the American College of Surgeons Oncology Group Trial Z0011. J Clin Oncol 2007;25:3657–63.
64. Liu CQ, Guo Y, Shi JY, et al. Late morbidity associated with a tumour-negative sentinel lymph node biopsy in primary breast cancer patients: a systematic review. Eur J Cancer 2009;45:1560–8.
65. Mitchell KB, Lin H, Shen Y, et al. DCIS and axillary nodal evaluation: compliance with national guidelines. BMC Surg 2017;17:12.
66. Fisher B, Costantino J, Redmond C, et al. Lumpectomy compared with lumpectomy and radiation therapy for the treatment of intraductal breast cancer. N Engl J Med 1993;328:1581–6.

67. Miller ME, Kyrillos A, Yao K, et al. Utilization of axillary surgery for patients with ductal carcinoma in situ: a report from the national cancer data base. Ann Surg Oncol 2016;23:3337–46.
68. Wapnir IL, Dignam JJ, Fisher B, et al. Long-term outcomes of invasive ipsilateral breast tumor recurrences after lumpectomy in NSABP B-17 and B-24 randomized clinical trials for DCIS. J Natl Cancer Inst 2011;103:478–88.
69. Donker M, Litière S, Werutsky G, et al. Breast-conserving treatment with or without radiotherapy in ductal carcinoma In Situ: 15-year recurrence rates and outcome after a recurrence, from the EORTC 10853 randomized phase III trial. J Clin Oncol 2013;31:4054–9.
70. Holmberg L, Garmo H, Granstrand B, et al. Absolute risk reductions for local recurrence after postoperative radiotherapy after sector resection for ductal carcinoma in situ of the breast. J Clin Oncol 2008;26:1247–52.
71. Wärnberg F, Garmo H, Emdin S, et al. Effect of radiotherapy after breast-conserving surgery for ductal carcinoma in situ: 20 years follow-up in the randomized SweDCIS trial. J Clin Oncol 2014;32:3613–8.
72. Goodwin A, Parker S, Ghersi D, et al. Post-operative radiotherapy for ductal carcinoma in situ of the breast. Cochrane Database Syst Rev 2013;(11):CD000563.
73. Sagara Y, Freedman RA, Vaz-Luis I, et al. Patient prognostic score and associations with survival improvement offered by radiotherapy after breast-conserving surgery for ductal carcinoma in situ: a population-based longitudinal cohort study. J Clin Oncol 2016;34:1190–6.
74. Wong JS, Chen YH, Gadd MA, et al. Eight-year update of a prospective study of wide excision alone for small low- or intermediate-grade ductal carcinoma in situ (DCIS). Breast Cancer Res Treat 2014;143:343–50.
75. Solin LJ, Gray R, Hughes LL, et al. Surgical excision without radiation for ductal carcinoma in situ of the breast: 12-year results from the ECOG-ACRIN E5194 study. J Clin Oncol 2015;33:3938–44.
76. McCormick B, Winter K, Hudis C, et al. RTOG 9804: a prospective randomized trial for good-risk ductal carcinoma in situ comparing radiotherapy with observation. J Clin Oncol 2015;33:709–15.
77. Polgár C, Fodor J, Major T, et al. Breast-conserving therapy with partial or whole breast irradiation: ten-year results of the Budapest randomized trial. Radiother Oncol 2013;108:197–202.
78. Rodríguez N, Sanz X, Dengra J, et al. Five-year outcomes, cosmesis, and toxicity with 3-dimensional conformal external beam radiation therapy to deliver accelerated partial breast irradiation. Int J Radiat Oncol Biol Phys 2013;87:1051–7.
79. Livi L, Meattini I, Marrazzo L, et al. Accelerated partial breast irradiation using intensity-modulated radiotherapy versus whole breast irradiation: 5-year survival analysis of a phase 3 randomised controlled trial. Eur J Cancer 2015;51:451–63.
80. Strnad V, Ott OJ, Hildebrandt G, et al. 5-year results of accelerated partial breast irradiation using sole interstitial multicatheter brachytherapy versus whole-breast irradiation with boost after breast-conserving surgery for low-risk invasive and in-situ carcinoma of the female breast: a randomised, phase 3, non-inferiority trial. Lancet 2016;387:229–38.
81. Israel PZ, Vicini F, Robbins AB, et al. Ductal carcinoma in situ of the breast treated with accelerated partial breast irradiation using balloon-based brachytherapy. Ann Surg Oncol 2010;17:2940–4.
82. Shah C, McGee M, Wilkinson JB, et al. Clinical outcomes using accelerated partial breast irradiation in patients with ductal carcinoma in situ. Clin Breast Cancer 2012;12:259–63.

83. Vicini F, Shah C, Ben Wilkinson J, et al. Should ductal carcinoma-in-situ (DCIS) be removed from the ASTRO consensus panel cautionary group for off-protocol use of accelerated partial breast irradiation (APBI)? A pooled analysis of outcomes for 300 patients with DCIS treated with APBI. Ann Surg Oncol 2013;20:1275–81.

84. Kamrava M, Kuske RR, Anderson B, et al. Outcomes of breast cancer patients treated with accelerated partial breast irradiation via multicatheter interstitial brachytherapy: the pooled registry of multicatheter interstitial sites (PROMIS) experience. Ann Surg Oncol 2015;22(Suppl 3):S404–11.

85. National Comprehensive Cancer Network (ONCCN). NCCN clinical practice guidelines in oncology, Breast Cancer (Version 2.2017). Available at: http://www.nccn.org/professionals/physician_gls/pdf/breast.pdf. Accessed July 20, 2016.

86. Allred DC, Anderson SJ, Paik S, et al. Adjuvant tamoxifen reduces subsequent breast cancer in women with estrogen receptor-positive ductal carcinoma in situ: a study based on NSABP protocol B-24. J Clin Oncol 2012;30:1268–73.

87. Lo AC, Truong PT, Wai ES, et al. Population-based analysis of the impact and generalizability of the NSABP-B24 study on endocrine therapy for patients with ductal carcinoma in situ of the breast. Ann Oncol 2015;26:1898–903.

88. Johnston SR. Endocrine treatment for ductal carcinoma in situ: balancing risks and benefits. Lancet 2016;387:819–21.

89. Llarena NC, Estevez SL, Tucker SL, et al. Impact of fertility concerns on tamoxifen initiation and persistence. J Natl Cancer Inst 2015;107 [pii:djv202].

90. Nichols HB, Bowles EJ, Islam J, et al. Tamoxifen initiation after ductal carcinoma in situ. Oncologist 2016;21:134–40.

91. Flanagan MR, Rendi MH, Gadi VK, et al. Adjuvant endocrine therapy in patients with ductal carcinoma in situ: a population-based retrospective analysis from 2005 to 2012 in the national cancer data base. Ann Surg Oncol 2015;22:3264–72.

92. Karavites LC, Kane AK, Zaveri S, et al. Tamoxifen acceptance and adherence among patients with ductal carcinoma in situ (DCIS) treated in a multidisciplinary setting. Cancer Prev Res (Phila) 2017;10:389–97.

93. Cuzick J, Sestak I, Cawthorn S, et al. Tamoxifen for prevention of breast cancer: extended long-term follow-up of the IBIS-I breast cancer prevention trial. Lancet Oncol 2015;16:67–75.

94. Early Breast Cancer Trialists' Collaborative Group (EBCTCG). Aromatase inhibitors versus tamoxifen in early breast cancer: patient-level meta-analysis of the randomised trials. Lancet 2015;386:1341–52.

95. Margolese RG, Cecchini RS, Julian TB, et al. Anastrozole versus tamoxifen in postmenopausal women with ductal carcinoma in situ undergoing lumpectomy plus radiotherapy (NSABP B-35): a randomised, double-blind, phase 3 clinical trial. Lancet 2016;387:849–56.

96. Forbes JF, Sestak I, Howell A, et al. Anastrozole versus tamoxifen for the prevention of locoregional and contralateral breast cancer in postmenopausal women with locally excised ductal carcinoma in situ (IBIS-II DCIS): a double-blind, randomised controlled trial. Lancet 2016;387:866–73.

97. Hudis CA. Trastuzumab–mechanism of action and use in clinical practice. N Engl J Med 2007;357:39–51.

98. Dahabreh IJ, Linardou H, Siannis F, et al. Trastuzumab in the adjuvant treatment of early-stage breast cancer: a systematic review and meta-analysis of randomized controlled trials. Oncologist 2008;13:620–30.

99. Rakovitch E, Nofech-Mozes S, Hanna W, et al. HER2/neu and Ki-67 expression predict non-invasive recurrence following breast-conserving therapy for ductal carcinoma in situ. Br J Cancer 2012;106:1160–5.

100. Borgquist S, Zhou W, Jirström K, et al. The prognostic role of HER2 expression in ductal breast carcinoma in situ (DCIS); a population-based cohort study. BMC Cancer 2015;15:468.

101. Williams KE, Barnes NL, Cramer A, et al. Molecular phenotypes of DCIS predict overall and invasive recurrence. Ann Oncol 2015;26:1019–25.

102. Noh JM, Lee J, Choi DH, et al. HER-2 overexpression is not associated with increased ipsilateral breast tumor recurrence in DCIS treated with breast-conserving surgery followed by radiotherapy. Breast 2013;22:894–7.

103. Di Cesare P, Pavesi L, Villani L, et al. The Relationships between HER2 overexpression and DCIS characteristics. Breast J 2017;23:307–14.

104. Poulakaki N, Makris GM, Battista MJ, et al. Hormonal receptor status, Ki-67 and HER2 expression: prognostic value in the recurrence of ductal carcinoma in situ of the breast? Breast 2016;25:57–61.

105. Holmes P, Lloyd J, Chervoneva I, et al. Prognostic markers and long-term outcomes in ductal carcinoma in situ of the breast treated with excision alone. Cancer 2011;117:3650–7.

106. Curigliano G, Disalvatore D, Esposito A, et al. Risk of subsequent in situ and invasive breast cancer in human epidermal growth factor receptor 2-positive ductal carcinoma in situ. Ann Oncol 2015;26:682–7.

107. Thorat MA, Wagner S, Jones LJ, et al. Prognostic and predictive relevance of HER2 status in ductal carcinoma in situ: results from the UK/ANZ DCIS trial. San Antonio Breast Cancer Symposium. San Antonio (TX), December 8–12, 2015. P3-07-02.

108. Estévez LG, Suarez-Gauthier A, García E, et al. Molecular effects of lapatinib in patients with HER2 positive ductal carcinoma in situ. Breast Cancer Res 2014;16:R76.

109. Kuerer HM, Buzdar AU, Mittendorf EA, et al. Biologic and immunologic effects of preoperative trastuzumab for ductal carcinoma in situ of the breast. Cancer 2011;117:39–47.

110. Siziopikou KP, Anderson SJ, Cobleigh MA, et al. Preliminary results of centralized HER2 testing in ductal carcinoma in situ (DCIS): NSABP B-43. Breast Cancer Res Treat 2013;142:415–21.

111. Boughey JC, Gonzalez RJ, Bonner E, et al. Current treatment and clinical trial developments for ductal carcinoma in situ of the breast. Oncologist 2007;12:1276–87.

112. Silverstein MJ, Poller DN, Waisman JR, et al. Prognostic classification of breast ductal carcinoma-in-situ. Lancet 1995;345:1154–7.

113. Silverstein MJ, Lagios MD, Craig PH, et al. A prognostic index for ductal carcinoma in situ of the breast. Cancer 1996;77:2267–74.

114. Silverstein MJ. The University of Southern California/Van Nuys prognostic index for ductal carcinoma in situ of the breast. Am J Surg 2003;186:337–43.

115. Silverstein MJ, Lagios MD. Choosing treatment for patients with ductal carcinoma in situ: fine tuning the University of Southern California/Van Nuys Prognostic Index. J Natl Cancer Inst Monogr 2010;2010:193–6.

116. Boland GP, Chan KC, Knox WF, et al. Value of the Van Nuys Prognostic Index in prediction of recurrence of ductal carcinoma in situ after breast-conserving surgery. Br J Surg 2003;90:426–32.

117. Altintas S, Lambein K, Huizing MT, et al. Prognostic significance of oncogenic markers in ductal carcinoma in situ of the breast: a clinicopathologic study. Breast J 2009;15:120–32.
118. Gilleard O, Goodman A, Cooper M, et al. The significance of the Van Nuys prognostic index in the management of ductal carcinoma in situ. World J Surg Oncol 2008;6:61.
119. MacAusland SG, Hepel JT, Chong FK, et al. An attempt to independently verify the utility of the Van Nuys Prognostic Index for ductal carcinoma in situ. Cancer 2007;110:2648–53.
120. Di Saverio S, Catena F, Santini D, et al. 259 Patients with DCIS of the breast applying USC/Van Nuys prognostic index: a retrospective review with long term follow up. Breast Cancer Res Treat 2008;109:405–16.
121. Early Breast Cancer Trialists' Collaborative Group (EBCTCG), Correa C, McGale P, Taylor C, et al. Overview of the randomized trials of radiotherapy in ductal carcinoma in situ of the breast. J Natl Cancer Inst Monogr 2010;2010: 162–77.
122. Mammary Fold Academic and Research Collaborative. Variation in the management of ductal carcinoma in situ in the UK: results of the mammary fold national practice survey. Eur J Surg Oncol 2016;42:1153–61.
123. Rudloff U, Jacks LM, Goldberg JI, et al. Nomogram for predicting the risk of local recurrence after breast-conserving surgery for ductal carcinoma in situ. J Clin Oncol 2010;28:3762–9.
124. Sweldens C, Peeters S, van Limbergen E, et al. Local relapse after breast-conserving therapy for ductal carcinoma in situ: a European single-center experience and external validation of the Memorial Sloan-Kettering Cancer Center DCIS nomogram. Cancer J 2014;20:1–7.
125. Wang F, Li H, Tan PH, et al. Validation of a nomogram in the prediction of local recurrence risks after conserving surgery for Asian women with ductal carcinoma in situ of the breast. J Clin Oncol 2014;26(11):684–91.
126. Collins LC, Achacoso N, Haque R, et al. Risk prediction for local breast cancer recurrence among women with DCIS treated in a community practice: a nested, case-control study. Ann Surg Oncol 2015;22:S502–8.
127. Yi M, Meric-Bernstam F, Kuerer HM, et al. Evaluation of a breast cancer nomogram for predicting risk of ipsilateral breast tumor recurrences in patients with ductal carcinoma in situ after local excision. J Clin Oncol 2012;30:600–7.
128. Benson JR, Wishart GC. Predictors of recurrence for ductal carcinoma in situ after breast-conserving surgery. Lancet Oncol 2013;14:e348–57.
129. Solin LJ, Gray R, Baehner FL, et al. Multigene expression assay to predict local recurrence risk for ductal carcinoma in situ of the breast. J Natl Cancer Inst 2013;105:701–10.
130. Rakovitch E, Nofech-Mozes S, Hanna W, et al. A population-based validation study of the DCIS Score predicting recurrence risk in individuals treated by breast-conserving surgery alone. Breast Cancer Res Treat 2015;152:389–98.
131. Hughes LL, Wang M, Page DL, et al. Local excision alone without irradiation for ductal carcinoma in situ of the breast: a trial of the Eastern Cooperative Oncology Group. J Clin Oncol 2009;27:5319–24.
132. Wood WC, Alvarado M, Buchholz DJ, et al. The current clinical value of the DCIS score. Oncology (Williston Park) 2014;28(Suppl 2):C2, 1–8, C3.
133. Raldow AC, Sher D, Chen AB, et al. Cost effectiveness of the oncotype DX DCIS score for guiding treatment of patients with ductal carcinoma in situ. J Clin Oncol 2016;34 [pii:JCO678532].

134. Matlock K, Lioyd JM, Carter WB, et al. Concordance of Van-Nuys prognostic index, Memorial Sloan Kettering Breast Cancer Nomogram and oncotype Dx DCIS scores in prediction of ductal carcinoma in situ (DCIS) recurrence risk. J Clin Oncol 2015;33:56.
135. Leonard C, Lei R, Antell A, et al. A comparison of models (physician, the Van Nuys prognostic index, the Memorial-Sloan-Kettering Cancer Center DCIS nomogram)to predict ipsilateral breast events in patients with ductal carcinoma in situ (DCIS) of the breast after breast-conserving surgery failed to replicate results of the oncotype DCIS recurrence score [abstract]. Cancer Res 2017;77. SABCS16-P1-11-02.
136. Altintas S, Toussaint J, Durbecq V, et al. Fine tuning of the Van Nuys prognostic index (VNPI) 2003 by integrating the genomic grade index (GGI): new tools for ductal carcinoma in situ (DCIS). Breast J 2011;17:343–51.
137. Francis A, Thomas J, Fallowfield L, et al. Addressing overtreatment of screen detected DCIS; the LORIS trial. Eur J Cancer 2015;51:2296–303.
138. Elshof LE, Tryfonidis K, Slaets L, et al. Feasibility of a prospective, randomised, open-label, international multicentre, phase III, non-inferiority trial to assess the safety of active surveillance for low risk ductal carcinoma in situ - the LORD study. Eur J Cancer 2015;51:1497–510.
139. The Alliance for Clinical Trials in Oncology Foundation. Principal Investigator: Hwang S. Comparison of operative versus medical endocrine therapy for low risk DCIS: the COMET trial. 2016. Available at: http://www.pcori.org/research-results/2016/comparison-operativeversus-medical-endocrine-therapy-low-risk-dcis-comet. Accessed July 20, 2016.
140. Lippey J, Spillane A, Saunders C. Not all ductal carcinoma in situ is created equal: can we avoid surgery for low-risk ductal carcinoma in situ? ANZ J Surg 2016;86:859–60.

Management of the Axilla in the Patient with Breast Cancer

Ko Un Park, MD, Abigail Caudle, MD, MS*

KEYWORDS

- Breast cancer • Sentinel lymph node • Nodal metastasis
- Axillary lymphadenectomy • Neoadjuvant chemotherapy

KEY POINTS

- Axillary nodal disease burden, which is critical to multidisciplinary treatment decision making, can be predicted with physical examination and axillary ultrasound and with fine-needle aspiration of suspicious-appearing nodes.
- Completion of axillary lymph node dissection may be omitted in select clinically node-negative patients undergoing breast-conserving surgery found to have 1 or 2 positive lymph nodes on sentinel lymph node dissection.
- Emerging data suggest that avoiding axillary node dissection may be appropriate in clinically node-positive patients who receive neoadjuvant chemotherapy.

INTRODUCTION

The presence of nodal metastasis is a key prognostic predictor in breast cancer with significant impacts on treatment planning.[1–3] The nodal status often determines the need for systemic therapy, the extent of surgery, reconstruction options, and the need for radiation after mastectomy. Historically, patients diagnosed with breast cancer underwent axillary node dissection (ALND) to stage the axilla. Advancements in diagnostic imaging and surgical technique, however, now allow for nonsurgical or minimally invasive approaches that help clinicians attain the same information with reduced morbidity. Beyond diagnosis, the use of ALND as a therapeutic modality has been re-examined, with the recognition that all patients with nodal disease may not require extensive axillary surgery. In the modern era, surgeons must have a thorough understanding of the impact of axillary disease on multidisciplinary therapy and surgical planning.

STAGING OF THE AXILLARY NODAL REGIONS

Nodal staging in breast cancer patients begins with physical examination of regional nodal basins, including axillary, infraclavicular, and supraclavicular regions. When

Disclosure Statement: The authors have no relevant financial disclosures.
Department of Breast Surgical Oncology, Division of Surgery, The University of Texas MD Anderson Cancer Center, 1515 Holcombe Boulevard, Unit 1434, Houston, TX 77030, USA
* Corresponding author.
E-mail address: ascaudle@mdanderson.org

Surg Clin N Am 98 (2018) 747–760
https://doi.org/10.1016/j.suc.2018.04.001
0039-6109/18/© 2018 Elsevier Inc. All rights reserved.

axillary adenopathy is identified, the clinician should take care to determine the size of palpable nodes and whether they appear to be matted. Unfortunately, physical examination is impacted by body habitus, making it highly unreliable with a false-negative rate (FNR) as high as 45%.[4] Because of this, ultrasound (US) has emerged as the preferred technique for nodal assessment before therapy. One benefit of US is that abnormal nodes can be assessed in the same setting with needle biopsy to allow for pathologic confirmation of disease. In a study from the authors' institution, axillary US with fine-needle aspiration (FNA) of abnormal nodes was found to have a sensitivity of 86.4%, specificity of 100%, and negative predictive value of 67%. The sensitivity increased to 93% in patients with metastatic deposits measuring greater than 5 mm compared with 44% when the largest focus was less than 5 mm.[5] In 1 study of 115 cases, the investigators reported on FNAs done by palpation alone (n = 66) and those done under US guidance (n = 49). The overall sensitivity was 65%; however, the sensitivity was higher (88%) in patients undergoing ALND, where the median metastatic focus was 1.5 cm, compared with a sensitivity of 16% in patients undergoing sentinel lymph node dissection (SLND), where the median focus was 0.25 cm. The investigators reported that 81.5% of the false-negative cases occurred when the metastatic focus was less than 1 cm.[6] Current National Comprehensive Cancer Network (NCCN) guidelines recommend pathologic confirmation of clinically palpable nodes using US-guided needle biopsy. As discussed later, there are also now recommendations to place clips to mark nodes with biopsy-confirmed disease.[7]

The American Joint Committee on Cancer staging system includes nodal staging based on clinical and pathologic evaluation.[3] Clinical staging includes nodes detected by examination or imaging and defines N1 as mobile ipsilateral level I and level II axillary lymph nodes; N2 as matted ipsilateral level I and level II nodes or clinically detected ipsilateral internal mammary node in the absence of level I or level II adenopathy; and N3a as ipsilateral infraclavicular (level III) adenopathy. If level I or level II adenopathy is present along with disease in ipsilateral internal mammary, it is categorized as N3b. Supraclavicular lymphadenopathy is defined as N3c. Pathologic LN staging is based on the location of involved nodes and the number.[8]

CLINICALLY NEGATIVE LYMPH NODE
Sentinel Lymph Node Dissection

The introduction of SLND for axillary staging in breast cancer was one of the most important contemporary advances in care, allowing for accurate staging while minimizing morbidity. Prior to the advent of SLND, patients routinely underwent ALND, thus exposing them to the risks of lymphedema, chronic pain, and sensory deficits.[9,10] Many of these patients did not have nodal metastasis yet suffered from the side effects of the surgery without oncologic benefit. SLND was first introduced for melanoma in the early 1990s,[11] however was quickly also validated for the use in breast cancer.[12-14] SLND is based on the concept that there is a specific drainage pattern for lymphatics of the breast. Evaluation of the sentinel nodes, or the first draining nodes for the breast, can predict the status of the remaining nodes.

There are now long-term survival data comparing SLND with ALND in patients with clinically node-negative breast cancer. In the National Surgical Adjuvant Breast and Bowel Project (NSABP) B-32 trial, 5611 patients were randomized to SLND plus ALND (group 1) or SLND with ALND only if positive nodes were identified (group 2) to assess oncologic outcomes. There were no differences seen in disease-free (82.4% vs 81.5%) or overall survival (91.8% vs 90.3%) rates at 8 years. The investigators concluded that SLND alone was an appropriate therapy when SLNs showed no disease.[15] Similarly, the smaller Axillary Lymphatic Mapping Against Nodal Axillary Clearance trial was a multi-institutional randomized study designed to compare arm and shoulder morbidity as well as quality of life in SLND with standard axillary treatment in clinically node-negative early breast cancer patients.[16] The trial demonstrated decreased incidence of lymphedema in the SLND arm (relative risk 0.37; 95% CI, 0.23–0.6) compared with standard axillary management. The sentinel node group also had lower drain usage, hospital stay, and a shorter time to return to normal activities with improved quality-of-life scores.[10,16] Thus, SLND is currently the standard approach for axillary staging in those with clinically negative axilla. If the SLNs are negative for metastasis, then a completion ALND is not required.[7]

Management of Positive Sentinel Lymph Nodes

With the incorporation of SLND, pathologists could focus on a smaller number of nodes and began to perform more detailed evaluation. This has led to a growing proportion of patients diagnosed with micrometastatic (defined as >0.2 mm but <2 mm)[3] or very low-volume nodal disease.[17] Although the standard practice at the time was to perform completion ALND when a positive node was identified regardless of the size of metastatic focus, clinicians began to question this approach.[18] A survey of the Surveillance, Epidemiology, and End Results database demonstrated that 16% of patients with a positive sentinel lymph node (SLN) did not undergo ALND between 1998 and 2004. Only 62% of those with microscopic metastasis underwent ALND.[19] Similarly, a report from the National Cancer Database showed that 20.8% of patients with a positive SLN treated between 1998 and 2005 did not undergo ALND.[20] Although there were no data at that time to support this practice, these studies showed that clinicians believed that ALND could be avoided in patients with small-volume disease.

The American College of Surgeons Oncology Group (ACOSOG) Z0011 trial was designed to determine if ALND was necessary in clinically node-negative patients who were found to have small-volume disease after SLND.

This multicenter, randomized, prospective trial enrolled clinically T1-2N0 breast cancer patients who underwent breast-conserving therapy (BCT) and were found to have 1 or 2 positive SLNs by hematoxylin-eosin (H&E) evaluation. Participants were randomized to either completion ALND or SLND alone without any additional axillary therapy and followed for locoregional and overall survival outcomes.[21,22] Although the planned accrual was 1900 patients, the trial closed early in 2004 with 891 patients due to slow enrollment and a low event rate. In the intent-to-treat analysis, there were 420 patients in the ALND arm and 436 in the SLND-only arm with similar patient and tumor characteristics between the 2 groups; 27% of the ALND group were found to have metastases in non-SLNs. In patients with micrometastatic disease, only 10% had additional positive lymph nodes. The first report of the trial showed no difference in local recurrence (3.6% ALND group vs 1.8% SLND group; $P = .11$), ipsilateral axillary recurrence (0.5% ALND vs 0.9% SLND; $P = .45$) or 5-year overall survival (91.9% ALND vs 92.5% SLND; $P = .24$). The trial concluded that ALND could be safely omitted in T1 or T2 tumors with clinically node-negative disease but with less than or equal to 2 positive SLNs. The investigators have recently reported updated results at a median follow-up of 9.3 years. The original findings remain in place, with only 1 additional regional recurrence occurring (in the SLND alone group). This translates into a 10-year cumulative incidence of locoregional recurrence of 5.3% with SLND alone versus 6.2% in the ALND group ($P = .36$).[23] The 10-year overall survival was 86.3% in the SLND group compared with 83.6% in the ALND cohort.[24]

Although the trial stated the addition of a third radiation field was not allowed, recent evaluation of treatment plans reveals inconsistencies.[25] Of the 605 patients with case report forms, 11% did not receive radiotherapy. One question that has been raised is the use of high tangents, which broadens coverage to less than or equal to 2 cm from the humeral head incorporating much of level I/II of the axilla. Although it was postulated that the SLND arm may have been more likely to have this addition to the radiation field,[26] an analysis of 142 patients with detailed records available showed that 50% (33/66) of ALND patients and 52.6% (40/76) of SLND patients received high tangent coverage. In addition, 18.9% (43/225) received regional nodal irradiation despite this prohibited in the protocol—22 in the ALND cohort and 21 in the SLND one.[25] There was no difference in disease-free survival, overall survival, or locoregional failure between those who were treated with nodal field irradiation and those who did not receive any radiotherapy.[24] These inconsistencies make it difficult to determine the optimal adjuvant radiation plan for patients who do not undergo ALND.

There were similar trials investigating the need for completion ALND from Europe. One of these was the International Breast Cancer Study Group 23-01 trial, a phase 3 noninferiority trial that evaluated the role of omitting ALND in patients who had positive SLNs limited to micrometastatic disease.[27] Patients were randomized to completion ALND or no ALND, and adjuvant radiation therapy was not specified. One of the most insightful aspects of this trial is that patients could undergo mastectomy or BCT; thus, the axillary region was not covered by radiation fields in all patients. In fact, 9% had mastectomy without radiation, and 17% had intraoperative partial radiation, which would not have provided axillary coverage. The regional recurrence rates were 2.4% (11/464) in the ALND arm and 2.8% (13/467) in the SLND-only arm. The 5-year disease-free survival was no different between the 2 groups (84.4% ALND vs 87.8% SLND-only arm; $P = .16$). The investigators concluded that patients with limited micrometastatic disease could safely omit further axillary surgery. The findings of this trial have recently been incorporated into NCCN guidelines, which recommend no further surgery for patients whose nodal disease is less than 2 mm.[28]

The European Organisation for Research and Treatment of Cancer 10981-22023, After Mapping of the Axilla, Radiotherapy or Surgery?, is another multicenter trial that randomized 1425 clinically node-negative patients with positive SLNs to ALND or axillary radiotherapy (ART).[29] At median 6.1 years' follow-up, the axillary recurrence rates were 0.54% in the ALND arm and 1.03% in the ART group. Like the other trials, there was no benefit to further axillary surgery. The 5-year axillary recurrence rates were 0.43% in the ALND group, 1.19% in the ART group, and 0.72% in the negative SLN group. There were no statistical differences in 5-year disease-free survival (86.9% ALND vs 82.7% ART; $P = .2$) or overall survival (93.3% ALND vs 92.5% ART; $P = .3$). One of the strong correlative aspects of this trial was the assessment of lymphedema rates by recording arm circumferences and clinical signs of lymphedema at baseline and at 1-year, 3-year, and 5-year intervals after surgery. Clinical signs of lymphedema were statistically more likely in the surgery group at 1 year (28% vs 15%; $P<.0001$), 3 years (23% vs 14%; $P = .003$), and 5 years (23% vs 11%; $P<.0001$). The proportion of patients with a greater than or equal to 10% increase in arm circumference was similar at 1 year (8% vs 6%; $P = .3$) and at 3 years (10% vs 6%; $P = .8$) but became statistically different at 5 years (13% vs 6%; $P = .0009$).

These trials have led to a significant practice changes in the United States and abroad. For instance, the MD Anderson Cancer Center convened a multidisciplinary discussion after publication of the ACOSOG Z0011 trial to decide how to incorporate these findings into practice.[30] In the first year after this discussion, the number of SLN-positive patients who underwent ALND dropped to 24% from 85% in the year before publication of the trial.[31] This paradigm shift has expanded with time, with a recent publication demonstrating that the number of SLN-positive patients who undergo

ALND has dropped further to 8% (4/48). In addition to cost savings from less surgery, the investigators showed that the use of intraoperative frozen section evaluation of SLNs has been abandoned, decreasing costs and operative times.[32] A report of greater than 74,000 patients from the National Cancer Database showed that the number of SLN-positive patients undergoing ALND dropped from 77% in 2009 (before publication of ACOSOG Z0011) to 44% in 2011.[33] It is likely that this number has further decreased with time. Omission of ALND in appropriate patients is now considered a quality metric for breast surgeons by the Society of Surgical Oncology and the American Society of Breast Surgeons.[34]

The Z0011 trial has brought considerable debate as to the utility of preoperative US of nodal regions. Some investigators argue that biopsy should not be performed if less than or equal to 2 suspicious nodes are seen in patients who would have otherwise meet Z0011 criteria because this would define them as clinically node positive, thus requiring ALND. One study compared patients with T1-2 tumors who had nodal metastasis identified by US with those who had disease found by SLND after a negative US. When looking at patients with less than or equal to 2 suspicious nodes seen on US, 45% had at least 3 positive nodes at surgery compared with 19% in the group that had nodal disease identified by SLND (P<.001). Patients with disease seen on US had more positive nodes (4.1 vs 2.2; P<.0001), larger foci of nodal metastases (13.8 mm vs 5.3 mm; P<.0001), and a higher incidence of extranodal extension (53% vs 24%; P<.0001).[35] A similar study showed that having greater than 1 abnormal node on imaging was associated with having greater than or equal to 3 positive nodes at surgery (68% vs 43%; P = .003).[36]

With the acceptance of ACOSOG Z0011 in patients undergoing BCT, there are no data regarding patients who undergo mastectomy, which has led to heterogeneity in practice.[37] There are trails ongoing to assess the value of added surgery in these patients.[38]

Isolated Tumor Cells

With the spread of SLND, pathologists had fewer nodes to review so the use of immunohistochemistry (IHC) became more popular. This allowed for the identification of isolated tumor cells (ITCs), defined as clusters of metastatic cells spanning less than or equal to 0.2 mm, single tumor cells, or clusters of less than 200 cells in a single cross-section.[3] The discovery of these extremely small metastases that were previously unrecognized by standard H&E evaluation left clinicians with a dilemma regarding how to manage these patients. The ACOSOG Z0010 was designed as a prospective observation trial that enrolled women who had negative SLNs by H&E staining. SLN blocks were then sent for central laboratory IHC staining to look for ITCs. Treating physicians were blinded to the IHC results (thus they treated everyone based on the negative H&E staining). Among the 3326 H&E negative nodes, 349 (10.5%) had IHC-positive SLNs. There was no difference in 5-year overall survival rates between IHC-negative and IHC-positive patients (95.7% vs 95.1%; P = .64).[39] Similarly, a subgroup analysis of NSABP B-32 showed that 15.9% of patients with H&E-negative SLNs had positive metastasis by IHC (11.1% ITCs, 4.4% micrometastases, and 0.4% macrometastases). Unlike the Z0010 study, 5-year overall survival rate was statistically significant in this study but the difference was very small (94.6% in IHC-positive patients vs 95.8% in IHC-negative patients; P = .03).[40] Thus, current NCCN guidelines do not recommend routine use of cytokeratin IHC to define lymph node involvement.

The 1 group where ITCs may be clinically relevant are those with lobular tumors. Because lobular cancer cells have noncohesive growth patterns, nodal metastases may present as widely dispersed ITCs.[41,42] In 1 study, 17% of patients with lobular tumors had additional positive nodes.[41] Many surgeons still consider ALND when ITCs are identified in patients with lobular tumors.[31]

Elderly Patients

In 2016, the Society of Surgical Oncology joined the American Board of Internal Medicine Foundation in their Choosing Wisely campaign. One of the recommendations included omitting the routine use of SLND in women greater than 70 years old with clinically node-negative, hormone receptor–positive breast cancer.[43] This recommendation was made based on the premise that elderly patients tend to have less aggressive, more indolent breast cancer and there is no significant difference in breast cancer mortality between patients undergoing ALND versus those who do not.[44,45] One of the studies supporting this recommendations is the Cancer and Leukemia Group B 9343 trial in which elderly patients with early-stage breast cancer undergoing BCT were randomized to adjuvant radiation with tamoxifen versus tamoxifen only.[44] In a 10-year follow-up, only 3% died from breast cancer, adjuvant radiation therapy after breast-conserving surgery did not alter survival, and local recurrence and axillary recurrence rates were low. Importantly, this trial was conducted before the widespread acceptance of SLND, so 60% of the participants had no surgical staging of the axilla. Thus these results could be based on classifying patients as node negative on clinical evaluation alone. The current NCCN guideline considers axillary staging by SLND optional in elderly patients with particularly favorable tumors, in whom decisions on adjuvant systemic treatment will not be affected by the results of axillary staging.[28]

Sentinel Lymph Node Dissection in Clinically Node-Negative Patients Receiving Neoadjuvant Chemotherapy

Neoadjuvant chemotherapy (NAC) is sometimes used in clinically node-negative patients based on either tumor size, patient desire for BCT, or tumor biology. There are multiple advantages to this approach, including in situ assessment of tumor response and tumor downstaging. There has been debate, however, as to when SLND should be performed in these patients. Although some investigators propose that SLND should be performed before initiation of chemotherapy to get complete nodal staging, others have proposed that this should be performed after chemotherapy in conjunction with the breast operation. By performing SLND at the completion of NAC, patients can have 1 operation that allows for evaluation of disease with consideration of response to therapy. Data from MD Anderson show that the SLN identification rate is only slightly better before NAC (98.7% surgery first vs 97.4% after NAC) with comparable FNRs (4.1% surgery first vs 5.8% NAC; $P = .4$).[46] After stratification for T category, patients with SLND performed after NAC had a lower probability of having a positive SLN (T1: 12.7% vs 19%, $P = .2$; T2: 20.5% vs 36.5%, $P<.0001$; and T3: 30.4% vs 51.4%, $P = .04$), with similar locoregional recurrence rates and disease-free and overall survival rates.[46] Comparable SLN identification rate before and after NAC has been corroborated with an evaluation of the Netherlands Cancer Registry, showing SLN identification rates of 98% when SLN was performed before NAC and 95% when performed after NAC. The proportion of patients with a positive SLN was higher when SLN was performed before NAC (45% vs 33%; $P = .006$).[47] Dual-tracer technique and surgeon depth of experience improve the success of SLN identification in this setting whereas dual-tracer technique and removal of greater than or equal to 2 SLNs are associated with a decreased FNR.[46]

CLINICALLY NODE-POSITIVE PATIENTS

Although there is much interest in minimizing axillary surgery, ALND remains the standard operation for patients with clinical disease identified by physical examination or imaging and confirmed with needle biopsy. It is also indicated in cases where an SLN cannot be identified or there is a contraindication to SLND, such as in inflammatory breast cancer. ALND allows for comprehensive staging of the axilla because all nodes are removed and can be evaluated. Standard ALND is an anatomic resection of the level I and II axillary regions with care to preserve the axillary vein, thoracodorsal neurovascular bundle, and the long thoracic nerve. Routine removal of the level III nodes is not indicated unless there is clinical evidence of their involvement.

Neoadjuvant Chemotherapy

Patients who are clinically node positive often receive NAC, which can eradicate nodal disease in 40% of patients.[48] Because the efficacy of systemic therapy has improved, however, especially with targeted agents, such as trastuzumab and pertuzumab, this proportion of patients achieving nodal pathologic complete response in some tumor biology subsets has also risen. The ACOSOG Z1071 trial reported nodal conversion rates of 21.1% in patients with hormone receptor–positive, HER2-negative tumors; 49.4% with triple-negative tumors; and 64.7% with HER2-positive tumors.[48] With increasingly high nodal conversion rates, clinicians have questioned the use of extensive axillary surgery in patients who have no residual nodal disease. Single-institution reports addressing the use of SLND in this population have shown FNRs ranging from 5% to 20%, limiting its use in this setting.[49–52] These reports are limited, however, by heterogeneity in surgical technique. Three large multi-Institutional prospective registry studies have recently been published evaluating the use of SLND in clinically node-positive patients who receive NAC, enrolling patients with clinical T1-4, N1-2, M0 breast cancer who receive NAC. After completion of chemotherapy, they underwent SLND followed by ALND so that the FNR of SLND could be determined.[53–55] Results are summarized in **Table 1**.

The ACOSOG Z0171 trial was designed to evaluate the FNR of SLND with a prespecified success threshold of 10%. Although the overall reported FNR of 12.6% (90% CI, 9.85%–16.05%) made this a negative trial, further evaluation of subsets provided valuable insights into the use of SLND in this setting. First, the importance of surgical technique was highlighted. Use of dual-tracer technique reduced the FNR to 10.8% compared with 20.3% when a single agent was used ($P = .05$). Also removal of greater than or equal to 3 SLNs improved the FNR to 9.1% compared with 21.1% when 2

Table 1 Trials evaluating sentinel lymph node dissection in clinically node-positive patients who receive neoadjuvant chemotherapy			
	ACOSOG Z1071[53,56]	SENTINA (Arm C)[55]	SN FNAC[54]
Number of patients	cN1 = 603 cN2 = 34	592	153
SLN identification rate	92.7%	87.8%	87.6%
Overall FNR	12.6%	14.2%	13.4%
FNR based on mapping agents			
One agent	20.3%	16%	16%
Dual agent	10.8%	8.6%	5.2%
FNR by number of SLNs			
1 SLN	31%	24.3%	18.2%
2 SLNs	21.1%	18.5%	≥2 SLNs = 4.9%
≥3 SLNs	9.1%	4.9%	—
FNR with IHC	8.7%	NA	8.4%

SLNs were removed or 31% when a single SLN was removed.[53] The use of IHC also showed benefit by reducing the FNR to 8.7%.[56] US alone was not predictive of nodal response. In 430 patients who had normalized nodes on US after NAC, 243 (56.5%) had residual pathologic disease. Alternatively, 28.2% (51/181) of patients with nodes that looked suspicious on USafter NAC had a nodal pathologic complete response.[57]

The SENTinel NeoAdjuvant (SENTINA) study is a 4-arm, multicenter European trial.[55] One of the arms (arm C) focused on clinically node-positive patients who converted to clinically node negative after NAC. One important difference in this trial is that the trial did not require pathologic confirmation of clinical nodal disease. Only 25% (149/592), however, underwent needle biopsy. The overall FNR was 14.2% but, similar to the ACOSOG Z1071 trial, surgical technique was critical. Dual-tracer mapping reduced the FNR to 8.6% compared with 16% with 1 agent. Removal of greater than or equal to 3 SLNs improved the FNR to 4.9% compared with 18.5% when 2 nodes were removed and 24.3% when only 1 node was removed.[55] Again, the use of US was not found helpful, with a sensitivity of 23.9% and negative predictive value of 50.3%.[58]

Lastly, the Sentinel Node biopsy Following NeoAdjuvant Chemotherapy in Biopsy Proven Node Positive Breast Cancer Study (SN FNAC) evaluated 145 clinical T0-T3, N1-2 patients undergoing SLND and ALND after NACT.[54] This trial was terminated early with 153 patients secondary to slow accrual and the recent publication of the Z1071 and SENTINA trials. In this trial, the use of IHC reduced the FNR to 8.4% from the overall FNR of 13.4%. Again, the use of dual-tracer technique (FNR 5.2% vs 16% with single agent) and removal of greater than or equal to 2 SLNs (FNR 4.9% vs 18.2% with 1 SLN) were important.

Specific Evaluation of Biopsied Nodes

One of the interesting findings from the ACOSOG Z1071 was that placement of a clip in nodes with biopsy-proved metastases may be useful. In that study, 170 patients had a clip placed in the lymph node containing metastases at the time of initial biopsy. In the 107 patients where the clipped node was retrieved as an SLN, the FNR was 6.8% (95% CI, 1.9%–16.5%).[59] A recent study from the authors' institution also showed utility in placing clips in lymph nodes with biopsy-proved metastases and ensuring removal of these nodes for evaluation. In the authors' study, the FNR for SLND alone was 10.1% (95% CI, 4.2–19.8). Evaluation of the clipped node alone had an FNR of 4.2% (95% CI, 1.4–9.5). When removal of all SLNs and the clipped node was assured, the FNR was reduced to 1.4% (95% CI, 0.03–7.3). In 23% of patients, the clipped node was not an SLN; therefore, evaluation of SLNs alone would have neglected the node with biopsy-confirmed disease.[60] This finding was also seen in the Z1071 trial, where the clipped node was an SLN in 63% (107/170) of those who had a clip placed and was definitely not an SLN in 20% (34/170) because it was found in the ALND specimen. The location of the clipped node is unknown in the remaining 17% (29/170) of patients. A study from University of Pittsburgh demonstrated that the clipped node was not an SLND in 27% (8/30) of cases,[61] whereas this proportion was 21% (3/14) in a study from Mayo Clinic.[62]

Specific evaluation of the node that has biopsy-confirmed disease is a logical addition to surgical staging after NAC; however, SLND alone does not always ensure this, as shown by the studies discussed previously. Therefore, a novel surgical technique called targeted axillary dissection was developed to ensure removal of the sentinel nodes as well as the clipped node.[63] The technique involves placing a clip in a node when needle biopsy confirms pathologic involvement. To selectively remove the clipped node at surgery, the clipped node is marked with an I^{125} seed under US guidance up to 5 days before surgery. The surgeon can then use a gamma probe to identify the node as well as the sentinel nodes for removal. In the first series published with this procedure, including 85 patients, the FNR was 2% (95% CI, 0.05–10.7).[60] Other groups have been evaluating this technique as well, including Diego and colleagues,[61] who reported on 29 patients with successful localization and removal of the clipped node in addition to sentinel node dissection. In the 11 patients with residual nodal disease, all had disease seen in the clipped node. A group from the Netherlands reported on marking axillary nodes with radioactive iodine seeds, which involves placing the seed at the time of initial biopsy before initiating chemotherapy.[64] They report an FNR of 7% in their first 100 patients.[65] To date, they have not published on this technique in addition to SLND; however, trials to assess this are ongoing.[66] The importance of evaluation of the clipped node is now seen by the addition of recommendations for placement of clips and ensured removal of the clipped nodes in the NCCN guidelines.[7]

These trials have led to considerable debate regarding the optimal management of clinically node-positive patients after NAC. Even without concerns about the FNR, there are no prospective data evaluating the oncologic safety of omitting ALND in these patients. Despite, this, many surgeons have incorporated the use of SLND with possible omission of ALND into their practice. A recent survey of the American Society of Breast Surgeons showed that 85% of respondents now offer SLND to at least some of their patients compared with 45% before publication of the trials. Technical factors considered critical for the technique included use of dual-tracer technique (86%), placement of clips with ensured removal (82%), and removal of greater than or equal to 2 nodes (70%); 67% said they routinely place clips in nodes with biopsy-confirmed disease. Of these, 71% localize the clipped node with a wire (73%), seed (13%), or other method (14%). In those who do not localize the clipped node, 82% confirm removal with radiograph.[67]

ONGOING CLINICAL TRIALS

Prospective, multicenter, randomized controlled trials provide the best evidence in answering questions regarding the management of breast cancer patients. The following trials were initiated to address some of these questions in clinically node-positive patients who receive NAC.

National Surgical Adjuvant Breast and Bowel Project B-51/Radiation Therapy Oncology Group 1304 Trial

NASBP B-51/Radiation Therapy Oncology Group 1304 trial is a randomized phase III study that began enrollment in 2013 (ClinicalTrials.gov identifier: NCT01872975). The main goal of the study is to evaluate the benefit of nodal radiation in clinically node-positive patients with a complete nodal response after NAC. Patients with clinical T1-T3 and biopsy-confirmed N1 disease are initially treated with standard anthracycline and/or taxane-based chemotherapy. After NAC, patients undergo axillary staging either by SLND alone, SLND with ALND, or ALND. Patients with no residual nodal disease are eligible to be randomized to no dedicated nodal radiation (chest wall and whole-breast radiotherapy are allowed) versus regional nodal irradiation. The primary endpoint of the study is recurrence-free interval with secondary endpoints, including overall survival, quality of life, toxicity, treatment adequacy, and molecular predictors of recurrence.

Alliance A11202 Trial

The Alliance A11202 trial is an option for patients with residual positive SLNs after NAC (ClinicalTrials.gov identifier: NCT01901094). Patients are randomized to ALND versus no further axillary surgery and all patients receive regional nodal irradiation. The primary endpoint of the study is recurrence. The secondary outcomes include survival, regional recurrence, lymphedema development, adequacy of radiation fields, and residual cancer burden.

SUMMARY

Accurate evaluation of axillary lymph nodes has significant impact on treatment decisions. Surgeons caring for breast cancer patients must understand the technical aspects of axillary staging techniques as well as which procedures are appropriate to provide adequate oncologic outcomes while limiting morbidity. Ongoing studies will further define the role of extensive axillary surgery in breast cancer patients.

REFERENCES

1. Carter C, Allen C, Henson D. Relation of tumor size, lymph node status, and survival in 24,740 breast cancer cases. Cancer 1989;63:181–7.
2. Beenken S, Urist M, Zhang Y, et al. Axillary lymph node status, but not tumor size, predicts locoregional recurrence and overall survival after mastectomy for breast cancer. Ann Surg 2003;237:732–8.
3. Amin MB, Edge S, Greene F, et al. AJCC cancer staging manual. 8th edition. New York: Springer; 2017.
4. Sacre R. Clinical evaluation of axillar lymph nodes compared to surgical and pathological findings. Eur J Surg Oncol 1986;12:169–73.
5. Krishnamurthy S, Sneige N, Bedi D, et al. Role of ultrasound-guided fine-needle aspiration of indeterminate and suspicious axillary lymph nodes in the initial staging of breast carcinoma. Cancer 2002;95:982–8.
6. Alkuwari E, Auger M. Accuracy of fine-needle aspiration cytology of axillary lymph nodes in breast cancer patients: a study of 115 cases with cytologic-histologic correlation. Cancer 2008;114:89–93.
7. National Comprehensive Cancer Network (NCCN) Clinical Practice Guidelines in Oncology: Breast, Version 2.2017, BINV-11. Available at: www.nccn.org. Accessed September 1, 2017.
8. Giuliano A, Connolly J, Edge S, et al. Breast cancer-major changes in the American Joint Committee on Cancer eighth edition cancer staging manual. CA Cancer J Clin 2017;67:290–303.
9. Lucci A, McCall A, beitsch P, et al. Surgical complications associated with sentinel lymph node dissection (SLND) plus axillary lymph node dissection compared with SLND alone in the American College of Surgeons Oncology Group Trial Z0011. J Clin Oncol 2007;25:3657–63.
10. Fleissig A, Fallowfield L, Langridge C, et al. Post-operative arm morbidity and quality of life. Results of the ALMANAC randomised trial comparing sentinel node biopsy with standard axillary treatment in the management of patients with early breast cancer. Breast Cancer Res Treat 2006;95:279–93.
11. Morton D, Wen D, Wong J, et al. Technical details of intraoperative lymphatic mapping for early stage melanoma. Arch Surg 1992;127:392–9.
12. Krag D, Weaver D, Ashikaga T, et al. The sentinel node in breast cancer–a multicenter validation study. N Engl J Med 1998;339:941–6.
13. Giuliano A, Kirgan D, Guenther J, et al. Lymphatic mapping and sentinel lymphadenectomy for breast cancer. Ann Surg 1994;220:391–9.

14. Veronesi U, Paganelli G, Viale G, et al. A randomized comparison of sentinel-node biopsy with routine axillary dissection in breast cancer. N Engl J Med 2003;349:546–53.
15. Krag D, Anderson S, Julian T, et al. Sentinel-lymph-node resection compared with conventional axillary-lymph-node dissection in clinically node-negative patients with breast cancer: overall survival findings from the NSABP B-32 randomised phase 3 trial. Lancet Oncol 2010;11:927–33.
16. Mansel R, Fallowfield L, Kissin M, et al. Randomized multicenter trial of sentinel node biopsy versus standard axillary treatment in operable breast cancer: the ALMANAC trial. J Natl Cancer Inst 2006;98:599–609.
17. Giuliano A, Dale P, Turner R, et al. Improved axillary staging of breast cancer with sentinel lymphadenectomy. Ann Surg 1995;222:394–9.
18. Lyman G, Giuliano A, Somerfield M, et al. American Society of Clinical Oncology guideline recommendations for sentinel lymph node biopsy in early-stage breast cancer. J Clin Oncol 2006;24:210–1.
19. Yi M, Giordano S, Meric-Bernstam F, et al. Trends in and outcomes from sentinel lymph node biopsy (SLNB) alone vs. SLNB with axillary lymph node dissection for node-positive breast cancer patients: experience from the SEER database. Ann Surg Oncol 2010;17(Suppl 3):343–51.
20. Bilimoria K, Bentrem D, Hansen N, et al. Comparison of sentinel lymph node biopsy alone and completion axillary lymph node dissection for node-positive breast cancer. J Clin Oncol 2009;27:2946–53.
21. Giuliano A, Hunt K, Ballman K, et al. Axillary dissection vs no axillary dissection in women with invasive breast cancer and sentinel node metastasis: a randomized clinical trial. JAMA 2011;305:569–75.
22. Giuliano A, McCall L, Beitsch P, et al. ACOSOG Z0011: a randomized trial of axillary node dissection in women with clincial T1-2 N0M0 breast cancer who have a positive sentinel node. J Clin Oncol 2010;28 [abstract: CRA506].
23. Giuliano A, Ballman K, McCall L, et al. Locoregional recurrence after sentinel lymph node dissection with or without axillary dissection in patients with sentinel lymph node metastases: long-term follow-up from the American College of Surgeons Oncology Group (Alliance) ACOSOG Z0011 randomized trial. Ann Surg 2016;264:413–20.
24. Giuliano A, Ballman K, McCall A, et al. Effect of axillary dissection vs no axillary dissection on 10-year overall survival among women with invasive breast cancer and sentinel node metastasis: the ACOSOG Z0011 (alliance) randomized clinical trial. JAMA 2017;318:918–26.
25. Jagsi R, Chadha M, Moni J, et al. Radiation field design in the ACOSOG Z0011 (alliance) trial. J Clin Oncol 2014;32:3600–6.
26. Haffty B, Hunt K, Harris J, et al. Positive sentinel nodes without axillary dissection: implications for the radiation oncologist. J Clin Oncol 2011;29:4479–81.
27. Galimberti V, Cole B, Zurrida S, et al. Axillary dissection versus no axillary dissection in patients with sentinel-node micrometastases (IBCSG 23-01): a phase 3 randomised controlled trial. Lancet Oncol 2013;14:297–305.
28. National Comprehensive Cancer Network (NCCN) Clinical Practice Guidelines in Oncology: Breast, Version 2017. Available at: www.nccn.org. Accessed August 22, 2018.
29. Donker M, van Tienhoven G, Straver M, et al. Radiotherapy or surgery of the axilla after a positive sentinel node in breast cancer (EORTC 10981-22023 AMAROS): a randomised, multicentre, open-label, phase 3 non-inferiority trial. Lancet Oncol 2014;15:1303–10.

30. Caudle A, Hunt K, Kuerer H, et al. Multidisciplinary considerations in the implementation of the findings from the American College of Surgeons Oncology Group (ACOSOG) Z0011 study: a practice-changing trial. Ann Surg Oncol 2011;19:2407–12.

31. Caudle A, Hunt K, Tucker S, et al. American College of Surgeons (ACOSOG) Z0011: impact on surgeon practice patterns. Ann Surg Oncol 2012;19:3144–51.

32. Weiss A, Mittendorf E, DeSnyder S, et al. Expanding implementation of ACOSOG Z0011 in surgeon practice. Clin Breast Cancer 2017 [pii:S1526-8209(17)30412-3].

33. Yao K, Liederbach E, Pesce C, et al. Impact of the American College of Surgeons Oncology Group Z0011 randomized trial on the number of axillary nodes removed for patients with early-stage breast cancer. J Am Coll Surg 2015;221: 71–81.

34. Landercasper J, Bailey L, Berry T, et al. Measures of appropriateness and value for breast surgeons and their patients: the American Society of Breast Surgeons Choosing Wisely (®) Initiative. Ann Surg Oncol 2016;23:3112–8.

35. Caudle A, Kuerer H, Le-Petross H, et al. Predicting the extent of nodal disease in early-stage breast cancer. Ann Surg Oncol 2014;21:3440–7.

36. Pilewskie M, Mautner S, Stempel M, et al. Does a positive axillary lymph node needle biopsy result predict the need for an axillary lymph node dissection in clinically node-negative breast cancer patients in the ACOSOG Z0011 era? Ann Surg Oncol 2016;23:1123–8.

37. FitzSullivan E, Bassett R, Kuerer H, et al. Outcomes of sentinel lymph node-positive breast cancer patients treated with mastectomy without axillary therapy. Ann Surg Oncol 2017;24:652–9.

38. van Roozendaal L, de Wilt J, van Dalen T, et al. The value of completion axillary treatment in sentinel node positive breast cancer patients undergoing a mastectomy: a Dutch randomized controlled multicentre trial (BOOG 2013-07). BMC Cancer 2015;15:610.

39. Giuliano A, Hawes D, Ballman K, et al. Association of occult metastases in sentinel lymph nodes and bone marrow with survival among women with early-stage invasive breast cancer. JAMA 2011;306:385–93.

40. Weaver D, Ashikaga T, Krag D, et al. Effect of occult metastases on survival in node-negative breast cancer. N Engl J Med 2011;364:412–21.

41. Mittendorf E, Sahin A, Tucker S, et al. Lymphovascular invasion and lobular histology are associated with increased incidence of isolated tumor cells in sentinel lymph nodes from early-stage breast cancer patients. Ann Surg Oncol 2008;15:3369–77.

42. Cserni G, Bianchi S, Vezzosi V, et al. The value of cytokeratin immunohistochemistry in the evaluation of axillary sentinel lymph nodes in patients with lobular breast carcinoma. J Clin Pathol 2006;59:518–22.

43. Oncology SoS. Choosing Wisely Campaign. Available at: www.choosingwisely.org/clinician-lists/sso-sentinel-node-biopsy-in-node-negative-women-70-and-over. Accessed October 22, 2017.

44. Hughes K, Schnaper L, Bellon J, et al. Lumpectomy plus tamoxifen with or without irradiation in women age 70 years or older with early breast cancer: long-term follow-up of CALGB 9343. J Clin Oncol 2013;31:2382–7.

45. Martelli G, Boracchi P, Ardoino I, et al. Axillary dissection versus no axillary dissection in older patients with T1N0 breast cancer: 15-year results of a randomized controlled trial. Ann Surg 2012;256:920–4.

46. Hunt K, Yi M, Mittendorf E, et al. Sentinel lymph node surgery after neoadjuvant chemotherapy is accurate and reduces the need for axillary dissection in breast cancer patients. Ann Surg 2009;250(4):558–66.

47. van der Heiden-ven der Loo M, de Munck L, Sonke G, et al. Population based study on sentinel node biopsy before or after neoadjuvant chemotherapy in clinically node negative breast cancer patients: identification rate and influence on axillary treatment. Eur J Cancer 2015;51:915–21.
48. Boughey J, McCall L, Ballman K, et al. Tumor biology correlates with rates of breast-conserving surgery and pathologic complete response after neoadjuvant chemotherapy for breast cancer: findings from the ACOSOG Z1071 (alliance) prospective multicenter clinical trial. Ann Surg 2014;260:608–14.
49. Alvarado R, Yi M, Le-Petross H, et al. The role for sentinel lymph node dissection after neoadjuvant chemotherapy in patients who present with node-positive breast cancer. Ann Surg Oncol 2012;19:3177–83.
50. Classe J, Bordes V, Campion L, et al. Sentinel lymph node biopsy after neoadjuvant chemotherapy for advanced breast cancer: results of Ganglion Sentinelle et Chimiotherapie Neoadjuvante, a French prospective multicentric study. J Clin Oncol 2009;27:726–32.
51. Newman E, Sabel M, Nees A, et al. Sentinel lymph node biopsy performed after neoadjuvant chemotherapy is accurate in patients with documented node-positive breast cancer at presentation. Ann Surg Oncol 2007;14:2946–52.
52. Balch G, Mithani S, Richards K, et al. Lymphatic mapping and sentinel lymphadenectomy after preoperative therapy for stage II and III breast cancer. Ann Surg Oncol 2003;10:616–21.
53. Boughey J, Suman V, Mittendorf E, et al. Sentinel lymph node surgery after neoadjuvant chemotherapy in patients with node-positive breast cancer: the ACOSOG Z1071 (alliance) clinical trial. JAMA 2013;310:1455–61.
54. Boileau JF, Poirier B, Basik M, et al. Sentinel node biopsy after neoadjuvant chemotherapy in biopsy-proven node-positive breast cancer: the SN FNAC study. J Clin Oncol 2015;33:258–64.
55. Kuehn T, Bauerfeind I, Fehm T, et al. Sentinel-lymph-node biopsy in patients with breast cancer before and after neoadjuvant chemotherapy (SENTINA): a prospective, multicentre cohort study. Lancet Oncol 2013;14:609–18.
56. Boughey J, Ballman K, Symmans W, et al. Methods impacting the false negative rate of sentinel lymph node surgery in patients presenting with node positive breast cancer (T0-T4,N1-2) who receive neoadjuvant chemotherapy – Results from a prospective trial – ACOSOG Z1071 (Alliance). Available at: http://eposter.abstractsonline.com/sabcs. Accessed January 31, 2015.
57. Boughey J, Ballman K, Hunt K, et al. Axillary ultrasound after neoadjuvant chemotherapy and its impact on sentinel lymph node surgery: results from the American College of Surgeons Oncology Group Z1071 Trial (Alliance). J Clin Oncol 2015;33:3368–93.
58. Schwentner L, Helms G, Neklijudova V, et al. Using ultrasound and palpation for predicting axillary lymph node status following neoadjuvant chemotherapy - Results from the multi-center SENTINA trial. Breast 2017;31:202–7.
59. Boughey J, Ballman K, Le-Petross H, et al. Identification and resection of clipped node decreases the false-negative rate of sentinel lymph node surgery in patients presenting with node-positive breast cancer (T0-T4, N1-N2) who receive neoadjuvant chemotherapy: results from ACOSOG Z1071 (Alliance). Ann Surg 2016;263:802–7.
60. Caudle A, Yang W, Krishnamurthy S, et al. Improved axillary evaluation following neoadjuvant therapy for patients with node-positive breast cancer using selective evaluation of clipped nodes: implementation of targeted axillary dissection. J Clin Oncol 2016;34:1072–8.

61. Diego E, McAuliffe P, Soran A, et al. Axillary staging after neoadjuvant chemo-therapy for breast cancer: a pilot study combining sentinel lymph node biopsy with radioactive seed localization of pre-treatment positive axillary lymph nodes. Ann Surg Oncol 2016;23:1549–53.

62. Nguyen T, KHieken T, Glazebrook K, et al. Localizing the clipped node in patients with node-positive breast cancer treated with neoadjuvant chemotherapy: early learning experience and challenges. Ann Surg Oncol 2017;24(10):3011–6.

63. Caudle A, Yang W, Mittendorf E, et al. Selective surgical localization of axillary lymph nodes containing metastases in patients with breast cancer: a prospective feasibility trial. JAMA Surg 2014;34:1072–8.

64. Straver M, Rutgers E, Rodenhuis S, et al. The relevance of breast cancer sub-types in the outcome of neoadjuvant chemotherapy. Ann Surg Oncol 2010;17:2411–8.

65. Donker M, Straver ME, Wesseling J, et al. Marking axillary lymph nodes with radioactive iodine seeds for axillary staging after neoadjuvant systemic treatment in breast cancer patients: the MARI procedure. Ann Surg 2015;261:378–82.

66. van Nijnatten T, Simons J, Smidt M, et al. A novel less-invasive approach for axil-lary staging after neoadjuvant chemotherapy in patients with axillary node-positive breast cancer by combining radioactive iodine seed localization in the axilla with the sentinel node procedure (RISAS): a dutch prospective multicenter validation study. Clin Breast Cancer 2017;17:399–402.

67. Caudle A, Bedrosian I, Milton D, et al. Use of sentinel lymph node dissection after neoadjuvant chemotherapy in patients with node-positive breast cancer at diag-nosis: practice patterns of American Society of breast surgeons members. Ann Surg Oncol 2017;24(10):2925–34.

Definition and Management of Positive Margins for Invasive Breast Cancer

Apoorve Nayyar, MBBS[a], Kristalyn K. Gallagher, DO[a],
Kandace P. McGuire, MD[b],*

KEYWORDS

- Breast-conserving surgery (BCS) • Negative margins • Reexcision • Margin width
- Recurrence

KEY POINTS

- Final margin status at breast-conserving surgery is the critical prognostic factor for ipsilateral breast tumor recurrence (IBTR).
- Negative (clear) margins reduce the risk of IBTR; wider margin widths do not further reduce this risk. No ink on tumor is adequate for optimal oncologic control.
- Positive margins require additional surgery.
- Additional margin resection (directed or shave) at primary lumpectomy significantly reduces the rate of positive margins.
- There is a current need for improved intraoperative assessment of the margin status to aid in complete resection.

INTRODUCTION

From the Halsted radical mastectomy to transcriptomics-based personalized therapy, the management of breast cancer has witnessed a massive evolution in the past 5 decades. The adoption of routine screening mammography, improved access to care, availability of radiation therapy, and development of robust systemic therapy options have all facilitated earlier diagnosis and the transition from mastectomy to breast-conserving surgery (BCS) for a select subset of patients. BCS entails complete tumor resection with a concentric margin of surrounding healthy tissue performed in a cosmetically acceptable manner. BCS portends a distinct advantage to the patient in

Disclosure: The authors have nothing to disclose.
[a] Division of Surgical Oncology, Lineberger Comprehensive Cancer Center, University of North Carolina at Chapel Hill, 170 Manning Drive, Chapel Hill, NC 27599, USA; [b] Section of Breast Surgery, Massey Cancer Center at Virginia Commonwealth University, West Hospital, 7th Floor West Wing, Box 980011, Richmond, VA 23298-0011, USA
* Corresponding author.
E-mail address: kandace.mcguire@vcuhealth.org

Surg Clin N Am 98 (2018) 761–771
https://doi.org/10.1016/j.suc.2018.03.008
0039-6109/18/© 2018 Elsevier Inc. All rights reserved.

the ability to preserve their breast while maintaining adequate oncologic control. However, the success of the BCS is predicated upon the ability to obtain tumor-free (negative) margins. What constitutes adequate negative margins has been a subject of much debate. This article discusses the current understanding and recent developments in the management of invasive breast cancer using BCS.

LOCAL THERAPY PARADIGM SHIFT: LESS IS MORE

For almost a century, the Halsted radical mastectomy, which included complete removal of breast tissue, underlying pectoralis muscles, and regional lymph nodes, was the procedure of choice for invasive breast cancer.[1] Improvements in understanding of the tumor biology and significant surgical morbidity associated with radical mastectomy led investigators from the National Surgical Adjuvant Breast and Bowel Project (NSABP) to conduct the NSABP-B04 (1971–1974) trial, which compared radical mastectomy to less extensive surgery (total mastectomy with or without radiation therapy).[2] To further minimize the extent of surgery, NSABP-B06 (1976–1984) and the European Organization for Research and Treatment of Cancer 10801 (1980–1986) trials were conducted to compare the outcomes of mastectomy with those of lumpectomy with radiation therapy and lumpectomy alone. Twenty-year follow-up results of these clinical trials established equivalent long-term disease-free and overall survival in patients receiving radical mastectomy, total mastectomy, or lumpectomy for invasive breast tumors.[3,4] The results of these trials established BCS with radiation therapy as the new "standard of care" for stage I/II breast cancer with the goal of optimal oncologic control and better cosmetic outcome in order to improve overall patient quality of life. In recent years, the use of neoadjuvant systemic therapy has facilitated the use of BCS for patients previously slated for mastectomy. The American College of Surgeons Oncology Group Z1031 and NSABP-B18 trials demonstrated the role of neoadjuvant endocrine therapy and chemotherapy in substantially increased use of lumpectomy as the surgical procedure over mastectomy.[5,6] Currently, about 60% to 75% of patients diagnosed with early stage breast cancer undergo BCS as their initial surgical treatment.[7–9]

MARGINS IN BREAST-CONSERVING SURGERY

The goal of optimally performed BCS is to achieve clear surgical margins during initial tumor resection while maintaining the natural shape of the breast. The status of surgical margins is determined microscopically by applying ink to the surface of the lumpectomy specimen and analyzing the closest distance between the inked lumpectomy edge and any cancerous tissue (invasive or ductal carcinoma in situ [DCIS]). The surgical margin status is one of the strongest predictors for local recurrence and guides the decision to reexcise.[10–12] On microscopic evaluation, the status of the margin can be (a) extensively positive, (b) focally positive, (c) close, and (d) negative (**Fig. 1**).

Extensively positive margins are defined as the presence of ink at the surface of the surgical specimen on either invasive cancer cells or DCIS and are a reflection of incomplete resection. Positive margins are strongly associated with a substantial increase in local recurrence risk than those with negative margins.[12–14] Focally positive margins, defined as tumor touching the inked margin over a length of 4 mm or less, are associated with a lower residual disease burden as compared with extensively positive margins.[15] Negative margins, initially defined by NSABP-B06 as no ink on invasive carcinoma or DCIS, have been shown to substantially decrease the risk of ipsilateral breast tumor recurrence (IBTR). Traditionally, negative but close margins have been described as margin width ≤2 mm from invasive carcinoma or DCIS. The appropriate

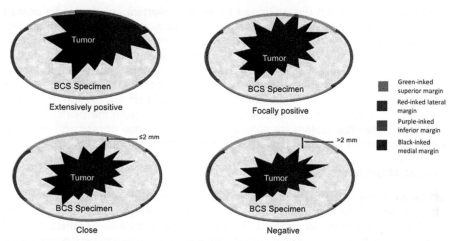

Fig. 1. Margin status at breast-conserving surgery.

management of close margins remained a subject of much debate until the release of Society of Surgical Oncology (SSO)–American Society for Radiation Oncology (ASTRO) Consensus Guideline on Margins for BCS, which established that wider margins width for invasive carcinoma do not lower the risk of IBTR as compared to "no ink on tumor."

The surgical decision for further treatment is based on the interpretation of the pathologic margin status reporting, which may be affected by variations in adequacy of pathologic margin status reporting practices. Currently, the College of American Pathologists (CAP) recommends documenting the distance to the closest negative margin, in addition to margin distance at all 6 specimen orientations. However, recent reports demonstrate wide variation in compliance with CAP guidelines, with more than a quarter of reports not meeting the minimal requirements of surgical margin reporting.[16] This variability in reporting is associated with variation in rates of reexcision and rates of mastectomy. Patients with maximally compliant reports tend to have lower rates of reexcision and mastectomy as compared with less compliant reports.[17]

PREDICTORS OF POSITIVE MARGINS

Given the need for additional surgery following positive margins at the index procedure and its subsequent impact on surgical morbidity, there has been considerable emphasis on identifying independent risk factors for positive margins. Knowledge of these risk factors is important for clinical management of the patient facilitating surgeons to better counsel patients about the risk for positive margins and to distinguish those patients who have a higher risk of local failure. The following multiple factors have been shown to be associated with a higher risk of positive margin status[18,19]:

- Age
- Larger tumor size
- Lobular histology
- Smaller breast size
- Tumor multifocality
- Extensive in situ component
- Receipt of surgical biopsy

Younger age has been demonstrated to be an important risk factor for margin positivity.[14,20] Method of tumor localization (needle localization vs palpation guided) once suggested as a factor for margin positivity has been demonstrated to have no effect on the margin status.[21] In a large prospective multi-institutional study conducted by Chagpar and colleagues,[22] it was shown that larger tumor size and lobular histology are associated with a greater likelihood of positive margins; however, the type of biopsy (needle/excisional) did not have an impact on margin status. Despite the conflicting evidence, it is important to note that, apart from the biopsy method, all other predicted risk factors are nonmodifiable. This avenue of research, although important for patient counseling, has little practice-changing impact.

SURGICAL MARGINS: HOW CLOSE IS TOO CLOSE?

The margin status at the index procedure is one of the strongest predictors for local (in-breast) recurrence and long-term survival. Initially investigated by Kurtz,[23] the rate of local recurrence in patients undergoing breast-conserving therapy (BCS followed by radiation therapy) with negative margins was shown to be 8% at 6 years, whereas that for positive margins was a staggering 24%. Subsequently, multiple studies have shown similar findings establishing unequivocally the association of positive margins with local recurrence (**Table 1**). Jobsen and colleagues[31] reported 5-year local recurrence rates to be 3.1% for negative and 5.6% positive margins, respectively. However, for women younger than 40 years of age, these rates were 8.4% in negative and 36.9% for positive margins, respectively, indicating the particular importance of clear margins for this subgroup of patients. A meta-analysis of 21 studies conducted by Houssami and colleagues[32] further showed a strong association of positive margin status with a higher likelihood of local recurrence than those with negative margins.[32] The association of positive margins (ink on tumor) with increased local recurrence risk has been long accepted, although the estimates of effect vary between the studies.[33–35] Significantly higher local failure rates are observed in those with positive margins that received no additional surgery, and it is established that local failure is associated with reduced survival. Therefore, reexcision to obtain clear "tumor-free" margins is an important intervention for all women with positive margins, for optimizing local disease control after BCS.

Table 1
Association of the margin status at definitive surgery with local recurrence

Study	Number of Patients (n)	Median Follow-up (mo)	Rates of Local Recurrence (%) Positive Margins	Negative Margins
Kurtz,[23] 1990	496	71	24	8
Solin et al,[24] 1990	697	58	7	2
Borger,[25] 1994	1026	66	16	2
Anscher et al,[10] 1993	259	60	10	2
Schnitt et al,[26] 1994	181	60	21	2
Spivack,[27] 1994	272	48	18.1	3.7
Smitt et al,[28] 1995	289	75	18	2
Heimann et al,[29] 1996	869	43	11	2
Gage et al,[11] 1996	343	109	16	2
Park et al,[12] 2000	533	127	27	7
Leong,[30] 2004	452	80	11.9	3.1

Multiple studies have corroborated the importance of obtaining negative margins for adequate oncologic resection and reducing the risk of local recurrence.[13,32]

Before the 2014 SSO-ASTRO Consensus guidelines for margins in BCS, significant variability existed among surgeons' opinion and practices on the amount of normal breast tissue that constitutes "optimal" negative margins, documented by multiple survey studies of practicing surgeons (**Table 2**). This lack of consensus for adequate margin width posed a dilemma for surgeons in choosing patients for additional surgery, leading to wide variations in reexcision rates nationally.

The rates of reexcision after initial BCS varied tremendously with reported rates ranging from 20% to 70% because of subjective assessment of the need for reexcision before SSO-ASTRO guidelines with a strong emphasis on achieving specific negative margin widths, with the belief that this reduces the risk of IBTR.[19,22,38,40–42] This quest for wider negative margin widths resulted in high rates of reexcision being performed for margins in which there is no ink on tumor.[42] In view of this significant variability in practice patterns for one of the most commonly performed procedures, SSO and ASTRO convened a multidisciplinary panel (Margins panel) in 2013 to critically review the literature and existing evidence for relationship of margin width and IBTR in invasive breast cancer. The panel conducted a systematic review and meta-analysis based on 33 eligible studies published between the years 1965 and 2013, including 28,162 patients with a median follow-up time of 79.2 months; 1506 (5.3%) patients had diagnosed IBTR. The results of the meta-analysis concluded that wider negative margin widths do not further lower the risk of IBTR and established "no ink on tumor" as the objective for BCS margins when surgery is followed by whole-breast radiation therapy. The study also shows a reduced rate of IBTR with the use of systemic therapy (chemotherapy or endocrine therapy). The panel recommended against the routine practice of obtaining wider margins than no ink on tumor for invasive breast cancer, even in the unusual circumstance of no systemic therapy.[13]

The results of this study, published in 2014, have been endorsed by American Society of Clinical Oncology (ASCO), SSO, and ASTRO as the recommended consensus guidelines for margins in BCS for invasive breast cancer. It is important to note that these guidelines are for invasive carcinomas only. For patients with DCIS alone (no invasive component), SSO-ASTRO-ASCO consensus guidelines, established in 2016,[43] recommend a margin width of 2 mm followed by whole-breast radiation therapy, as discussed in Ashlyn S. Everett and colleagues' article, "The Evolving Role of Post-Mastectomy Radiation Therapy," in this issue. The

Table 2
Variation in surgeons' opinion on adequate margin width for optimal oncologic control

| Study | Number of Surgeons (n) | Margin Width Described as "Adequate" by Surgeons Performing BCS (%) | | | |
		"No Ink on Tumor"	1–2 mm	≥5 mm	≥10 mm
Taghian et al,[36] 2005	1137 (702 NA, 431 EO)	45.9, 27.6 (NA, EO)	29.2, 20 (NA, EO)	20, 36.1 (NA, EO)	4.9, 16.3 (NA, EO)
Blair et al,[37] 2009	351	15	78 (28 1 mm, 50 2 mm)	12	3
Azu et al,[38] 2010	312	11	42	28	19
Lovrics et al,[39] 2012	591	39	43 (14 1 mm, 29 2 mm)	18	—

Abbreviations: EO, European surgeons; NA, North American surgeons.

publication and adoption of these consensus statements is significant step toward quality improvement in breast cancer surgery by implementing evidence-based consistency with the potential to reduce unwarranted reexcision procedures and the associated significant physical, psychological, and financial implications for the patient.

INTRAOPERATIVE MARGIN ASSESSMENT

Considering the impact of margin status on overall disease outcome, it is prudent to adopt practices that enable complete resection of the tumor in order to obtain negative margins. Several techniques have been investigated and practiced in this regard; however, currently no real-time intraoperative microscopic margin assessment technique exists as the "standard of care" to analyze lumpectomy margins. Conventionally, intraoperative frozen section analysis (IFSA), intraoperative touch prep cytology (IOTPC), radiofrequency spectroscopy (RF), and radiography have been used for intraoperative evaluation of the margin. IFSA is a relatively simple procedure with high sensitivity and specificity and has been shown to be useful in reducing the rates of positive margins.[44] However, increased operative time, costs, and inability of IFSA to be performed over the entire specimen margin limit its use as an efficient and effective assessment tool. In contrast, IOTPC can assess the entire surface area relatively quickly; however, the inability of IOTPC to evaluate the cells below the surface limits its utility. Radiography and RF suffer from low sensitivity and specificity due to an inability to adequately identify diffuse microscopic lesions. However, because of wide availability and low cost, specimen radiography still remains standard in many practices.

Newer techniques, such as optical coherence tomography (OCT), intraoperative ultrasound, radio-guided occult lesion localization (ROLL), and electromagnetic margin probes, are constantly evolving as tools for adequate margin assessment.[45,46] Intraoperative specimen radiography used to visualize the eccentric location of the tumor, or a preoperatively placed clip, facilitates the surgeon to remove additional tissue, if required. Similarly, intraoperative ultrasonography allows for adequate visualization of lesions and has been demonstrated to reduce the rate of positive margins significantly as compared with wire-guided resection.[47] However, it is imperative to be cognizant of the fact that many lesions, especially DCIS, may not be visible on ultrasound. For sonographically occult lesions, a biopsy clip can be placed preoperatively to assist in localization and excision of such lesions. A major limitation of the biopsy clip is the high rate of clip migration, as shown by Klein and colleagues.[48] Techniques such as ROLL entail the placement of a radioactive seed under imaging guidance, which is later localized at the time of the surgery using a hand-held gamma probe. A comparative analysis of wire-guided, ultrasound-guided, and radio-guided localization techniques demonstrated ultrasound-guided localization to be superior to others in obtaining adequate margins and reducing the rates of positive margins.[49] These real-time multidimensional high-resolution imaging techniques can assist the surgeon in accurately identifying the margin status intraoperatively, which may decrease the need for reexcision.

There is a growing body of evidence suggesting a role of additional margin resection (directed or shave) at the time of initial procedure in reducing rates of positive margins. Intraoperative assessment by the surgeon of the wall of the resection cavity from standard lumpectomy, done either by palpation or by ultrasound guidance, can yield additional disease. A study conducted by Guidroz and colleagues[50] demonstrated that subjective assessment and excision of additional directed margins during primary lumpectomy led to decreased need for additional surgery. The role of routine cavity shave margins is currently evolving, because multiple studies have shown reduction in rate of positive margins and the need for additional surgery. Cavity shave margins refer to removing additional tissue circumferentially around the resection cavity from primary lumpectomy. A large prospective randomized controlled trial conducted by Chagpar and colleagues[51] revealed more than 50% reduction in the rate of positive margins and subsequently halved the rates of additional surgery as compared with standard partial mastectomy performed with or without resection of additional selective margins. Multiple retrospective studies have corroborated these findings with most reporting a 40% to 50% decrease in rates of reexcision when additional cavity shave margins were taken during the primary surgery.[52–54] In addition, routine cavity shave resection has been shown to detect additional disease in some patients who were expected to have negative margins, for example, multifocal disease being found on cavity shave resection. A few studies have compared the cosmetic outcomes in patients undergoing cavity shave resection with those that did not and reported better cosmetic outcomes with routine cavity shave margins. However, this is likely related to lesser volume of the breast resected and surgeon skill set. Additional margin resection, whether directed or shave during the primary lumpectomy, significantly reduces the rates of positive margins.

ADDITIONAL SURGERY/OUTCOMES

The finding of positive margins (ink on tumor) warrants additional surgery for margin clearance. The choice of additional surgery, whether margin reexcision or mastectomy, depends on a combination of tumor and patient factors. The average time to the second surgery is 24 to 30 days after the index surgery.[55] Currently, about 65% of patients with positive margins receive reexcision as the additional surgery with the rest choosing either unilateral or bilateral mastectomy with or without reconstruction.[55] The adoption of the SSO-ASTRO consensus guidelines has facilitated a dramatic decline in the rates of reexcision from the previous 20% to 70% range to about 13% to 23%.[55–58] The implications of additional surgery however are multifold, physical and psychological stress of return to the operating room, associated surgical morbidity, longer hospital stay, and higher likelihood of complications, such as infections, hematomas, seromas, and fat necrosis. According to a recent report by Metcalfe and colleagues,[56] infections within the first 3 months were twice as likely in patients undergoing repeat breast surgery than those who underwent single BCS only. The 2-year infection rate for patients receiving additional surgery is about 15.3%, which is comparable to the 2-year infection rate of mastectomy (15.7%), resulting in reduced benefit of BCS to this subset of patient population. The need for repeat surgery delays the initiation of adjuvant therapy, which could have potential oncologic implications. A recent study by Vandergrift and colleagues[59] showed reexcision surgery prolonged the time to initiation of adjuvant therapy by 2.1 weeks, reflecting the importance of targeted efforts to minimize preventable causes of delay in treatment. Along with physical and psychological burden, additional surgery also poses a significant financial burden, both for the health care system and for the patient. The total health care costs are on an average $16,072 to $26,026 higher in those receiving repeat breast surgery, and reducing the rates of reexcision surgery represents an opportunity for potential health care costs reduction in breast cancer.[56,57,60]

SUMMARY

BCS is the standard of care for early stage breast cancer with excellent patient-reported outcomes, cosmesis, and long-term disease control. Complete resection of the tumor is critical for preventing breast cancer recurrence. The current recommendations of "no ink on tumor" for surgical margins supplemented with adjuvant therapy for invasive breast cancer provide excellent oncologic control reflecting the tremendous progress in breast cancer care. The road ahead presents opportunities to develop and implement precise real-time margin assessment intraoperatively to minimize the need and subsequent implications of additional surgery affecting the patient's quality of life.

REFERENCES

1. Halsted WS. I. The results of operations for the cure of cancer of the breast performed at the Johns Hopkins Hospital from June, 1889, to January, 1894. Ann Surg 1894;20(5):497–555.
2. Fisher B, Wolmark N, Redmond C, et al. Findings from NSABP Protocol No. B-04: comparison of radical mastectomy with alternative treatments. II. The clinical and biologic significance of medial-central breast cancers. Cancer 1981;48(8): 1863–72.
3. Fisher B, Anderson S, Bryant J, et al. Twenty-year follow-up of a randomized trial comparing total mastectomy, lumpectomy, and lumpectomy plus irradiation for the treatment of invasive breast cancer. N Engl J Med 2002;347(16):1233–41.
4. Litière S, Werutsky G, Fentiman IS, et al. Breast conserving therapy versus mastectomy for stage I–II breast cancer: 20 year follow-up of the EORTC 10801 phase 3 randomised trial. Lancet Oncol 2012;13(4):412–9.
5. Ellis MJ, Suman VJ, Hoog J, et al. Randomized phase II neoadjuvant comparison between letrozole, anastrozole, and exemestane for postmenopausal women with estrogen receptor–rich stage 2 to 3 breast cancer: clinical and biomarker outcomes and predictive value of the baseline PAM50-based intrinsic subtype—ACOSOG Z1031. J Clin Oncol 2011;29(17):2342–9.
6. Fisher B, Brown A, Mamounas E, et al. Effect of preoperative chemotherapy on local-regional disease in women with operable breast cancer: findings from National Surgical Adjuvant Breast and Bowel Project B-18. J Clin Oncol 1997; 15(7):2483–93.
7. Kummerow KL, Du L, Penson DF, et al. Nationwide trends in mastectomy for early-stage breast cancer. JAMA Surg 2015;150(1):9–16.
8. Lee MC, Rogers K, Griffith K, et al. Determinants of breast conservation rates: reasons for mastectomy at a comprehensive cancer center. Breast J 2009; 15(1):34–40.
9. McGuire KP, Santillan AA, Kaur P, et al. Are mastectomies on the rise? A 13-year trend analysis of the selection of mastectomy versus breast conservation therapy in 5865 patients. Ann Surg Oncol 2009;16(10):2682–90.
10. Anscher MS, Jones P, Prosnitz LR, et al. Local failure and margin status in early-stage breast carcinoma treated with conservation surgery and radiation therapy. Ann Surg 1993;218(1):22–8.
11. Gage I, Schnitt SJ, Nixon AJ, et al. Pathologic margin involvement and the risk of recurrence in patients treated with breast-conserving therapy. Cancer 1996; 78(9):1921–8.
12. Park CC, Mitsumori M, Nixon A, et al. Outcome at 8 years after breast-conserving surgery and radiation therapy for invasive breast cancer: influence of margin status and systemic therapy on local recurrence. J Clin Oncol 2000;18(8): 1668–75.

13. Moran MS, Schnitt SJ, Giuliano AE, et al. Society of Surgical Oncology–American Society for Radiation Oncology consensus guideline on margins for breast-conserving surgery with whole-breast irradiation in stages I and II invasive breast cancer. Int J Radiat Oncol Biol Phys 2014;88(3):553–64.
14. Aziz D, Rawlinson E, Narod SA, et al. The role of reexcision for positive margins in optimizing local disease control after breast-conserving surgery for cancer. Breast J 2006;12(4):331–7.
15. Vos EL, Gaal J, Verhoef C, et al. Focally positive margins in breast conserving surgery: predictors, residual disease, and local recurrence. Eur J Surg Oncol 2017; 43(10):1846–54.
16. Persing S, James TA, Mace J, et al. Variability in the quality of pathology reporting of margin status following breast cancer surgery. Ann Surg Oncol 2011;18(11): 3061–5.
17. Persing S, Jerome MA, James TA, et al. Surgical margin reporting in breast conserving surgery: does compliance with guidelines affect re-excision and mastectomy rates? Breast 2015;24(5):618–22.
18. Smitt MC, Horst K. Association of clinical and pathologic variables with lumpectomy surgical margin status after preoperative diagnosis or excisional biopsy of invasive breast cancer. Ann Surg Oncol 2007;14(3):1040–4.
19. Waljee JF, Hu ES, Newman LA, et al. Predictors of re-excision among women undergoing breast-conserving surgery for cancer. Ann Surg Oncol 2008;15(5): 1297–303.
20. van Deurzen CHM. Predictors of surgical margin following breast-conserving surgery: a large population-based cohort study. Ann Surg Oncol 2016;23(Suppl 5): 627–33.
21. Atkins J, Mushawah FA, Appleton CM, et al. Positive margin rates following breast-conserving surgery for stage I–III breast cancer: palpable versus nonpalpable tumors. J Surg Res 2012;177(1):109–15.
22. Chagpar AB, Martin RCG 2nd, Hagendoorn LJ, et al. Lumpectomy margins are affected by tumor size and histologic subtype but not by biopsy technique. Am J Surg 2004;188(4):399–402.
23. Kurtz JM. Why are local recurrences after breast-conserving therapy more frequent in younger patients? J Clin Oncol 1990;8(4):591–8.
24. Solin LJ, Fowble BL, Schultz DJ, et al. The significance of pathologic margins of tumor excision on the outcome of patients treated with definitive irradiation for early stage breast cancer. Int J Radiat Oncol Biol Phys 1990;19(Supplement 1):130.
25. Borger J. Risk factors in breast-conservation therapy. J Clin Oncol 1994;12(4): 653–60.
26. Schnitt SJ, Abner A, Gelman R, et al. The relationship between microscopic margins of resection and the risk of local recurrence in patients with breast cancer treated with breast-conserving surgery and radiation therapy. Cancer 1994; 74(6):1746–51.
27. Spivack B. Margin status and local recurrence after breast-conserving surgery. Arch Surg 1994;129(9):952–7.
28. Smitt MC, Nowels KW, Zdeblick MJ, et al. The importance of the lumpectomy surgical margin status in long term results of breast conservation. Cancer 1995;76(2):259–67.
29. Heimann R, Powers C, Halpem HJ, et al. Breast preservation in stage I and II carcinoma of the breast. The University of Chicago experience. Cancer 1996; 78(8):1722–30.

30. Leong C. Effect of margins on ipsilateral breast tumor recurrence after breast conservation therapy for lymph node-negative breast carcinoma. Cancer 2004; 100:1823–32.
31. Jobsen JJ, van der Palen J, Ong F, et al. The value of a positive margin for invasive carcinoma in breast-conservative treatment in relation to local recurrence is limited to young women only. Int J Radiat Oncol Biol Phys 2003;57(3):724–31.
32. Houssami N, Macaskill P, Marinovich ML, et al. Meta-analysis of the impact of surgical margins on local recurrence in women with early-stage invasive breast cancer treated with breast-conserving therapy. Eur J Cancer 2010;46(18): 3219–32.
33. Morrow M, Strom EA, Bassett LW, et al. Standard for breast conservation therapy in the management of invasive breast carcinoma. CA Cancer J Clin 2002;52(5): 277–300.
34. Schwartz GF, Veronesi U, Clough KB, et al. Consensus conference on breast conservation. J Am Coll Surg 2006;203(2):198–207.
35. Biglia N, Ponzone R, Bounous VE, et al. Role of re-excision for positive and close resection margins in patients treated with breast-conserving surgery. Breast 2014;23(6):870–5.
36. Taghian A, Mohiuddin M, Jagsi R, et al. Current perceptions regarding surgical margin status after breast-conserving therapy: results of a survey. Ann Surg 2005;241(4):629–39.
37. Blair SL, Thompson K, Rococco J, et al. Attaining negative margins in breast-conservation operations: is there a consensus among breast surgeons? J Am Coll Surg 2009;209(5):608–13.
38. Azu M, Abrahamse P, Katz SJ, et al. What is an adequate margin for breast-conserving surgery? Surgeon attitudes and correlates. Ann Surg Oncol 2010; 17(2):558–63.
39. Lovrics PJ, Gordon M, Cornacchi SD, et al. Practice patterns and perceptions of margin status for breast conserving surgery for breast carcinoma: National Survey of Canadian General Surgeons. Breast 2012;21(6):730–4.
40. Sanchez C, Brem RF, McSwain AP, et al. Factors associated with re-excision in patients with early-stage breast cancer treated with breast conservation therapy. Am Surg 2010;76(3):331–4.
41. Miller AR, Brandao G, Prihoda TJ, et al. Positive margins following surgical resection of breast carcinoma: analysis of pathologic correlates. J Surg Oncol 2004; 86(3):134–40.
42. McCahill LE, Single RM, Aiello Bowles EJ, et al. Variability in reexcision following breast conservation surgery. JAMA 2012;307(5):467–75.
43. Morrow M, Van Zee KJ, Solin LJ, et al. Society of Surgical Oncology-American Society for Radiation Oncology-American Society of Clinical Oncology consensus guideline on margins for breast-conserving surgery with whole-breast irradiation in ductal carcinoma in situ. Pract Radiat Oncol 2016;6(5):287–95.
44. Olson TP, Harter J, Munoz A, et al. Frozen section analysis for intraoperative margin assessment during breast-conserving surgery results in low rates of re-excision and local recurrence. Ann Surg Oncol 2007;14(10):2953–60.
45. Nguyen FT, Zysk AM, Chaney EJ, et al. Intraoperative evaluation of breast tumor margins with optical coherence tomography. Cancer Res 2009;69(22):8790–6.
46. Haloua MH, Volders JH, Krekel NMA, et al. Intraoperative ultrasound guidance in breast-conserving surgery improves cosmetic outcomes and patient satisfaction: results of a multicenter randomized controlled trial (COBALT). Ann Surg Oncol 2016;23(1):30–7.

47. Rahusen FD, Bremers AJA, Fabry HFJ, et al. Ultrasound-guided lumpectomy of nonpalpable breast cancer versus wire-guided resection: a randomized clinical trial. Ann Surg Oncol 2002;9(10):994–8.
48. Klein RL, Mook JA, Euhus DM, et al. Evaluation of a hydrogel based breast biopsy marker (HydroMARK(R)) as an alternative to wire and radioactive seed localization for non-palpable breast lesions. J Surg Oncol 2012;105(6):591–4.
49. Krekel N, Zonderhuis BM, Stockmann H, et al. A comparison of three methods for nonpalpable breast cancer excision. Eur J Surg Oncol 2011;37:109–15.
50. Guidroz JA, Larrieux G, Liao J, et al. Sampling of secondary margins decreases the need for re-excision after partial mastectomy. Surgery 2011;150(4):802–9.
51. Chagpar AB, Killelea BK, Tsangaris TN, et al. A randomized, controlled trial of cavity shave margins in breast cancer. N Engl J Med 2015;373(6):503–10.
52. Kobbermann A, Unzeitig A, Xie X-J, et al. Impact of routine cavity shave margins on breast cancer re-excision rates. Ann Surg Oncol 2011;18(5):1349–55.
53. Marudanayagam R, Singhal R, Tanchel B, et al. Effect of cavity shaving on reoperation rate following breast-conserving surgery. Breast J 2008;14(6):570–3.
54. Unzeitig A, Kobbermann A, Xie XJ, et al. Influence of surgical technique on mastectomy and reexcision rates in breast-conserving therapy for cancer. Int J Surg Oncol 2012;2012:725121.
55. Morrow M, Abrahamse P, Hofer TP, et al. Trends in reoperation after initial lumpectomy for breast cancer. JAMA Oncol 2017;3(10):1352–7.
56. Metcalfe LN, Zysk AM, Yemul KS, et al. Beyond the margins—economic costs and complications associated with repeated breast-conserving surgeries. JAMA Surg 2017;152(11):1084–6.
57. Pataky R, Baliski CR. Reoperation costs in attempted breast-conserving surgery: a decision analysis. Curr Oncol 2016;23(5):314–21.
58. Jiwa N, Ayyar S, Provenzano E, et al. The impact of a change in margin width policy on rates of re-excision following breast conserving surgery (BCS). Eur J Surg Oncol 2016;42(5):S33.
59. Vandergrift JL, Niland JC, Theriault RL, et al. Time to adjuvant chemotherapy for breast cancer in national comprehensive cancer network institutions. J Natl Cancer Inst 2013;105(2):104–12.
60. Singer L, Brown E, Lanni T. Margins in breast conserving surgery: the financial cost & potential savings associated with the new margin guidelines. Breast 2016;28(Supplement C):1–4.

Future Developments in Neoadjuvant Therapy for Triple-Negative Breast Cancer

Lakisha Moore-Smith, MD, PhD[a], Andres Forero-Torres, MD[b],
Erica Stringer-Reasor, MD[c],*

KEYWORDS

- Neoadjuvant chemotherapy • Early stage breast cancer
- Triple-negative breast cancer • Targeted therapy

KEY POINTS

- Triple-negative breast cancer (TNBC) is an aggressive subtype in which there are limited treatment options.
- The mainstay systemic treatment of TNBC is chemotherapy.
- Using neoadjuvant chemotherapy will help identify novel effective therapies in the treatment of TNBC.
- Prioritizing neoadjuvant clinical trials that use molecular-based profiling may aid in improving patient outcomes in TNBC.

INTRODUCTION

Breast cancer is the leading cause of cancer for women living in the United States, with more than 200,000 new cases diagnosed annually.[1] Triple-negative breast cancer (TNBC) develops in about 15% to 20% of breast cancers and disproportionately affects African American, Hispanic, premenopausal women and BRCA1-mutation carriers.[2] TNBC is a breast tumor subtype that is hormone receptor (HR)–negative, expressing less than 1% of estrogen, progesterone, and human epidermal growth factor receptor 2, as determined through immunohistochemistry staining. Generally, this subtype is more aggressive at presentation, associated with larger size, higher grade, and frequent nodal involvement. As a result of these characteristics, the rate of distant metastasis and risk of recurrence in the first 2 to 3 years following definitive treatment are high.[3,4]

Disclosure Statement: The authors have nothing to disclose.
[a] Department of Medicine, Brookwood Baptist Health – Princeton, 833 Princeton Avenue, POB III Suite 200, Birmingham, AL 35211-1311, USA; [b] Department of Medicine, Division of Hematology Oncology, University of Alabama at Birmingham, 1720 2nd Avenue South, NP 2517, Birmingham, AL 35294-3300, USA; [c] Department of Medicine, Division of Hematology Oncology, University of Alabama at Birmingham, 1720 2nd Avenue South, NP 2501, Birmingham, AL 35294-3300, USA
* Corresponding author.
E-mail address: esreasor@uabmc.edu

Surg Clin N Am 98 (2018) 773–785
https://doi.org/10.1016/j.suc.2018.04.004
0039-6109/18/© 2018 Elsevier Inc. All rights reserved.

Over the past 2 decades, significant milestones have been achieved in the detection and treatment of breast cancer. Despite progress, locally advanced, highly aggressive breast cancers such as TNBC have significantly lower responses to therapy.[5] In addition, retrospective data from the Surveillance Epidemiology and Results (SEER) categorizing breast cancer by molecular subtypes reported significantly lower 4-year survival in TNBC (77%) compared with HR+/HER2− (92.5%), HR+/HER2+ (90.3%), and HR−/HER2+ (82.7%).[6] Breast cancer is a very heterogeneic disease; therefore, designing drugs that target molecular pathways, as well as identifying microenviromental changes that may contribute to TNBC intrinsic subtypes, may help improve survival in a subset of patients.[7]

NEOADJUVANT THERAPY

Patients with TNBC have limited treatment options, most of which consist of chemotherapy; the mainstay systemic treatments of TNBC are anthracycline- and taxane-based regimens.[4] Platinum-based therapies have been used but are yet to receive approval by national guidelines as first-line therapy. Adjuvant-based therapies have improved relapse-free survival (RFS) and overall survival (OS) in early stage TNBC.[8] Most recently, neoadjuvant chemotherapy has quickly become a reasonable alternative to adjuvant chemotherapy for patients with early stage, operable breast cancer. Upfront systemic therapy before surgery has many advantages. For example, this approach allows clinicians to evaluate real-time tumor response to treatment and can increase the success rate of breast-conserving surgery. If a measurable response is achieved, the necessity for a complete axillary lymph node dissection is decreased,[9] thereby reducing morbid side effects, such as lymphedema, arm paresthesia, chronic pain, adhesive capsulitis, postmastectomy syndrome, and arm immobility.[10–12] High-grade tumors, such as TNBC, are typically more responsive to preoperative chemotherapy. However, the TNBC subtype has overall higher relapse rates compared with hormone-positive breast cancers; a phenomenon coined the "triple-negative paradox."[13]

Currently, there are multiple trials using neoadjuvant therapy not only to assess tumor response but also to use this platform to evaluate mechanisms of resistance and develop diagnostic assays to contribute to individualized therapy planning. Results from recent clinical trials have shown that patients whose breast tumors achieve a pathologic complete response (pCR) defined as no residual cancer in the breast or lymph nodes (ypT0/is and ypN0) following neoadjuvant therapy have improved survival outcomes. In contrast, the outcome for patients with residual disease posttreatment is poor.[14] It is estimated that one-third of patients diagnosed with TNBC achieve a pCR with standard neoadjuvant chemotherapy.[15] Translational trials, such as I-SPY 1 and 2 trials (investigation of serial studies to predict patient response with imaging and molecular analysis), are an adaptive approach for the application of biomarker-driven neoadjuvant therapies in women with locally advanced, high-risk invasive breast cancer to improve tumor response.[16,17] Thus the identification of molecular targets will lead to the optimization of therapies, thereby improving future outcomes for patients with TNBC.

TRIPLE-NEGATIVE BREAST CANCER MOLECULAR SUBTYPE

Although there are many ongoing studies to assess possible TNBC molecular targets, no clinically relevant biomarker has been identified to date. One constraint to finding a specific target is the inherent heterogeneity within the TNBC subtype initially described by Perou and colleagues.[17] Since this publication, many groups have further genomically classified TNBC, including investigators at Vanderbilt (Lehmann group) and Baylor.[18–20] Lehmann and colleagues[4,18] identified 6 subtypes of TNBC based on molecular profiling:

2 basal-like (BL1 and BL2), 2 mesenchymal (M and mesenchymal stem-like [MSL]), 1 immunomodulary, luminal androgen receptor (LAR), and 1 unstable subtype. In a similar study, a group at Baylor found only 4 subtypes by assimilating messenger RNA and DNA profiling—the LAR, mesenchymal, basal-like immunosuppressed, and basal-like immune activated.[20] A third gene expression profile assay PAM50 has been clinically relevant in predicting disease recurrence and response to treatment.[19] This assay identified 4 predominant subtypes of TNBC: basal-like, mesenchymal, immune-enriched, and LAR. Although variations exist between the studies, collectively these data suggest that within TNBC, there seems to be clusters sharing similar genetic expression profiles, mostly composed of basal-like subtypes.[4] Identification of these subtypes and their gene expression patterns, based on molecular profiling, have been instrumental in elucidating potential therapeutic targets. For example, basal-like tumors have been associated with mutations in DNA damage response pathways. Two agents, platinum salts such as cisplatin and poly (ADP-ribose) polymerase 1 (PARP) inhibitors that target mutations in these pathways, have emerged as potential therapies for these tumors.[21] Mesenchymal subtypes are characterized by upregulation of cell differentiation and growth factor signaling pathways. Wnt, Notch, MET, and mTOR are intracellular targets under investigation for the treatment of the mesenchymal subtype. In a few clinical trials, the immunomodulatory subtype has shown the best response to current chemotherapy agents. In addition, modulation of immune checkpoint inhibitors for treatment of these tumor subtypes is currently under investigation. Lastly, the LAR subtype is characterized by androgen signaling and is thought to be the poorest responder to current chemotherapy regimens. Greater knowledge acquisition will lead to a better understanding of these molecular mechanisms, resulting in the development of targeted therapeutics for tumors shown to have a poor prognosis based on current therapeutics. Gulcalp and colleagues reported a phase II trial using bicalutamide, an androgen receptor (AR) blocker in patients with AR-positive TNBC, which showed a clinical benefit rate of 19% [95% CI, 7-39%] and median PFS was 12 weeks [95% CI, 11-22 weeks].[22] A second study in AR-positive TNBC reported a CBR of 25% (95%CI, 17-33%) and median survival of 12.7 months in the intention-to-treat population, supporting the use of AR blockage in the LAR subtype.[23] A study by Masuda and colleagues,[24] which evaluated response rates between different TNBC subtypes, reported an overall pathologic complete response (pCR) rate of 28% with neoadjuvant taxane and anthracycline-based regimens. However, pCR rates differed substantially by subtypes. The highest pCR rate (52%) was observed in the BL1 subtype. By contrast, the pCR rate was lower in patients with the BL2, MSL, and LAR subtypes (0%, 23%, and 10%, respectively).[14] Furthermore, Echavarria and colleagues[25] observed similar results in a multivariant analysis of a nonrandomized trial of neoadjuvant carboplatin AUC 6 and docetaxel 75mg/m^2 for six cycles with an overall pCR rate of 44%, in which the BL1 subtype observed with the highest pCR of 65.6%, followed by BL2 (47.4%), MSL (36.4%), and LAR (21.4%). Biomarkers under ongoing investigation include vascular endothelial growth factor (VEGF), interleukin 8, epithelial growth factor receptor (EGFR), insulin-like growth factor–binding protein, c-Kit, c-Met, programmed cell death-ligand 1 (PD-L1), PIK3CA, pAKT/S6/p4E-BP1, PTEN, ALDH1, PIK3CA/AKT/mTOR, BRCA1, TP53, and Ki-67.[26] Although some biomarkers hold more promise than others, we will briefly discuss neoadjuvant trials that target a few of these pathways for the treatment of TNBC.

Bevacizumab

Bevacizumab is a monoclonal antibody targeting VEGF-A. VEGF-A protein is shown to be involved with tumor angiogenesis and is associated with an increased risk of metastatic disease. Bevacizumab is currently approved by Food and Drug Administration for the treatment of colon, lung, brain, and eye cancers. Bear and colleagues[9] examined breast cancer response to bevacizumab (anti-VEGF therapy) when added to chemotherapy; a study in which 1206 patients were recruited and 244 tumors identified as hormone-receptor negative. The patients were randomized to receive neoadjuvant therapy that consisted of docetaxel 100 mg/m^2 on day 1; docetaxel 75 mg/m^2 on day 1 plus capecitabine 825 mg/m^2 twice a day on days 1 to 14; or docetaxel 75 mg/m^2 on day 1 plus gemcitabine (1000 mg/m^2 on days 1 and 8 for 4 cycles), with all regimens followed by treatment with doxorubicin–cyclophosphamide for 4 cycles (**Table 1**). Patients were also randomly assigned to receive or not to receive bevacizumab 15 mg/kg of body weight for the first 6 cycles of chemotherapy. Bevacizumab's effect was more pronounced in HR-positive tumors (15.1% without bevacizumab vs 23.2% with bevacizumab, $P = .007$) when compared with HR-negative tumors (47.1% without bevacizumab vs 51.5% with bevacizumab, $P = .34$). The rate of pCR in the breast was significantly increased when bevacizumab was added to the docetaxel/capecitabine regimen (36.1% vs 23.5%, $P = .009$), but not when the monoclonal antibody was added to the docetaxel/gemcitabine regimen (35.8% vs 27.6%, $P = .10$) or the docetaxel regimen (31.6% vs 33.7%, $P = .75$). Unfortunately, the data are pooled and no subset analysis (HR + vs HR−) was performed. This study also reported that the addition of bevacizumab was associated with increased toxicity, specifically decreased wound healing and left ventricular heart dysfunction. A second trial, the CALGB 40603 study, evaluated 443 patients with stage II to III TNBC who received paclitaxel 80 mg/m^2 once per week for 12 weeks, followed by doxorubicin plus cyclophosphamide once every 2 weeks (ddAC) for 4 cycles, and were randomly assigned to concurrent carboplatin area under curve (AUC) 6 once every 3 weeks for 4 cycles and/or bevacizumab 10 mg/kg once every 2 weeks for 9 cycles. The authors concluded that for patients with TNBC treated with bevacizumab in the neoadjuvant setting, there was increased pCR 59% vs 48% ($P = .0089$) within the breast, but ≥ grade 3 toxicities, such as neutropenia, thrombocytopenia, infection, and post-op complications, were increased[15] (see **Table 1**). In addition, improvement in RFS and OS was not demonstrated. These studies consistently show that the addition of bevacizumab increases complication rates and does not reduce the recurrence rates in TNBC. Based on these results, bevacizumab is not recommended for neoadjuvant therapy in patients with TNBC.

Sunitinib

TNBC has been shown to overexpress EGFR, known as HER1.[27] EGFR overexpression was associated with a lower 10-year survival rate for patients with TNBC.[26] Sunitinib is a multi-target oral tyrosine kinase inhibitor approved for use in renal cell carcinoma[28] and gastrointestinal stromal tumors. It has been shown to have downregulatory effects on multiple signaling pathways, including EGFR, VEGF, platelet-derived growth factor, KIT, and RET, which all play important roles in angiogenesis and breast cancer development. A randomized Phase II trial assessed sunitinib monotherapy in heavily pretreated patients with advanced TNBC. When compared with standard chemotherapies, sunitinib resulted in a response rate of 3% in patients with TNBC[29] and 7% response rate in the chemotherapy arm (one-sided $P = .962$). A Phase I/II study using neoadjuvant sunitinib 25 mg daily administered weekly with paclitaxel 70 mg/m^2 on days 1, 8, and 15 and carboplatin AUC 5 on day 1. Fifty-four patients were enrolled and 41 received treatment in the Phase II portion with a primary endpoint of pCR. Thirty-four patients were evaluated with a pCR of 35% (see **Table 1**). Moreover, significant toxicities, including myelosuppression, fatigue, rash, and mucositis resulted in numerous dose reductions and/or omissions of paclitaxel and carboplatin treatments.[30] Based on the evidence and/or lack of evidence to support its use, sunitinib is not recommended for treatment of TNBC.

Table 1
Clinical trials: neoadjuvant therapy for invasive breast cancer

Author, Year	Trial Name/Type	Country	# of Analyzed Participants	Tumor Stage	Adjuvant Therapy	Treatment Duration	Primary Endpoints	Outcomes	Toxicities
Rugo et al,[42] 2016	I-SPY 2 Phase II RCT	United States	60	Stage II–III	PTX ± carboplatin ± veliparib followed by ddAC	Weekly paclitaxel × 12 wk ± carboplatin weekly ± veliparib twice daily by mouth followed by ddAC	pCR	51% with the addition of veliparib and carboplatin vs 26% control	Increased grade 3/4 toxic effects in veliparib plus carboplatin group (neutropenia, thrombocytopenia, and anemia)
Nanda et al,[38] 2017	I-SPY 2 Phase II RCT	United States	69	Stage II–III	PTX ± pembrolizumab followed by ddAC	Weekly PTX × 12 wk ± pembrolizumab every 3 wk × 12 wk followed by ddAC	pCR	pCR 60% vs 20% in the control arm	Grade 3–5 toxicity noted in pembrolizumab arm, including colitis, adrenal insufficiency, fatigue, vomiting, febrile neutropenia, and anemia
Sikov et al,[15] 2015	CALGB 40603	United States	443	Stage II–III	PTX + ddAC ± carboplatin ± BEV	Once weekly PTX × 12 wk followed ddAC and randomized to concurrent carboplatin once every 3 wk × 4 cycles and/or BEV every 2 wk × 9 cycles	pCR	pCR breast 60% vs 46% (P = .0018) in the carboplatin group; pCR breast 59% vs 48% (P = .0089) in BEV group	Significant grade 3/4 neutropenia, thrombocytopenia, bleeding, hypertension. Patients assigned to carboplatin and/or BEV were more likely to skip doses or discontinue

(continued on next page)

Table 1
(continued)

Author, Year	Trial Name/Type	Country	# of Analyzed Participants	Tumor Stage	Adjuvant Therapy	Treatment Duration	Primary Endpoints	Outcomes	Toxicities
Llombart-Cussac et al,[44] 2015	SOLTI NeoPARP – Phase II RCT	Spain, France, and Germany	141	Stage II–IIIA	PTX + iniparib	Once weekly PTX × 12 wk + iniparib (once a week or twice weekly)	pCR	pCR in 3 arms: 21% vs 22% vs 19%	Grade 3/4 neutropenia in the twice-weekly iniparib plus PTX
Yardley et al,[30] 2015	Phase I/II Trial	United States	34	Stage II–III	PTX + carboplatin + sunitinib	PTX days 1, 8, and 15 of 28 d cycle, carboplatin on day 1, daily sunitinib × 6 cycles	pCR	pCR 35%	Grade 3/4 myelosuppression, fatigue, rash, and mucositis. 27% discontinued sunitinib due to toxicity
Cancello et al,[48] 2015	Phase II Trial	Italy	34	Stage II–III	ECF + paclitaxel + oral CP	ECF once every 21 d × 4 cycles PTX (days 1,8, and 15 every 28 d) and CP daily × 12 wk	pCR cCR	pCR 56% cCR + partial response in 91%	Grade 3 adverse events included leukopenia, neutropenia, anemia, and stomatitis
Bear et al,[9] 2012	NSABP B-40—Phase III RCT	United States	244	Stage II–III	DTX ± capecitabine or gemcitabine followed by AC ± BEV	DTXI every 3 wk × 4 cycles, gemcitabine days 1 and 8 every 3 wk × 4 cycles capecitabine days 1–14 every 3 wk, AC every 3 wk × 4 cycles, BEV every 3 wk × 6 cycles	pCR	pCR 47% vs 51.5%; P = .34 in BEV arm	Grade 3/4 toxicities increased hand-foot syndrome, mucositis hypertension, fatigue, and neutropenia

von Minckwitz et al,[45] 2014	GeparSixto; GBG 66	Germany	158	Stage II–III	BEV + PTX + liposomal doxorubicin ± carboplatin	PTX weekly days 1 and 8 every 22 d × 18 wk, doxorubicin weekly days 1 and 8 every 22 d × 18 wk, BEV every 3 wk × 18 wk, carboplatin weekly × 18 wk	pCR	53% vs 36% (P = .005) with Carboplatin	Grade 3/4 neutropenia, anemia, thrombocytopenia, and diarrhea
Sharma et al,[46] 2017	Combined analysis of two cohorts	2 Sites: Kansas and Spain	190	Stage I–III	Carboplatin + DTX	Carboplatin and DTX every 3 wk × 6 cycles	pCR and RCB	pCR 59% vs 56% in BRCA mutant vs BRCA wildtype	Grade 3 or 4 toxicities (28%), including leukopenia, neutropenia, fatigue, peripheral neuropathy, nausea, diarrhea

Abbreviations: BEV, bevacizumab; cCR, clinical complete response; CP, cyclophosphamide; ddAC, dose-dense adriamycin and cyclophosphamide; DTX, docetaxel; ECF, epirubicin and cisplatin and 5-fluorouracil; pCR, pathologic complete response; PTX, paclitaxel; RCT, randomized control trial; wks, weeks.

Pembrolizumab

The role of checkpoint inhibitors continues to be controversial in breast cancer treatment and has gained more attention with the emergence of PD-L1. PD-L1 is a new target that has revolutionized the fields of metastatic melanoma[31–33] and non-small cell lung cancer[34–36] and has shown significant improvement in DFS and OS for these cancers. Programmed cell death protein 1 (PD-1) is expressed on the surface of T cells. PD-L1 is one of the ligands of PD-1, which plays a role in immune modulation and is found on many different tumor types. Ligation of PD-L1 with PD-1 inhibits T-cell proliferation, cytokine production, and cytolytic activity, leading to inactivation of T cells. Through upregulation of PD-L1 and other adaptive immune-resistance mechanisms, tumors are able to use this pathway to evade the antitumor immune response.[13] Higher levels of PD-L1 expression have been found in TNBC compared with other breast cancer subtypes, thus PD-1 has potential to be a molecular target in breast cancer treatment. A recent Phase 1b trial[38] used the high-affinity, anti–PD-1 antibody pembrolizumab 10 mg/kg intravenously every 2 weeks in PD-L1 expressing metastatic TNBC. The overall survival in patients on pembrolizumab monotherapy was 18.5% with a median response time of 17.9 weeks, suggesting a potential role of PD-L1 as a predictive TNBC biomarker in tailoring immune checkpoint therapy.[37] The most common treatment-related side effects were nausea, fatigue, arthralgia, and myalgia. Furthermore, an ongoing Phase II study in the I-SPY 2 clinical research program evaluated standard neoadjuvant chemotherapy in combination with pembrolizumab for 4 cycles. This combination tripled the pCR rate in multiple subtypes of HER2-negative breast cancer, specifically a pCR rate of 60% with pembrolizumab/chemotherapy compared with 20% with standard chemotherapy alone in TNBC[38] (see **Table 1**). Standard chemotherapy is defined as taxol weekly for 12 weeks followed by ddAC. PD-1 and PD-L1 expression in TNBC has been associated with better DFS.[39] Because of the significant responses reported by Nanda and colleagues, this regimen will graduate to a Phase III study.

Onartuzumab

Onartuzumab is a monoclonal antibody directed against hepatic growth factor receptor, c-Met. Dieras and colleagues[40] examined metastatic TNBC treated with the addition of the c-Met inhibitor, onartuzumab, alongside bevacizumab or paclitaxel. The addition of inhibitor did not improve patients' progression-free survival or OS. A meta-analysis by Yan and colleagues[41] demonstrated that c-Met overexpression increases the risk of recurrence in TNBC. Therefore, c-Met may function as a prognostic biomarker in TNBC, but additional studies are necessary to confirm the efficacy of this potential target.

Veliparib

PARP inhibitors block DNA single-strand break repair, which can lead to death of BRCA (breast cancer susceptibility gene)-deficient cells or may potentiate the effects of some chemotherapy agents, independent of BRCA status.[26] Preclinical models have demonstrated that veliparib, an oral, potent inhibitor of PARP 1/2, significantly heightens the antineoplastic effect of carboplatin. Carboplatin and veliparib, in combination with weekly paclitaxel followed by ddAC, demonstrated an outcome improvement of women with TNBC in the Phase III I-SPY 2 trial (see **Table 1**). pCR in the TNBC population was 51% (95% Bayesian probability interval [PI], 36%–66%) in the veliparib-carboplatin group versus 26% (95% PI, 9%–43%) in the control group of paclitaxel weekly for 12 weeks followed by ddAC.[14,42,43] In addition, the SOLTI

NeoPARP Phase II randomized trial of neoadjuvant paclitaxel 80 mg/m^2 weekly with iniparib (given once weekly 11.2 mg/kg on day 1 or twice weekly 5.6 mg/kg days 1 and 4) for 12 weeks.[44] Primary endpoint was pCR in the breast, which was similar between all three groups: 21%, 22%, 19%, respectively. Grade 3/4 neutropenia was observed in the twice-weekly iniparib group. Otherwise, there were no differences in serious adverse event among the groups. These results do not support further evaluation of PARP inhibitors plus paclitaxel in early stage TNBC.

CHEMOTHERAPY

Although studies involving new molecular targets are under intense investigation, there is also a large area of research focusing on the identification of patients who respond to current chemotherapies often used for metastatic breast cancer treatment. As mentioned earlier, platinum agents are a promising chemotherapeutic option for neoadjuvant TNBC therapy, because they exploit the loss of DNA repair proteins commonly seen in TNBC basal subtype patients. The aim of the GeparSixto trial was to assess the additional effect of neoadjuvant carboplatin with taxane-based therapy on pCR in a subset of patients with stage II–III TNBC. The taxane-based therapy contained paclitaxel 80 mg/m^2 weekly days 1 and 8 every 22 days for 18 weeks, pegylated liposomal doxorubicin 20 mg/m^2 once weekly days 1 and 8 every 22 days for 18 weeks, and bevacizumab 15 mg/kg intravenously every 3 weeks for 18 weeks in which patients were randomized 1:1 for the addition of carboplatin AUC 2 weekly. Of 158 patients with TNBC, 84 (53.2%, 54.4–60.9) patients achieved pCR with carboplatin, compared with 58 (36.9%, 95% CI 29.4–44.5) of 157 without ($P = .005$)[45] (see **Table 1**). The pCR rate was significantly higher in patients treated with carboplatin (58.7%) than in patients treated without carboplatin (37.9%).[45] Another randomized study, CALGB40603, assessed the addition of carboplatin AUC 6 every 3 weeks for four cycles or bevacizumab every 2 weeks for 9 cycles to backbone chemotherapy of weekly paclitaxel for 12 weeks, followed by dose-dense doxorubicin-cyclophosphamide as neoadjuvant treatment of patients with TNBC versus standard neoadjuvant chemotherapy.[15] Using one-sided P values, the addition of either carboplatin (60% vs 44%; $P = .0018$) or bevacizumab (59% vs 48%; $P = .0089$) significantly increased pCR breast. Moreover, the addition of carboplatin (54% vs 41%; $P = .0029$) significantly raised pCR in both breast and axilla.[15] Sharma and colleagues[46] evaluated 190 patients with stage I–III TNBC treated with neoadjuvant carboplatin AUC 6 + docetaxel 75 mg/m^2 every 3 weeks for 6 cycles. The overall pCR and RCB 0 + 1 rates were 55% and 68%, correspondingly. pCR in patients with BRCA-associated and wild-type TNBC were 59% and 56%, respectively ($P = .83$). On multivariable analysis, stage III disease was the only factor associated with a lower likelihood of achieving a pCR (see **Table 1**). Moreover, 28% of patients observed in the study experienced grade 3 or 4 toxicities from the regimen. In a similar randomized Phase II study, Alba and colleagues[47] combined epirubicin plus cyclophosphamide chemotherapy, followed by docetaxel with or without carboplatin AUC 6 given every 21 days in basal-like breast cancers. Disappointingly, the prespecified primary endpoint of improvement in pCR rates (defined as pCR in breast) was not met, with analogous pCR rates in breast and axilla of 30% in both treatment arms.

Various other taxane-based chemotherapy regimens have been evaluated in which toxicities outweighed response. In a study by Cancello and colleagues,[48] patients were treated with epirubicin and cisplatin and 5-fluorouracil (epirubicin and cisplatin on day 1 with low-dose 5-fluorouracil in continuous infusion every 21 days for 4 cycles), followed by paclitaxel (90 mg/m^2 on days 1, 8, and 15 every 28 days for 3 cycles), in combination with metronomic oral cyclophosphamide 50 mg daily for 12 weeks in TNBC (HER2-negative, estrogen receptor– and progesterone receptor–negative defined as <10%). The mean difference between the percentage of Ki-67 positive cells evaluated in surgical resection specimens and in pretreatment tumor core biopsy was 41% (95% confidence interval [CI], 30–51; P<.0001) for the entire population and 22% (95% CI, 7–38; P = .0097) in patients who did not achieve pCR. Clinical and partial responses were reached in 31 patients (91%) with 19 patients (56%; 95% CI, 35–70) having a pCR. Stable disease was observed in 3 patients and 0 patient had progressive disease. Notable grade ≥3 hematological adverse events were observed, including neutropenia (38%), leukopenia (9%), and anemia (3%) of participants (see **Table 1**).

Oral chemotherapy regimens have been evaluated as well. For example, capecitabine is a chemotherapy drug presently used for metastatic breast cancer; however, its role in the neoadjuvant setting is unclear because of conflicting reports.[49] A meta-analysis of eight studies comprising 9302 patients showed that addition of capecitabine to standard chemotherapy was associated with significantly improved DFS in TNBC versus non-TNBC (HR 0.72 vs 10.01, interaction P = .02) as well as increased the grade 3/4 toxicity of diarrhea and hand foot syndrome.[49] Investigators postulated that capecitabine may have an improved effect in the neoadjuvant setting, in contrast to the low response rates seen with metastatic TNBC.

Although anthracycline-based therapies have been the most promising treatment of TNBC, because of toxicities, some patients are unable to tolerate this regimen. One group performed a retrospective analysis to determine the efficacy of nonanthracycline-based regimens in the neoadjuvant setting, specifically platinum-containing regimens. Of the 10 patients with TNBC included in the study, 6/10 (60%) had a pCR (breast and lymph nodes) and 7/10 (70%) had a pCR-breast.[43] Overall, no recurrences were observed in the patients who had a pCR during a 25-month follow-up period. These results are promising because high pCR were observed with a tolerable toxicity profile.

SUMMARY

TNBC is a very aggressive form of breast cancer with a higher risk of mortality and morbidity compared with HR positive subtypes. The recurrence rate is significantly higher in the first 3 years following treatment, even in small (≤2 cm) tumors. As such, researchers have focused on new therapeutic target development that can potentially improve DFS and OS in this high-risk patient population. Currently patients with TNBC are treated with a combination of taxane- and anthracycline-based regimens. Unlike patients with HR-positive breast cancer, there are no US FDA-approved targeted therapies for TNBC. New studies have uncovered the presence of distinct, intrinsic genotypic profiles within the larger subtype of TNBC, which may be used to predict chemotherapy response. Neoadjuvant chemotherapy is now being used as an adaptive approach in TNBC to help predict tumor response across various regimens with the desired goal to improve patient outcome. New targets such as VEGF, PD-L1, EGFR, and PARP are presently under investigation and may potentially be used as prognostic indicators, therapeutic targets, and/or pharmacogenomic markers. There continues to be unmet needs to develop agents targeting these pathways and apply a robust screening model for responses to newer targeted therapies. However, groups such as the I-SPY research program and the Translational Breast Cancer Research Consortium (TBCRC), which focus on the treatment of highly-aggressive breast cancers, are making great strides. Because response rates are dismal and recurrences are high with standard chemotherapy approaches, molecular-based profiling is a methodology that must be used universally to result in impactful, positive outcomes in TNBC.

REFERENCES

1. Siegel RL, Miller KD, Jemal A. Cancer statistics, 2017. CA Cancer J Clin 2017; 67(1):7–30.
2. Carey LA, Perou CM, Livasy CA, et al. Race, breast cancer subtypes, and survival in the Carolina Breast Cancer Study. JAMA 2006;295(21):2492–502.
3. Dent R, Trudeau M, Pritchard KI, et al. Triple-negative breast cancer: clinical features and patterns of recurrence. Clin Cancer Res 2007;13(15 Pt 1):4429–34.
4. Ahn SG, Kim SJ, Kim C, et al. Molecular classification of triple-negative breast cancer. J Breast Cancer 2016;19(3):223–30.
5. Kinne DW, Butler JA, Kimmel M, et al. Estrogen receptor protein of breast cancer in patients with positive nodes. High recurrence rates in the postmenopausal estrogen receptor-negative group. Arch Surg 1987;122(11):1303–6.
6. Howlader N, Cronin KA, Kurian AW, et al. Differences in breast cancer survival by molecular subtypes in the United States. Cancer Epidemiol Biomarkers Prev 2018 [pii:cebp.0627.2017].
7. Prat A, Perou CM. Deconstructing the molecular portraits of breast cancer. Mol Oncol 2011;5(1):5–23.
8. Berry DA, Cirrincione C, Henderson IC, et al. Estrogen-receptor status and outcomes of modern chemotherapy for patients with node-positive breast cancer. JAMA 2006;295(14):1658–67.
9. Bear HD, Tang G, Rastogi P, et al. Bevacizumab added to neoadjuvant chemotherapy for breast cancer. N Engl J Med 2012;366(4):310–20.
10. Kuehn T, Klauss W, Darsow M, et al. Long-term morbidity following axillary dissection in breast cancer patients–clinical assessment, significance for life quality and the impact of demographic, oncologic and therapeutic factors. Breast Cancer Res Treat 2000;64(3):275–86.
11. McCredie MR, Dite GS, Porter L, et al. Prevalence of self-reported arm morbidity following treatment for breast cancer in the Australian Breast Cancer Family Study. Breast 2001;10(6):515–22.
12. Olson JA Jr, McCall LM, Beitsch P, et al. Impact of immediate versus delayed axillary node dissection on surgical outcomes in breast cancer patients with positive sentinel nodes: results from American College of Surgeons Oncology Group Trials Z0010 and Z0011. J Clin Oncol 2008;26(21):3530–5.
13. Anders CK, Abramson V, Tan T, et al. The evolution of triple-negative breast cancer: from biology to novel therapeutics. Am Soc Clin Oncol Educ Book 2016;35: 34–42.
14. Castrellon AB, Pidhorecky I, Valero V, et al. The role of carboplatin in the neoadjuvant chemotherapy treatment of triple negative breast cancer. Oncol Rev 2017; 11(1):324.
15. Sikov WM, Berry DA, Perou CM, et al. Impact of the addition of carboplatin and/or bevacizumab to neoadjuvant once-per-week paclitaxel followed by dose-dense doxorubicin and cyclophosphamide on pathologic complete response rates in stage II to III triple-negative breast cancer: CALGB 40603 (alliance). J Clin Oncol 2015;33(1):13–21.
16. Esserman LJ, Berry DA, Cheang MC, et al. Chemotherapy response and recurrence-free survival in neoadjuvant breast cancer depends on biomarker profiles: results from the I-SPY 1 TRIAL (CALGB 150007/150012; ACRIN 6657). Breast Cancer Res Treat 2012;132(3):1049–62.
17. Perou CM, Sorlie T, Eisen MB, et al. Molecular portraits of human breast tumours. Nature 2000;406(6797):747–52.

18. Lehmann BD, Bauer JA, Chen X, et al. Identification of human triple-negative breast cancer subtypes and preclinical models for selection of targeted therapies. J Clin Invest 2011;121(7):2750–67.

19. Lehmann BD, Pietenpol JA. Identification and use of biomarkers in treatment strategies for triple-negative breast cancer subtypes. J Pathol 2014;232(2):142–50.

20. Burstein MD, Tsimelzon A, Poage GM, et al. Comprehensive genomic analysis identifies novel subtypes and targets of triple-negative breast cancer. Clin Cancer Res 2015;21(7):1688–98.

21. Watkins JA, Irshad S, Grigoriadis A, et al. Genomic scars as biomarkers of homologous recombination deficiency and drug response in breast and ovarian cancers. Breast Cancer Res 2014;16(3):211.

22. Gucalp A, Tolaney S, Isakoff SJ, et al. Phase II trial of bicalutamide in patients with androgen receptor-positive, estrogen receptor-negative metastatic breast cancer. Clin Cancer Res 2013;19(19):5505–12.

23. Traina TA, Miller K, Yardley DA, et al. Enzalutamide for the treatment of androgen receptor-expressing triple-negative breast cancer. J Clin Oncol 2018;36(9):884–90.

24. Masuda H, Baggerly KA, Wang Y, et al. Differential response to neoadjuvant chemotherapy among 7 triple-negative breast cancer molecular subtypes. Clin Cancer Res 2013;19(19):5533–40.

25. Echavarria I, Lopez-Tarruella S, Picornell A, et al. Pathological response in a triple-negative breast cancer cohort treated with neoadjuvant carboplatin and docetaxel according to Lehmann's refined classification. Clin Cancer Res 2018;24(8):1845–52.

26. Fleisher B, Clarke C, Ait-Oudhia S. Current advances in biomarkers for targeted therapy in triple-negative breast cancer. Breast Cancer (Dove Med Press) 2016;8:183–97.

27. Foulkes WD, Smith IE, Reis-Filho JS. Triple-negative breast cancer. N Engl J Med 2010;363(20):1938–48.

28. Motzer RJ, Hutson TE, Cella D, et al. Pazopanib versus sunitinib in metastatic renal-cell carcinoma. N Engl J Med 2013;369(8):722–31.

29. Curigliano G, Pivot X, Cortes J, et al. Randomized phase II study of sunitinib versus standard of care for patients with previously treated advanced triple-negative breast cancer. Breast 2013;22(5):650–6.

30. Yardley DA, Shipley DL, Peacock NW, et al. Phase I/II trial of neoadjuvant sunitinib administered with weekly paclitaxel/carboplatin in patients with locally advanced triple-negative breast cancer. Breast Cancer Res Treat 2015;152(3):557–67.

31. Robert C, Ribas A, Wolchok JD, et al. Anti-programmed-death-receptor-1 treatment with pembrolizumab in ipilimumab-refractory advanced melanoma: a randomised dose-comparison cohort of a phase 1 trial. Lancet 2014;384(9948):1109–17.

32. Robert C, Schachter J, Long GV, et al. Pembrolizumab versus Ipilimumab in Advanced Melanoma. N Engl J Med 2015;372(26):2521–32.

33. Hamid O, Robert C, Daud A, et al. Safety and tumor responses with lambrolizumab (anti-PD-1) in melanoma. N Engl J Med 2013;369(2):134–44.

34. Garon EB, Rizvi NA, Hui R, et al. Pembrolizumab for the treatment of non-small-cell lung cancer. N Engl J Med 2015;372(21):2018–28.

35. Sul J, Blumenthal GM, Jiang X, et al. FDA approval summary: pembrolizumab for the treatment of patients with metastatic non-small cell lung cancer whose tumors express programmed death-ligand 1. Oncologist 2016;21(5):643–50.

36. Reck M, Rodriguez-Abreu D, Robinson AG, et al. Pembrolizumab versus chemotherapy for PD-L1-positive non-small-cell lung cancer. N Engl J Med 2016; 375(19):1823–33.
37. Nanda R, Chow LQ, Dees EC, et al. Pembrolizumab in patients with advanced triple-negative breast cancer: phase Ib KEYNOTE-012 study. J Clin Oncol 2016;34(21):2460–7.
38. Nanda R, Liu MC, Yau C, et al. Pembrolizumab plus standard neoadjuvant therapy for high-risk breast cancer: results from I-SPY 2. Paper presented at the ASCO annual meeting held at Chicago (IL), June 5, 2017 [abstract: 506].
39. Li X, Wetherilt CS, Krishnamurti U, et al. Stromal PD-L1 expression is associated with better disease-free survival in triple-negative breast cancer. Am J Clin Pathol 2016;146(4):496–502.
40. Dieras V, Campone M, Yardley DA, et al. Randomized, phase II, placebo-controlled trial of onartuzumab and/or bevacizumab in combination with weekly paclitaxel in patients with metastatic triple-negative breast cancer. Ann Oncol 2015;26(9):1904–10.
41. Yan S, Jiao X, Zou H, et al. Prognostic significance of c-Met in breast cancer: a meta-analysis of 6010 cases. Diagn Pathol 2015;10:62.
42. Rugo HS, Olopade OI, DeMichele A, et al. Adaptive randomization of veliparib-carboplatin treatment in breast cancer. N Engl J Med 2016;375(1):23–34.
43. Shinde AM, Zhai J, Yu KW, et al. Pathologic complete response rates in triple-negative, HER2-positive, and hormone receptor-positive breast cancers after anthracycline-free neoadjuvant chemotherapy with carboplatin and paclitaxel with or without trastuzumab. Breast 2015;24(1):18–23.
44. Llombart-Cussac A, Bermejo B, Villanueva C, et al. SOLTI NeoPARP: a phase II randomized study of two schedules of iniparib plus paclitaxel versus paclitaxel alone as neoadjuvant therapy in patients with triple-negative breast cancer. Breast Cancer Res Treat 2015;154(2):351–7.
45. von Minckwitz G, Schneeweiss A, Loibl S, et al. Neoadjuvant carboplatin in patients with triple-negative and HER2-positive early breast cancer (GeparSixto; GBG 66): a randomised phase 2 trial. Lancet Oncol 2014;15(7):747–56.
46. Sharma P, Lopez-Tarruella S, Garcia-Saenz JA, et al. Efficacy of neoadjuvant carboplatin plus docetaxel in triple-negative breast cancer: combined analysis of two cohorts. Clin Cancer Res 2017;23(3):649–57.
47. Alba E, Chacon JI, Lluch A, et al. A randomized phase II trial of platinum salts in basal-like breast cancer patients in the neoadjuvant setting. Results from the GEICAM/2006-03, multicenter study. Breast Cancer Res Treat 2012;136(2): 487–93.
48. Cancello G, Bagnardi V, Sangalli C, et al. Phase II study with epirubicin, cisplatin, and infusional fluorouracil followed by weekly paclitaxel with metronomic cyclophosphamide as a preoperative treatment of triple-negative breast cancer. Clin Breast Cancer 2015;15(4):259–65.
49. Natori A, Ethier JL, Amir E, et al. Capecitabine in early breast cancer: a meta-analysis of randomised controlled trials. Eur J Cancer 2017;77:40–7.

Inflammatory Breast Cancer
What to Know About This Unique, Aggressive Breast Cancer

Arjun Menta[a], Tamer M. Fouad, MD[b,c], Anthony Lucci, MD[b,d],
Huong Le-Petross, MD[b,e], Michael C. Stauder, MD[b,f],
Wendy A. Woodward, MD, PhD[b,f], Naoto T. Ueno, MD, PhD[b,g],
Bora Lim, MD[b,g],*

KEYWORDS

- Inflammatory breast cancer • Trimodality care • Clinical trials • Breast changes

KEY POINTS

- Inflammatory breast cancers have unique characteristics that are not typical presentation of breast cancers.
- Inflammatory breast cancer carries features that can be easily confused with other skin diseases, such as infection (mastitis or cellulitis), and often are attempted to be treated with antibiotics.
- Delayed diagnosis of inflammatory breast cancer can result in a dismal clinical outcome; therefore, it is critical to make a timely and accurate diagnosis at the beginning.
- Trimodality care regardless of response is appropriate in all stage III and most stage IV cases: chemotherapy, surgery, and radiation.
- Direct and efficient referral system via networking in community can facilitate this process of accurate and timely diagnosis and treatment of inflammatory breast cancer.

The authors have nothing to disclose.
[a] The University of Texas at Austin, 110 Inner Campus Drive, Austin, TX 78705, USA; [b] Morgan Welch Inflammatory Breast Cancer Research and Clinic Program, The University of Texas MD Anderson Cancer Center, 1515 Holcombe Boulevard, Houston, TX 77030, USA; [c] Department of Medical Oncology, The National Cancer Institute, Cairo University, Cairo 11796, Egypt; [d] Breast Surgical Oncology, The University of Texas MD Anderson Cancer Center, 1515 Holcombe Boulevard, Houston, TX 77030, USA; [e] Breast Diagnostic Imaging, The University of Texas MD Anderson Cancer Center, 1515 Holcombe Boulevard, Houston, TX 77030, USA; [f] Radiation Oncology, The University of Texas MD Anderson Cancer Center, 1515 Holcombe Boulevard, Houston, TX 77030, USA; [g] Breast Medical Oncology, The University of Texas MD Anderson Cancer Center, 1515 Holcombe Boulevard, Houston, TX 77030, USA
* Corresponding author. The University of Texas MD Anderson Cancer Center, 1515 Holcombe Boulevard, Unit 1354, Houston, TX 77030.
E-mail address: blim@mdanderson.org

Surg Clin N Am 98 (2018) 787–800
https://doi.org/10.1016/j.suc.2018.03.009
0039-6109/18/© 2018 Elsevier Inc. All rights reserved.

INCIDENCE, MORTALITY, AND RISK FACTORS
Incidence of Inflammatory Breast Cancer

Inflammatory breast cancer (IBC) is a rare form of breast cancer that accounts for only about 2% to 4% of all breast cancer cases in the United States.[1] Despite its low incidence, IBC contributes to 7% of breast cancer–caused mortality.[2] Based on the data from the Surveillance, Epidemiology, and End Results (SEER) program of National Cancer Institute, the diagnosis of IBC between 1973 and 2002 has increased at an annual rate of between 1.23% and 4.35% per year, which is a much higher rate of increase than the incidence of overall breast cancer diagnosis, which is 0.42%. In Western Africa, or Egypt, this occurrence is as high as 10%, and this justifies a collective international effort to better understand the distinctive biological, clinical aspect of IBC as well as to discover novel targets for this unique and rare disease entity. The first scientific documentation of IBC was noted in the eighteenth century by St. Charles, as a female patient with a red and swollen breast.[3]

Risk Factors of Inflammatory Breast Cancer

High body mass index continues to be recognized as an independent risk factor of IBC.[4] No association with inherited genetic mutations or family history has been clearly demonstrated. Less established and yet possible risk factors that need investigation are the viral infections or chronic inflammation as either causative event for the occurrence of IBC or mediators of the specific pathobiology of IBC, which may explain some racial and regional differences.[5,6] The association between the exposure to certain types of viral infection or chronic inflammation has been suggested and needs to be further studied.

Histopathologic Definition of Inflammatory Breast Cancer

Scattered tumor emboli on biopsy or surgical specimen and dermal lymphatic invasion are key histopathologic findings of IBC.[7,8] About 75% of IBC tumor samples exhibit dermal lymphatic invasion and thereby aid in making the diagnosis, but this is neither required nor suffices for the diagnosis of IBC.[9] The scattered distribution of tumor often as emboli throughout the breast contributes to the difficulty in detecting this disease on mammogram. The relative proportion of breast cancer molecular subtypes is different between IBC and non-IBC. In IBC, the incidence of hormone receptor (HR) -positive subtype is relatively lower, and both HER2-positive and triple-negative breast cancer (TNBC) are higher: 40% of HER2-positive, and 30% in TNBC than non-IBC.[10] A recent retrospective review of 659 patients with IBC showed that about 4.5% IBC showed lobular type lower compared with 10% in all breast cancer. Most tumors are modified nuclear grade 3. All subtypes across showed 62% to 68% 3-year overall survival (OS). This also applies to the HR-positive IBC. Same stage HR positive IBC has significantly worse prognosis compared to HR positive non-IBC.[11] Histologic type of lobular versus ductal did not affect survival.[12]

CURRENT CLINICAL DIAGNOSIS OF INFLAMMATORY BREAST CANCER
Clinical Diagnosis

Rapid changes in the skin overlying the affected breast (erythema, edema, and peau d'orange affecting a large area of breast) and pathologic evidence of invasive carcinoma are basic elements for the diagnosis of IBC. Changes of skin or underlying mass occur within 3 to 6 months, offering an important point to distinguish IBC from noninflammatory locally advanced breast cancer.[13] In some cases, skin can be the only site of disease. The current American Joint Committee on Cancer (AJCC) guideline defines IBC as a separate "clinico-pathologic entity" with the erythema and edema occupying at least one-third of the breast, that can extend to the whole breast and across to the contralateral breast involving mediastinum, upper extremities, and neck area.[14] A typical case of IBC is depicted in **Fig. 1**.

International expert panel recommended diagnosis guideline of IBC is summarized in **Table 1**.[13] Note the difference in description of onset in the international consensus of erythema, edema, and OR peau d'orange versus the AJCC staging that requires erythema. This diagnosis criteria based on skin changes highlights that at times a patient may not have classically "red" skin but clearly may have skin symptoms consistent with IBC. It is particularly true among women with darker skin tones. Baseline laboratory tests that need to be performed at diagnosis include routine laboratory tests like complete blood count and SMA-12, tumor markers, for example, cancer antigen 15-3 and CEA, which can help assess patients at the initial diagnosis, in support of staging.[15] Local imaging with mammogram and ultrasound (US), complete staging with imaging modality, with more recent emphasis on highly sensitive PET/computed tomography (CT) utilization, is important (covered in later discussion).

Breast Imaging

For locoregional imaging in diagnosis of IBC, mammography and US remain the current standard of care. The baseline mammography imaging can reveal information like microcalcifications, architectural distortion, trabecular thickening, and global skin thickening.[16] Because of the painful inflamed breast-limiting optimal compression required for mammography and the increased mammographic density from global edema obscuring visualization of an underlying breast mass, mammography detects 68% of a primary breast lesion compared 94% with US and 98% with MRI.[17] The actual primary breast lesion may not be detected on imaging in all cases with only diffuse skin thickening seen; however, the lack of an imaging-detected breast mass does not exclude the diagnosis of IBC. Mammography is still recommended to provide screening of the contralateral breast.[16]

US can detect a solid mass, parenchymal changes, or skin thickening in patients with IBC better than mammography, with reported sensitivity of 92% to 96%.[18,19] About one-third of patients had tumor emboli in dermis confirmed by histopathologic

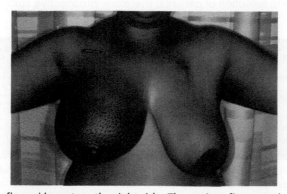

Fig. 1. Swollen, inflamed breast on the right side. The patient first noted a small red patch, which soon spread within a 4-week period of time. Biopsy testing confirmed invasive ductal carcinoma. The patient was treated at Morgan Welch Inflammatory Breast Cancer Clinic at the University of Texas MD Anderson Cancer Center.

Table 1	
Diagnosis guideline of inflammatory breast cancer based on expert consensus	
Minimum criteria required for the diagnosis of IBC	
Onset	Rapid onset of breast erythema, edema and/or peau d'orange, with or without an underlying breast mass
Duration	History of such findings no more than 6 mo, mostly within 3 mo
Extent	Erythema and/or edema occupying at least 1/3 of whole breast
Pathology	Pathologic confirmation of invasive carcinoma
Pathologic specimen diagnosis	
Parenchyma	Core biopsy-proven invasive carcinoma
Skin	Any suspicious lesions should be biopsied with at least 2 skin punch biopsies
Biomarker	Same procedure for ER/PR and HER2 as in non-IBC

examination.[18] Many have confirmed axillary lymph node involvement better detected by US.[19] Breast MRI and molecular breast imaging (MBI) show higher sensitivity in the detection of invasive breast cancers, including IBC.[20] These modalities provide better visualization of the breast lesions and additional information associated with skin thickening, such as skin enhancement, skin nodules, or tumoral emboli, than conventional modalities like mammography or US (**Fig. 2**).

PET/Computed Tomography Scan

In recent years, accumulating data showed the benefit of PET/CT scan over CT scan and bone scan as a staging modality. For example, a study of 111 patients with IBC who were evaluated with PET/CT scan showed higher detection of lymph node metastasis.[17] This "upstaging" phenomenon was associated with longer progression-free survival,[21] followed by other papers to support similar findings.[22,23] Reviewing the PET/CT in IBC at MD Anderson revealed up to 10% of IBC cases will have contralateral lymph nodes as the only site of M1 disease, potentially a locally controllable dissemination.[24] Another utilization of PET/CT in the IBC is the ability to monitor treatment response. In a study of 53 patients with IBC, the changes in PET/CT during neoadjuvant therapy predicted long-term outcome of patients. This clinical benefit seen in trials is likely due to selection of patients; therefore, prospective study is necessary to

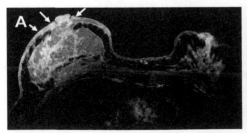
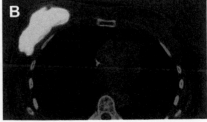

Fig. 2. A 76-year-old woman with a self-palpated left breast mass, and core biopsy revealed triple-negative inflammatory breast carcinoma. (A) Contrast-enhanced breast MRI examination showed multicentric breast lesions with diffuse skin thickening and skin enhancement/lesions (*arrows*) secondary to biopsy-proven dermal tumor emboli. (B) PET/CT image revealed multicentric hypermetabolism throughout the right breast related to the IBC.

validate such benefit. It is not known whether upstaging from stage III to IV impacts the OS of patients, whereas the initial stage can predict the long-term outcome of patients and need to studied.[23,25]

CURRENT TREATMENT OF INFLAMMATORY BREAST CANCER
General Approach for Stage III Inflammatory Breast Cancer

Both National Comprehensive Cancer Network (NCCN) guidelines and the international IBC expert guidelines recommend intensive therapy for patients with primary IBC to achieve best local control and survival outcome, via trimodality approach: systemic therapy, surgery, and radiation therapy (**Fig. 3**). In the preguideline era, when IBC was treated mainly with surgery and with or without adjuvant radiation therapy, the 5-year survival was only 5%.[26] In a large case series composed of 495 patients that were treated with radical mastectomy from 1935 to 1942, the median survival of patients was 19 months.[27] Anthracycline use was introduced in the treatment of IBC since 1974 at MD Anderson.[28] Then, the presurgical introduction of the systemic therapy (neoadjuvant therapy) approach using anthracycline as a backbone was accepted as a standard of care for IBC.[29] Subsequently, taxane was added to anthracycline-based regimen, showing additional benefit in the neoadjuvant setting.[30] However, without proper locoregional management by surgery and radiation, the response to systemic therapy is not durable in stage III IBC.[31]

There are several critical practice points the authors recommend for appropriate local control in IBC patients: they do not recommend skin-sparing mastectomy, or immediate reconstruction, simultaneous contralateral mastectomy unless the contralateral breast is also involved. All these practices can minimize the immediate recurrence-related treatment delay/complication, and longer-term better cosmetic outcome as well. Local therapy, including both surgery and radiation therapy, is indicated in most cases, and this is recommended in the setting wherein there is no complete resolution of the cancer.

Preoperative Systemic Chemotherapy

Neoadjuvant anthracycline-based chemotherapy for IBC was first introduced in the 1970s. Anthracycline-based combination therapy followed by surgery and adjuvant radiotherapy was proven to be efficacious in several prospective clinical trials.[32] Chemotherapy regimens are similar to the ones used for non-IBC patients. From a

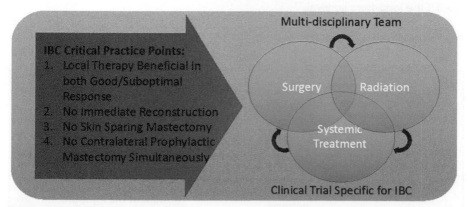

Fig. 3. Critical practice points of IBC.

retrospective MD Anderson data review collected over 20 years, anthracycline-based chemotherapy in IBC patients resulted in 40% OS in 5 years, and 33% in 10 years.[30] Anthracycline containing triplet regimen, including 5-fluorouracil, showed similar efficacy in survival in a retrospective analysis of 68 patients.[33] Furthermore, taxane-based combination chemotherapy was also effective as neoadjuvant treatment of IBC patients, showing median survival of 46 months.[34] The same investigators also showed the addition of paclitaxel to FAC regimen (5-fluorouracil, Adriamycin, and cyclophosphamide) in IBC improved benefit. However, this benefit was more prominent in the subset of HR-negative IBC patients.[35] At MD Anderson, taxane treatment followed by anthracycline-containing regimen is the standard regimen for IBC neoadjuvant therapy. Historical rates of pathological complete response are summarized in **Table 2**. Although both HR-positive and TNBC IBC undergo the same anthracycline-and taxane-based chemotherapy, if IBC overexpresses HER-2/*neu*, double-HER2 targeting therapy is combined similar to treatment of non-IBC. If the patient does not achieve meaningful clinical response after routine neoadjuvant chemotherapy treatment, additional neoadjuvant chemotherapy might be recommended before surgery. If there are available neoadjuvant therapy clinical trials, patients with IBC are strongly recommended to enroll into clinical trials to optimize clinical outcomes. Clinical evaluation of response to chemotherapy is performed based on the RECIST response criteria by medical examination and radiological assessment every 6 to 12 weeks. In addition, baseline and repeated medical photography are extremely useful in monitoring skin changes, such as erythema and edema.[36] Current and upcoming available clinical trials for neoadjuvant therapy in IBC at the MD Anderson, Dana Farber, and other major IBC treatment centers are summarized in **Table 3**, along with other trials available in different settings.

The success of systemic therapy in stage III IBC is measured by the pathologic response to the therapy. Patients who achieved pathologic complete response (pCR) have significantly improved outcomes compared with patients who did not.[37] A historical collection of patient IBC data showed that the pCR rate in stage III IBC was about 15.2%; it is slightly different among molecular subtype groups. The pCR rate of HR-positive/HER2-negative subtype and HR-negative/HER2-positive subtype was 7.3% and 30.6%, respectively. Triple-negative IBC showed about 18.6% pCR rate. Although there are small differences, pCR in patients with IBC is lower compared with stage and molecular subtype-matched non-IBC breast cancers. More importantly, pCR has been shown to be a predictive marker of survival in IBC. Contrastingly, from non-IBC HR-positive breast cancer, the pCR in HR-positive IBC also was able to predict the long-term survival.[11]

Based on most recent survival analysis of stage IV patients, with median follow-up of 4.7 years of IBC patients between 1987 to 2012, the median survival of patients with

Table 2
Summary of pathologic complete response rate in inflammatory breast cancer patients, data collected from 1989 to 2011, at the MD Anderson Cancer Center in comparison with noninflammatory breast cancer historical data

	TNBC, %	ER+/HER2−	ER+/HER2+, %	ER−HER2+, %
Historic pCR rate of IBC	12	7.4%	30	15
Historic pCR rate of non-IBC	30–40	7%–16%, but not clearly related to worse clinical outcome	35	40–60

Table 3
Clinical trials portfolio for inflammatory breast cancer that are currently open for accrual as of February 2018

Neoadjuvant	Adjuvant	Metastatic	Metastatic Maintenance
Bevacizumab + FEC followed by adjuvant therapy by docetaxel ± trastuzumab phase 2 (NCT01880385)	A study of anti-PD-1 (pembrolizumab) + hormonal therapy in HR-positive localized IBC patients with non-pCR to neoadjuvant chemotherapy phase 2 (NCT02971748)	Nintedanib for HER2-negative IBC phase 2 (NCT02389764)	Pembrolizumab single-agent maintenance phase 2 (NCT02411656)
Eribulin followed by AC phase 2 (NCT02623972)		T-VEC phase 2 (NCT02658812)	
Carboplatin + nab-paclitaxel phase 2 (NCT01525966)		Olaparib and radiotherapy in inoperable breast cancer (NCT02227082)	
Paclitaxel + trastuzumab + pertuzumab phase 2 (NCT01796197)		Romidepsin + abraxane phase 1/2 (NCT01938833)	
Ruxolitinib + chemo phase 1/2 (NCT02041429)		Study of triple combination of atezolizumab + cobimetinib + eribulin (ACE) in patients with chemotherapy resistant recurrent/metastatic IBC phase 2 (NCT03202316)	
3HT with Taxol for HER2-positive IBC, and neratinib + taxol for HR–positive IBC in neoadjuvant setting phase 1/2 (NCT03101748)			

IBC versus that of non-IBC was 2.27 versus 3.40 years ($P = .0128$).[38] This significantly lower survival of patients with IBC remains to be significant regardless of molecular subtype and tumor stage.[39] In previous analysis of 68 stage III IBC patients with median follow-up greater than 10 years, 4-year median survival ranged from 5 months to 14.7 months. The OS rate at 5 years and 10 years were 44% and 32%, respectively.[33] Collectively, the survival of patients with IBC is lower than same stage, same molecular subtype of patients with non-IBC.

Surgery

Surgical treatment, in the form of a modified radical mastectomy, needs to be offered to those patients who have at least a partial response to neoadjuvant systemic therapy.[40] Patients with developing disease progression during primary systemic therapy are generally not candidates for surgery at this point; they are offered additional local and systemic therapeutic options, with the exception of some limited cases whereby salvage therapy is indicated (discussed later). Surgery to prevent morbid local spread in patients switching systemic therapies should be watched closely to not lose the window of operability when this control is desired.

The surgical goal for treatment of patients with IBC is the complete removal to pathologically negative margins. Removal of all involved areas in the skin is strongly recommended, because the remnant cells within the skin can further manifest as a recurrence of disease.

Patients with IBC commonly present with detectable lymph node involvement, including the infraclavicular lymph nodes. Sentinel node mapping is not recommended for IBC patients, because it has not proved to be accurate in this population,[41] and axillary node dissection is recommended.

Although advances in the treatment of non-IBC have gradually focused more on breast-conserving operation with sentinel node biopsy, more extensive surgery in the form of mastectomy with axillary node dissection is still the optimal method of surgery in patients with IBC.[42] Skin-sparing approaches, including placement of a tissue expander, are discouraged to avoid leaving disease behind. Immediate reconstruction further compromises radiation planning. Contralateral mastectomy should be delayed until reconstruction if desired so as not to incur side effects from an elective surgery that reduces the timeliness of the oncologic care for the IBC.

Radiation Therapy

Consistent with current NCCN guidelines for breast cancer,[26] the authors' institutional approach to the management of IBC includes radiation therapy, after chemotherapy, and surgery as a major and necessary treatment modalities. Preoperative radiation therapy for IBC has previously been shown to have high complication rates, and the benefit to the patient who is not a surgical candidate is debatable. However, radiation techniques have progressed substantially since these reports, and this may be considered when surgery is not feasible or for local control without surgery.

Postmastectomy radiation, including the chest wall, undissected high axilla (level III), supraclavicular, and internal mammary lymph nodes, is the standard of care.[43] Medical photography at diagnosis can ensure all affected skin areas are covered with radiation. It is important to treat the field with large radiation coverage in patients with IBC, given involvement of skin and dermal lymphatic system at presentation. Radiation therapy for IBC often involves crossing midline to provide adequate margin on the medial scar.

Contralateral nodal basins should always be imaged before beginning systemic therapy, and consideration should be given to bilateral therapy in selected cases whereby metastases are limited to the contralateral regional nodes or breast. In addition, postoperative changes to blood flow and lymphatic drainage can allow progression to the contralateral breast, lymph node areas, or the skin of the upper abdomen. Anecdotally, many treatment failures are seen at the most medial aspect of the surgical scar or within the contralateral skin and lymph nodes. Inadequate coverage of this area can promote progression and recurrence in these areas.[44,45]

Dose escalation in IBC is critical to prevent local recurrence, more so than non-IBC patients.[45] Twice-daily treatment, as well as radiosensitizer combination with radiation, may help to lower the local failure rate in young patients and women with inadequate response to therapy.[46] Boost targets are dependent on sites of initially involved gross disease. If there is no N3 nodal disease at presentation, only the chest wall flaps are included in the boost field to cover the entire mastectomy surgical bed. If any N3 nodes were involved at presentation, that nodal bed is included in the boost field.

Importance of a Multidisciplinary Team Approach

Although trimodality therapy is critical in the treatment of IBC, the adaptation of multimodality therapy ranged from 58.4% to 73.4% annually in IBC patients who were diagnosed between 1998 and 2010 who had local resection. For this study, patients without all 3 modality treatments were associated with a lower 5- and 10-year OS.[47] Based on the analysis of 107 patients with stage III IBC, only 25.8% received treatment concordant with NCCN guidelines.[48]

From the same analysis, IBC patients receiving guideline-based treatment survived longer with a statistically significant difference. The same trends were observed between 2003 guidelines and 2013 guidelines.

Among 10,197 patients with nonmetastatic IBC from 1998 to 2010 analyzed by SEER data, the rate of utilization of full trimodality fluctuated between 58.4% and 73.4%. Patients who had trimodality showed the best overall survival (including reported 5 and 10 years survivals), compared to patients who had only one or two modalities of therapy.[47] Therefore, the authors at the MD Anderson IBC Clinic make every effort for a newly diagnosed patient with IBC to be evaluated by the multidisciplinary team consisting of a medical oncologist, surgeon, and radiation oncologist.

The multidisciplinary team approach is critical in the care of patients with IBC (**Fig. 3**). Timely referral of patients to an expert can also be a critical matter in urgent treatment initiation of this rare disease, improved understanding of disease biology, and collaboration with IBC-specific education program and advocacy.

Management of Stage IV

Approximately one-third of patients with IBC present with metastatic disease at diagnosis (stage IV), whereas most patients ultimately develop distant relapse.[49–51] Several clinical trials tried to address the question of benefit in local therapy in patients with stage IV IBC and non-IBC, including the ECOG E2108 study, hoping to address currently available conflicting results, although this is not directly targeted to the IBC population only.[52,53] Akay and colleagues compared the OS of patients presenting with stage IV IBC (n = 218) with those presenting with stage IV non-IBC (n = 1454). Patients with IBC were associated with significantly shorter OS compared with non-IBC (2.3 vs 3.4 years; $P = .004$) (hazard ratio = 1.33; 95% confidence interval: 1.05-1.69).[54] Importantly, local therapy in stage IV IBC also has shown benefit. When local therapy was combined, the outcome was the best: based on review of a total of 172 cases of metastatic IBC, with all patients undergoing chemotherapy, but with or without local therapy, with stratification of response to chemotherapy. Both 5-year OS and distant progression-free survival (DPFS) and local control evaluation showed that among 172 patients total, 79 patients (46%) were able to undergo surgery. Both OS (47% vs 30% with P<.0001) and DPFS were better (10% vs 3% with P<.0001) with patients who underwent surgery. Addition of radiation therapy to the surgery improved this OS and DPFS (OS rate: 50% vs 25% vs 14%, respectively; DPFS rate: 32% vs 18% vs 15%, both P<.0001). Interestingly, this survival advantage remained even after stratification with response to chemotherapy, and the benefit of surgery plus radiation therapy remained after multivariate analysis. Intact local control at the last follow-up in patients who underwent surgery and radiation was 4-fold higher compared with patients who only had chemotherapy (81% vs 18%; P<.0001), independent of chemotherapy itself. Given significant morbidity related to the skin involvement of IBC, this higher rate of local control also offered clinical benefit.[38] Based on this significant difference, patients with stage IV IBC are strongly encouraged to consult for whether undergoing aggressive local therapy is appropriate. However, one should note that although this large case analysis study showed benefit of local therapy in patients who had poor response to chemotherapy, the possibility of a "window of opportunity" to have salvage local control surgery is not always possible. When cancer is refractory to chemotherapy, patients quickly recur (median recurrence within 5 months) with all patients further developing metastasis or death.[55] Moreover, a tailored trial to validate this in prospective manner is warranted, to facilitate the compliance of this approach in a broader community setting practice.

CLINICAL TRIALS FOR PATIENTS WITH INFLAMMATORY BREAST CANCER

Since 2009, more than 50 publications specifically aimed to determine the biology of IBC have been published with active studies ongoing. The major knowledge gap is that the following have yet to be found: (1) IBC-specific treatment or (2) IBC-specific diagnosis tool. Clinical trials that are specific to IBC are critical to improving patient treatment and outcome. Clinical trials for localized IBC need to use innovative strategies to develop a novel combination to induce higher pCR. Identifying new molecular targets and investigating the impact of novel agents and treatment approaches in IBC are critical. At the national level, patients with IBC are encouraged to enroll in clinical trials, including phase 1 trials when possible. More effort needs to be channeled toward adherence to diagnosis and treatment guidelines at the community level by reaching out and engaging with community oncologists and researchers (see **Table 1**).

SUMMARY AND FUTURE DIRECTION

IBC is a rare but deadly disease. Timely and accurate diagnosis based on a high index of suspicion, followed by guideline-based trimodality treatment, including chemotherapy-based neoadjuvant approach to induce best response and aggressive local therapy, is a basic requirement. A team approach, using team science to understand both the tumor and the microenvironment that are distinct in IBC, a team of clinicians to improve rapid initial management necessary referral of patients, a team of advocates, and an educational team are crucial to enhance community-based understanding of IBC. Last, a team approach is required to improve the standard of care for diagnosis and treatment based on the most updated understanding of IBC. These strategies are keys to a better understanding of the biological mechanisms that promote the aggressiveness of this disease and subsequently reduce the mortality of patients with IBC.

REFERENCES

1. Chang S, Parker SL, Pham T, et al. Inflammatory breast carcinoma incidence and survival: the surveillance, epidemiology, and end results program of the National Cancer Institute, 1975-1992. Cancer 1998;82(12):2366–72.
2. Hance KW, Anderson WF, Devesa SS, et al. Trends in inflammatory breast carcinoma incidence and survival: the surveillance, epidemiology, and end results program at the National Cancer Institute. J Natl Cancer Inst 2005;97(13):966–75.
3. Ellis DL, Teitelbaum SL. Inflammatory carcinoma of the breast. A pathologic definition. Cancer 1974;33(4):1045–7.
4. Goldner B, Behrendt CE, Schoellhammer HF, et al. Incidence of inflammatory breast cancer in women, 1992-2009, United States. Ann Surg Oncol 2014; 21(4):1267–70.
5. El-Shinawi M, Mohamed HT, Abdel-Fattah HH, et al. Inflammatory and non-inflammatory breast cancer: a potential role for detection of multiple viral DNAs in disease progression. Ann Surg Oncol 2016;23(2):494–502.
6. Levine PH, Hashmi S, Minaei AA, et al. Inflammatory breast cancer clusters: a hypothesis. World J Clin Oncol 2014;5(3):539–45.
7. Bonnier P, Charpin C, Lejeune C, et al. Inflammatory carcinomas of the breast: a clinical, pathological, or a clinical and pathological definition? Int J Cancer 1995; 62(4):382–5.
8. Manfrin E, Remo A, Pancione M, et al. Comparison between invasive breast cancer with extensive peritumoral vascular invasion and inflammatory breast carcinoma: a clinicopathologic study of 161 cases. Am J Clin Pathol 2014;142(3): 299–306.
9. Charpin C, Bonnier P, Khouzami A, et al. Inflammatory breast carcinoma: an immunohistochemical study using monoclonal anti-pHER-2/neu, pS2, cathepsin, ER and PR. Anticancer Res 1992;12(3):591–7.
10. Li J, Gonzalez-Angulo AM, Allen PK, et al. Triple-negative subtype predicts poor overall survival and high locoregional relapse in inflammatory breast cancer. Oncologist 2011;16(12):1675–83.
11. Masuda H, Brewer TM, Liu DD, et al. Long-term treatment efficacy in primary inflammatory breast cancer by hormonal receptor- and HER2-defined subtypes. Ann Oncol 2014;25(2):384–91.
12. Raghav K, French JT, Ueno NT, et al. Inflammatory breast cancer: a distinct clinicopathological entity transcending histological distinction. PLoS One 2016;11(1): e0145534.
13. Dawood S, Merajver SD, Viens P, et al. International expert panel on inflammatory breast cancer: consensus statement for standardized diagnosis and treatment. Ann Oncol 2011;22(3):515–23.
14. Edge S, Byrd D, Compton C. AJCC cancer staging handbook. 7th edition. New York: American Joint Committee on Cancer, Springer; 2010.
15. Martinez-Trufero J, de Lobera AR, Lao J, et al. Serum markers and prognosis in locally advanced breast cancer. Tumori 2005;91(6):522–30.
16. Yamauchi H, Woodward WA, Valero V, et al. Inflammatory breast cancer: what we know and what we need to learn. Oncologist 2012;17(7):891–9.
17. Le-Petross HT, Cristofanilli M, Carkaci S, et al. MRI features of inflammatory breast cancer. AJR Am J Roentgenol 2011;197(4):W769–76.
18. Abeywardhana DY, Nascimento VC, Dissanayake D, et al. Review of ultrasound appearance in inflammatory breast cancer: a pictorial essay. J Med Imaging Radiat Oncol 2016;60(1):83–7.

19. Gunhan-Bilgen I, Ustun EE, Memis A. Inflammatory breast carcinoma: mammographic, ultrasonographic, clinical, and pathologic findings in 142 cases. Radiology 2002;223(3):829–38.

20. O'Connor MK. Molecular breast imaging: an emerging modality for breast cancer screening. Breast Cancer Manag 2015;4(1):33–40.

21. Niikura N, Odisio BC, Tokuda Y, et al. Latest biopsy approach for suspected metastases in patients with breast cancer. Nat Rev Clin Oncol 2013;10(12):711–9.

22. Champion L, Lerebours F, Cherel P, et al. (1)(8)F-FDG PET/CT imaging versus dynamic contrast-enhanced CT for staging and prognosis of inflammatory breast cancer. Eur J Nucl Med Mol Imaging 2013;40(8):1206–13.

23. Champion L, Lerebours F, Alberini JL, et al. 18F-FDG PET/CT to predict response to neoadjuvant chemotherapy and prognosis in inflammatory breast cancer. J Nucl Med 2015;56(9):1315–21.

24. Woodward WA, Koav E, Tajkar V. Radiation therapy for inflammatory breast cancer: technical considerations and diverse clinical scenarios. Breast Cancer Mmanagement 2013. [Epub ahead of print].

25. Carkaci S, Sherman CT, Ozkan E, et al. (18)F-FDG PET/CT predicts survival in patients with inflammatory breast cancer undergoing neoadjuvant chemotherapy. Eur J Nucl Med Mol Imaging 2013;40(12):1809–16.

26. Bozzetti F, Saccozzi R, De Lena M, et al. Inflammatory cancer of the breast: analysis of 114 cases. J Surg Oncol 1981;18(4):355–61.

27. Haagensen CD, Stout AP. Carcinoma of the breast. III. Results of treatment, 1935-1942. Ann Surg 1951;134(2):151–72.

28. Krutchik AN, Buzdar AU, Blumenschein GR, et al. Combined chemoimmunotherapy and radiation therapy of inflammatory breast carcinoma. J Surg Oncol 1979; 11(4):325–32.

29. Pisansky TM, Schaid DJ, Loprinzi CL, et al. Inflammatory breast cancer: integration of irradiation, surgery, and chemotherapy. Am J Clin Oncol 1992;15(5): 376–87.

30. Ueno NT, Buzdar AU, Singletary SE, et al. Combined-modality treatment of inflammatory breast carcinoma: twenty years of experience at M. D. Anderson Cancer Center. Cancer Chemother Pharmacol 1997;40(4):321–9.

31. Buzdar AU, Singletary SE, Booser DJ, et al. Combined modality treatment of stage III and inflammatory breast cancer. M.D. Anderson Cancer Center experience. Surg Oncol Clin N Am 1995;4(4):715–34.

32. Dawood S, Ueno NT, Cristofanilli M. The medical treatment of inflammatory breast cancer. Semin Oncol 2008;35(1):64–71.

33. Baldini E, Gardin G, Evagelista G, et al. Long-term results of combined-modality therapy for inflammatory breast carcinoma. Clin Breast Cancer 2004;5(5):358–63.

34. Cristofanilli M, Buzdar AU, Sneige N, et al. Paclitaxel in the multimodality treatment for inflammatory breast carcinoma. Cancer 2001;92(7):1775–82.

35. Cristofanilli M, Singletary ES, Hortobagyi GN. Inflammatory breast carcinoma: the sphinx of breast cancer research. J Clin Oncol 2004;22(2):381–3 [author reply 383].

36. Walshe JM, Swain SM. Clinical aspects of inflammatory breast cancer. Breast Dis 2005;22:35–44.

37. Hennessy BT, Gonzalez-Angulo AM, Hortobagyi GN, et al. Disease-free and overall survival after pathologic complete disease remission of cytologically proven inflammatory breast carcinoma axillary lymph node metastases after primary systemic chemotherapy. Cancer 2006;106(5):1000–6.

38. Fouad TM, Kogawa T, Liu DD, et al. Overall survival differences between patients with inflammatory and noninflammatory breast cancer presenting with distant metastasis at diagnosis. Breast Cancer Res Treat 2015;152(2):407–16.

39. Anderson WF, Chu KC, Chang S. Inflammatory breast carcinoma and noninflammatory locally advanced breast carcinoma: distinct clinicopathologic entities? J Clin Oncol 2003;21(12):2254–9.

40. Kell MR, Morrow M. Surgical aspects of inflammatory breast cancer. Breast Dis 2005;22:67–73.

41. Stearns V, Ewing CA, Slack R, et al. Sentinel lymphadenectomy after neoadjuvant chemotherapy for breast cancer may reliably represent the axilla except for inflammatory breast cancer. Ann Surg Oncol 2002;9(3):235–42.

42. Fleming RY, Asmar L, Buzdar AU, et al. Effectiveness of mastectomy by response to induction chemotherapy for control in inflammatory breast carcinoma. Ann Surg Oncol 1997;4(6):452–61.

43. Walker GV, Niikura N, Yang W, et al. Pretreatment staging positron emission tomography/computed tomography in patients with inflammatory breast cancer influences radiation treatment field designs. Int J Radiat Oncol Biol Phys 2012; 83(5):1381–6.

44. Takiar V, Akay CL, Stauder MC, et al. Predictors of durable no evidence of disease status in de novo metastatic inflammatory breast cancer patients treated with neoadjuvant chemotherapy and post-mastectomy radiation. Springerplus 2014;3:166.

45. Woodward WA. Postmastectomy radiation therapy for inflammatory breast cancer: is more better? Int J Radiat Oncol Biol Phys 2014;89(5):1004–5.

46. Bristol IJ, Woodward WA, Storm EA, et al. Locoregional treatment outcomes after multimodality management of inflammatory breast cancer. Int J Radiat Oncol Biol Phys 2008;72(2):474–84.

47. Rueth NM, Lin HY, Bedrosian I, et al. Underuse of trimodality treatment affects survival for patients with inflammatory breast cancer: an analysis of treatment and survival trends from the National Cancer Database. J Clin Oncol 2014; 32(19):2018–24.

48. Denu RA, Hampton JM, Currey A, et al. Influence of patient, physician, and hospital characteristics on the receipt of guideline-concordant care for inflammatory breast cancer. Cancer Epidemiol 2015;40:7–14.

49. Wingo PA, Jamison PM, Young JL, et al. Population-based statistics for women diagnosed with inflammatory breast cancer (United States). Cancer Causes Control 2004;15(3):321–8.

50. Elias EG, Vachon DA, Didolkar MS, et al. Long-term results of a combined modality approach in treating inflammatory carcinoma of the breast. Am J Surg 1991; 162(3):231–5.

51. Curcio LD, Rupp E, Williams WL, et al. Beyond palliative mastectomy in inflammatory breast cancer–a reassessment of margin status. Ann Surg Oncol 1999;6(3): 249–54.

52. Badwe R, Hawaldar R, Nair N, et al. Locoregional treatment versus no treatment of the primary tumour in metastatic breast cancer: an open-label randomised controlled trial. Lancet Oncol 2015;16(13):1380–8.

53. Harris E, Barry M, Kell MR. Meta-analysis to determine if surgical resection of the primary tumour in the setting of stage IV breast cancer impacts on survival. Ann Surg Oncol 2013;20(9):2828–34.

54. Akay CL, Ueno NT, Chisholm GB, et al. Primary tumor resection as a component of multimodality treatment may improve local control and survival in patients with stage IV inflammatory breast cancer. Cancer 2014;120(9):1319–28.

55. Belliere-Calandry A, Benoit C, Dubois S, et al. Salvage concomitant chemoradiation therapy for non-metastatic inflammatory breast cancer after chemotherapy failure. Cancer Radiother 2015;19(8):739–45 [in French].

The Evolving Role of Postmastectomy Radiation Therapy

Check for updates

Ashlyn S. Everett, MD[a], Jennifer F. De Los Santos, MD[b],
Drexell Hunter Boggs, MD[a],*

KEYWORDS

- Postmastectomy • Radiation • Regional nodes • Chest wall
- Neoadjuvant chemotherapy

KEY POINTS

- Recommendations for radiation therapy for breast cancer in the postmastectomy setting are evolving as surgical modalities and systemic therapies improve.
- In appropriately selected patients, postmastectomy radiation therapy shows improved locoregional control, disease-free survival, and overall survival.
- Although some clinical situations mandate radiation therapy, indications for radiation therapy for intermediate-risk patients remain controversial and require further clinical study.

INTRODUCTION
Background

In 2017, breast cancer remained the most diagnosed malignancy in women and the second most common cause of cancer death.[1] Appreciation of the molecular and genetic characteristics of breast tumors and their impact on tumor behavior has radically changed the treatment of breast cancer. As new therapies emerge, breast cancer outcomes are steadily improving, with 5-year relative survival improving from 60% to 92.2% in the past 50 years and death rates falling on average 1.8% annually since 2005 (**Fig. 1**).[2] These gains in breast cancer survival are largely attributed to improved chemotherapeutic agents, including cytotoxic agents in the anthracycline and taxane families, targeted agents like trastuzumab, and immunotherapies including pembrolizumab. Adequate locoregional control (LRC) with surgery and radiation therapy,

The authors have nothing to disclose.
[a] Department of Radiation Oncology, University of Alabama at Birmingham, Hazelrig Salter Radiation Oncology Center, 1700 6th Avenue South, Birmingham, AL 35233, USA; [b] Department of Radiation Oncology, University of Alabama at Birmingham, The Kirklin Clinic at Acton Road, 2145 Bonner Way, Birmingham, AL 35243, USA
* Corresponding author.
E-mail address: dboggs@uabmc.edu

Surg Clin N Am 98 (2018) 801–817
https://doi.org/10.1016/j.suc.2018.03.010
0039-6109/18/© 2018 Elsevier Inc. All rights reserved.

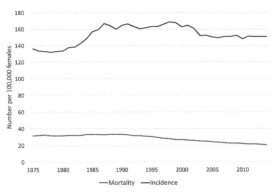

Fig. 1. Female breast cancer incidence and mortality trends, 1975 to 2014. (*Adapted from* Howlader N, NA, Krapcho M, et al. SEER cancer statistics review, 1975-2014. Secondary SEER cancer statistics review, 1975-2014 posted to the SEER web site, April 2017. 2017; with permission.)

however, continues to play an important role in managing breast cancer; therefore, practicing surgeons should have an appreciation for the role of postmastectomy radiation therapy (PMRT).

Radiation therapy is known to reduce locoregional failures in breast cancer by a factor of two-thirds by targeting tissues potentially harboring microscopic disease, or regions not addressed by surgery.[3] Randomized trials continue to show PMRT improves LRC and disease-free survival (DFS) and overall survival (OS) benefit in selected patients.[4–10] Current indications for PMRT include primary tumor greater than 5 cm, skin or chest wall invasion, and lymph node metastasis, although there are certain subgroups of patients where PMRT remains controversial.[11] Understanding the historical significance of PMRT and its evolution over the past 30 years will assist clinicians with determining its current and future role in the management of locally advanced breast cancers. This article reviews 3 designated historic eras of breast cancer therapy (**Fig. 2**), summarizes the retrospective, prospective, and randomized data supporting PMRT during each time period and discusses clinical questions under investigation that will shape the future of breast cancer treatment.

Pretaxane era: prior to 1998
Early randomized trials: National Surgical Adjuvant Breast and Bowel Project B-02 and National Surgical Adjuvant Breast and Bowel Project B-04 The earliest randomized

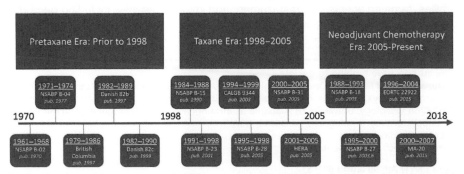

Fig. 2. Timeline of breast cancer therapy eras and relevant clinical trials, as discussed in this article.

trials investigating PMRT demonstrated LRC benefit but failed to show improved OS.[12,13] After organization of the National Surgical Adjuvant Breast and Bowel Project (NSABP), breast cancer research in large, multi-institutional trials began. In NSABP B-02, Fisher and colleagues[13] randomized patients to Halstead radical mastectomy (RM) alone or to surgery followed by radiation (**Table 1**). PMRT was delivered to 35 Gy to 45 Gy to the regional lymphatics (the axillary apex, supraclavicular fossa, and the internal mammary chain), with omission of the chest wall and the dissected axilla. Results showed patients in the radiation arm had improved LRC but higher distant failures, likely due to inadequate systemic therapy, and no improved survival. During this era, clinicians began to appreciate breast cancer deaths were often due to distant disease, suggesting a systemic disease process that was not adequately controlled by locoregional therapies alone.

The NSABP B-04 trial randomized clinically lymph node-negative patients to RM (including axillary dissection) versus total mastectomy (TM) with or without radiation therapy; women with clinically node-positive disease were randomized to RM with or without PMRT (see **Table 1**). Radiation was delivered to the chest wall (50 Gy in 25 fractions) and internal mammary and supraclavicular nodes (45 Gy in 25 fractions), and an additional boost was given to the midaxilla in the setting of node-positive disease. For node-negative patients, locoregional failure was statistically higher in the TM arm compared with the RM or TM plus PMRT groups. Despite this higher rate of locoregional failure, DFS and OS were unchanged for patients who had RM versus less extensive surgery due to high distant failure rates.[14] In node-positive patients, the addition of RT after RM did not seem to improve LRC, OS, or DFS. This is not surprising given the 41% to 43% risk of distant disease failure that largely dictated prognosis.

Table 1
Results of the National Surgical Adjuvant Breast and Bowel Project B-02 and National Surgical Adjuvant Breast and Bowel Project B-04 trials

Trial (n = Patients)	Treatment Arms	LF (%) (P-Value)	RF (%) (P-Value)	Disease-Free Survival (%) (P Value)	Overall Survival (%) (P Value)	Conclusion
NSABP B-02 (n = 1163)	HM + RT	7.8	0.6	50.6	56	PMRT improved
	HM + TSPA	5.9	8.5	50.2	62	RF, with more
	HM + Placebo	15.4	3.4	50.2	62	DF; no DFS or
		NS	SS	NS	NS	OS benefit
NSABP B-04 (n = 1765)	N0:					PMRT improves
	TM + RT	1	4	13	19	LF, RF for N0;
	TM	7	6	19	25	no benefit
	RM	5	4	19	25	in N+
		(P = .002)	(P = .002)	(P = .65)	(P = .68)	
	N+:					
	RM	8	8	11	14	
	TM + RT	3	3	10	14	
		(P = .67)	(P = .67)	(P = .20)	(P = .49)	

Abbreviations: HM, Halsted mastectomy; LF, local failure; NS, not significant; RF, regional failure; RT, radiation therapy; SS, statistically significant; TSPA, thiotepa.

Adapted from Fisher B, Slack NH, Cavanaugh PJ, et al. Postoperative radiotherapy in the treatment of breast cancer: results of the NSABP clinical trial. Ann Surg 1970;172(4):716; and Fisher B, Jeong JH, Anderson S, et al. Twenty-five-year follow-up of a randomized trial comparing radical mastectomy, total mastectomy, and total mastectomy followed by irradiation. N Engl J Med 2002;347(8):570; with permission.

In these early studies, the benefit of PMRT was largely negated due to lack of adequate systemic therapy controlling metastatic disease, as shown by the high rates of distant failures. In addition, these older studies investigating PMRT used antiquated (now obsolete) radiation field design and technologies that increased the toxicity of treatment and likely offset treatment benefit given the equivalent or worse survival.[3,15] Thus, radiation was largely abandoned with data showing PMRT did not improve survival and with valid concerns regarding increased risks of treatment-related complications.

More contemporary randomized trials: Danish and British Columbia trials The Danish Breast Cancer Cooperative Trials 82b and 82c were the first large clinical trials incorporating adjuvant systemic therapy and PMRT. The Danish 82b trial enrolled 1708 premenopausal patients with high-risk features after TM with partial axillary node dissection and then randomized patients to cyclophosphamide, methotrexate, and 5-fluorouracil (CMF) chemotherapy with or without radiation.[5] The Danish 82c trial included 1375 high risk postmenopausal women randomized to tamoxifen alone or tamoxifen with PMRT after TM with partial axillary node dissection.[6] High-risk features on both trials included any number of positive axillary lymph nodes, tumor size greater than 5 cm, and/or invasion of the skin or pectoral fascia. PMRT in both trials was delivered to a total dose of 48 Gy in 22 fractions or 50 Gy in 25 fractions, targeting the chest wall and ipsilateral regional lymphatics (including the supra/infraclavicular, axillary, and internal mammary nodes between the first 4 intercostal spaces). At 10 years of follow-up, these trials demonstrated statistically improved locoregional failure (LRF), DFS, and OS in the radiation arms **(Table 2)**.[4–6] The benefit of radiation was seen across all groups, including patients with 1 to 3 positive lymph nodes.[16]

Critics of these trials question their relevance to modern-era therapy, given their use of first-generation chemotherapy with CMF, and potentially suboptimal axillary dissection, with a median of only 7 axillary nodes removed. In addition, tamoxifen was given for only 1 year, which was later proved inferior to 5 years and subsequently 10 years of adjuvant treatment.[17,18] Despite these criticisms, the Danish trials established PMRT as standard of care for high-risk breast cancers, defined as patients with tumors over 5 cm, positive axillary lymph nodes, invasion of the skin, or invasion of the chest wall. These findings were also confirmed by a smaller randomized trial from British Columbia (see **Table 2**).[7]

Table 2
Results of 3 randomized trials of postmastectomy radiation therapy

Trial (n = Patients)	Treatment Arms	LRF (%) (P Value)	Disease-Free Survival (%) (P Value)	Overall Survival (%) (P Value)	Conclusion
Danish 82b (n = 1708)	CMF vs CMF + PMRT	32 9	34 48 (P<.001)	45 54 (P<.001)	PMRT improved all outcomes
Danish 82c (n = 1375)	TAM vs TAM + PMRT	35 8 (P<.001)	24 36 (P<.001)	36 45 (P = .03)	PMRT improves all outcomes
British Columbia (n = 318)	CMF vs CMF + PMRT	28 10 (P<.001)	30 48 (P = .001)	37 47 (P = .03)	PMRT improves all outcomes

Abbreviations: CMF, cyclophosophaminde, methotrexate, fluorouracil; LRF, locoregional failure; TAM, tamoxifen.
Data from Refs.[4–7]

The Early Breast Cancer Trialists Collaborative Group (EBCTCG) published an updated meta-analysis, including 8135 patients from 22 randomized trials to further define the role of PMRT.[19] Women evaluated were those enrolled on eligible randomized trials between 1964 and 1986, who received mastectomy and axillary surgery, and were randomized to radiation therapy to the chest wall and regional lymph nodes or observation. Most patients (72%) had pathologically node-positive (pN+) disease, and 90% to 95% of women received some form of systemic therapy. Results showed patients received LRC and OS benefit with PMRT regardless of the extent of axillary surgery. Accounting for adjuvant chemotherapy and tamoxifen use, PMRT decreased recurrences and improved breast cancer survival, likely driven by the node-positive patients. In the pathologically node-negative (pN0) women, the risk of LRF after axillary dissection (44%) was merely 1.4% and not improved by radiation; in fact, mortality increased with PMRT in this cohort. In contrast, women with pN0 disease who underwent axillary sampling alone (55%) had LRF of 16.3%, which improved to 3.3% with PMRT without impacting survival. Given the limitations of this meta-analysis (outdated chemotherapy, antiquated radiation techniques, and lower detection of early stage breast cancers), the EBCTCG concluded the absolute benefit may be smaller but the proportional benefit of PMRT may be increased with modern chemotherapy and improved radiation technologies. The role of PMRT for a subset of intermediate-rusk to high-risk patients (T1-2 primary tumors and 1–3 positive lymph nodes) remained controversial.

Key points for treatment in the pretaxane era: before 1998

- TM replaced RM

- Radiation therapy improved LRC and OS in the absence of adequate systemic therapy

- PMRT indicated for
  ○ Tumors greater than 5 cm
  ○ Skin or chest wall invasion
  ○ Positive lymph nodes

- PMRT NOT indicated for
  ○ Node-negative disease with primary tumor less than 5 cm

Taxane era: 1998 to 2005
First-generation systemic therapies Prior to the 1990s, systemic therapies for treatment of breast cancer included alkylating agents and antimetabolite agents, commonly a regimen of cyclophosphamide, methotrexate, and 5-fluorocil (CMF) that improved OS and DFS compared with no chemotherapy.[20] Tamoxifen was approved by the Food and Drug Administration for use in the metastatic setting in 1977 and incorporated into clinical trials as adjuvant therapy in the 1980s. Tamoxifen quickly became standard of care, with early trials showing improved outcomes.[14] A worldwide meta-analysis performed by the EBCTCG evaluated women treated with tamoxifen and/or chemotherapy across 194 randomized trials confirmed a survival benefit at 15 years with use of tamoxifen and chemotherapy in early-stage breast cancer, with or without positive lymph nodes.[10]

Anthracyclines Doxorubicin was introduced as a chemotherapeutic agent for breast cancer and incorporated into the NSABP B-15 and B-23 trials, which compared 4 cycles of doxorubicin and cyclophosphamide (AC) with 6 cycles of CMF and found no DFS or OS improvement (**Table 3**).[21,22] Because the AC regimen duration (12 weeks) was many weeks shorter than the CMF regimen (24 weeks), AC was frequently incorporated into clinical use. Unfortunately, the anthracycline regimen was also found to

Table 3
Results of randomized clinical trials investigating chemotherapeutic regimens

Trial (NO or N+) (n = Pts)	Treatment Arms	LRC (%) (P value)	Disease-Free Survival (%) (P value)	Overall Survival (%) (P value)	Conclusion
Milan (N+) (n = 386)	CMF vs No chemo	14 15	29 22	25 16	28 y f/u. DFS and OS improved with CMF
B-15 (pN+) (n = 2194)	AC × 4 vs CMF × 6	NR	62 62 (P = .5)	(P = .8)	3 y f/u. No difference in outcomes; duration tx shorter with AC
B-23 (ER- and pN0) (n = 2008)	AC × 4 vs AC × 4 + TAM vs CMF × 6 vs CMF × 6 + TAM	NR	87 87 88 87 (P = .96)	90 90 89 89 (P = .8)	No difference in outcomes; AC is preferred with shorter duration tx, TAM not effective in ER-tumors
C9344 (pN+) (n = 3121)	AC × 4 vs AC × 4 + T × 4	NR	65 70 (P = .001)	77 80 (P = .006)	T improved DFS and OS. No benefit with dose-escalating doxorubicin
B-28 (pN+) (n = 3060)	AC × 4 vs AC × 4 + T × 4	7.6 6.5 (P = .056)	72 76 (P = .006)	85 85 (P = .46)	5 y f/u. T improved DFS but not OS. Toxicity acceptable
HERA (HER2+) (n = 5099)	1 y H vs 2 y H vs Observation	1.6 3.0	69 69 63 (P<.001)	79 80 73 (P<.001)	11 y f/u. 25% relative increase in DFS and OS. No benefit for a 2nd y of traztuzumab
B-31 (HER2+) (n = 2101)	AC × 4 + T × 4 or 12 vs AC × 4 + T × 4 or 12 + H	NR	73.7 85.7 (P<.001)	85.6 93.0 (P<.001)	2 y f/u. 50% relative reduction in DFS, 40% relative reduction in OS

Abbreviations: H, trastuzumab; N+, node positive; N0, node negative; NR, not reported; TAM, tamoxifen.
Data from Refs.[21–29]

cause congestive heart failure, requiring a lifetime dose restriction to minimize the risks of cardiac toxicity from 20% to 4%.[23]

Taxanes In 1971, a natural compound, paclitaxel (T), was discovered to have antitumor activity, but it was difficult to administer secondary to its physical properties. Eventually, a soluble form of the drug allowed for its widespread clinical use. After approval for metastatic disease in 1994, taxanes were investigated in the adjuvant setting on several randomized trials. The Intergroup/CALGB 9344 trial enrolled 3121 patients with node-positive disease and investigated the benefit of adding 4 cycles of T to the standard 4 cycles of AC. The addition of T significantly improved OS and DFS (see **Table 3**).[24] The NSABP B-28 clinical trial similarly investigated the role of 4 cycles of T after 4 cycles of AC, and demonstrated improvement in DFS without improvement in OS.[25] Based on the results of these clinical trials, T was approved for adjuvant use in breast cancer in 1998.

HER2/neu-targeted therapies Among the breast cancer phenotypes, HER2/neu amplified breast tumors historically had poor outcomes relative to estrogen positive tumors, until the development of trastuzumab. In 2005, publication of 2 clinical trials demonstrated significant improvement of recurrences, DFS and OS with the addition of trastuzumab to standard adjuvant chemotherapy (see **Table 3**).[26–29] A second HER2-targeted agent, pertuzumab, was later shown to DFS in high-risk pN0 or any node-positive HER2-amplified breast cancer.[30] Ongoing trials are evaluating new HER2-targeted therapies, but these drugs are not recommended for routine use at this time.

A meta-analysis by the EBCTCG evaluated various chemotherapy regimens and demonstrated that taxane-plus-anthracycline based chemotherapy reduced breast cancer mortality by one-third, with a parallel decrease in overall mortality.[31] These benefits were seen independent of age, lymph node status, tumor size, tumor grade, ER status, or tamoxifen use. Current trials are evaluating specific tumor markers or genomic profiles that may direct individualized treatment recommendations, selecting those patients with greatest benefit from chemotherapy and/or radiotherapy.

Key points for treatment in the taxane era: 1998 to 2005

- Anthracycline and taxane-based chemotherapy reduced breast cancer mortality by one-third

- Traztuzumab improved outcomes for HER2+ disease

- PMRT generally used for
  - Tumors greater than 5 cm
  - Skin or chest wall invasion
  - Four or more positive lymph nodes

- PMRT NOT indicated for
  - Node negative disease with primary less than 5 cm
  - 1 to 3 positive lymph nodes (later disputed)

Neoadjuvant chemotherapy era: 2005 to 2017

Rationale for neoadjuvant chemotherapy Despite improved systemic therapies, patients with locally advanced disease have higher rates of recurrence. A new treatment paradigm hoped to improve outcomes: chemotherapy given prior to surgery, or neoadjuvant chemotherapy (NCT). In 2 separate randomized trials (NSABP B-17 and NSABP B-23), however, this approach did not improve survival.[32,33] NCT does have several advantages, including allowing clinicians to initiate systemic therapy without delay; treating micrometastatic disease early; monitor in vivo tumor response to treatment; downstage tumors to prevent morbid surgery; and determine valuable prognostic information. In patients younger than age 50, NCT may have survival benefit and patients should be referred to medical oncology to discuss the risks and benefits of this approach, or have consultation with a multidisciplinary team.

Postmastectomy radiation therapy in the era of neoadjuvant chemotherapy In some patients, NCT have pathologic complete responses (pCRs), so clinicians again began considering the role of PMRT. The randomized data showing the benefit of PMRT incorporated adjuvant systemic therapy, thus leaving some doubt regarding its use after NCT. Some physicians argue recommendations for PMRT should consider response to NCT, given available retrospective data. Pooled analysis of 1947 mastectomy patients on the NSABP B-18 and B-27 trials (both prohibited PMRT) reported an overall 12.6% locoregional recurrence rate (LRR). Tumors greater than 5 cm, clinically node positive (cN+) disease, and ypN+ disease after mastectomy were predictors of recurrence.[34] This study also reported LRR above 10% for patients with 1 to 3 lymph nodes involved, which increased with the number of residual positive nodes. Although these data are not randomized, it offers some insight into recurrence risk, without having more robust trial results available.

Similarly, a single institution retrospective series of 542 patients with nonmetastatic, noninflammatory breast disease treated with doxorubicin-based NCT, mastectomy, and axillary lymph node dissection (ALND) demonstrated reduced recurrence rates with PMRT despite more advanced disease in the control group. Radiation also improved survival in specific cohorts: cT3 tumors, greater than stage III disease, and 4 or more involved nodes.[35] Another study from the same institution demonstrated a recurrence and survival benefit to PMRT in the setting of a pCR in stage III patients (33% vs 3% LRR).[35,36]

A recent NCDB analysis of patients with cN+ disease treated with NCT and surgery found an OS benefit to PMRT with ypN0 and ypN+ disease.[37] Some oncologists suggest that patients with ypN0 and no residual primary tumor are low risk and do not warrant PMRT. Patients with ypN0 and residual breast disease after NCT and mastectomy represent an intermediate-risk group of patients, and those with high risk factors, including young age, increased extent residual disease, ER-subtype, and close/positive margins, warrant consideration of PMRT.[38] Current guidelines recommend using maximal pretreatment stage to counsel patients regarding PMRT[39]; however, forthcoming data from the NSABP B-51/RTOG1304 study may show benefit to tailoring adjuvant radiation recommendations based on treatment response.[40]

Recent radiotherapy trials: radiation for 1 to 3 positive lymph nodes Prior randomized trials showed an undeniable benefit of PMRT in patients with more than 4 lymph nodes positive (LN+); however, radiating patients with 1 to 3 LN+ remained controversial. In 2015, results from the MA-20 and European Organisation for Research and Treatment of Cancer (EORTC) 22922 randomized trials helped define the role of regional nodal irradiation (RNI) for patients with 1 LN+ to 3 LN+.[8,9] The MA-20 study included only patients with lumpectomy; however, the EORTC included 24% mastectomy patients. Results from both trials demonstrated a significant benefit to RNI with improved LRC and DFS. The MA-20 trial failed to demonstrate survival benefit; however, a prespecified analysis of the ER/PR negative patients demonstrated a stronger DFS benefit than suggested by regional control in this subgroup. The EORTC trial showed improved OS and BCSS with RNI, plus DFS and BCSS benefit persisted in patients with 1 to 3 LN+, solidifying the value of PMRT even in patients with low burden nodal disease.

Recent trials also confirm the role of radiation therapy in patients with T3N0 disease. Previously, the Danish PMRT trials argued that patients with large tumors (>5 cm) would benefit from radiotherapy. Retrospective data from MD Anderson have also shown that patients with large tumors (>4 cm) and aggressive subtypes (estrogen receptor [ER]−) have higher risk of locoregional failure.[35,41] The EORTC trial included node negative patients with central or medial tumors; the MA-20 trial enrolled patients with high-risk features and node-negative disease. In both groups, the DFS and LRC benefits remained significant.

Key points to neoadjuvant chemotherapy era

- NCT does not improve survival; however, patients younger than 50 should be considered for NCT (possible survival advantage)
- PMRT recommendations should be based on maximal pretreatment staging
- The MA-20 and EORTC trials show benefit to radiation for all patients with node positive disease, especially those with high-risk features (T3; grade 3; lymphovascular space invasion [LVSI]; ER−)

The modern era: radiation targets, techniques, and toxicity

Radiation targets and techniques

Historical perspective Just as chemotherapies have advanced significantly in the past 30 years, so too have radiation techniques. Until the 1990s, radiation fields were designed using 2-D imaging and anatomic landmarks and calculated with limited computer capability. Radiation fields during this era were often large, and included more normal tissues (**Fig. 3**). Individual fields were customized using physical blocks, hand-crafted using heavy metals, which required increased labor to fabricate and exchange blocks for each field of treatment with every patient. These treatment techniques also limited physicians' ability to create conformal radiation fields that minimized dose to normal structures near the target volume, thereby increasing potential morbidity of treatment.

The CT scanner debuted in 1972, but it was many years before CT and 3-D became standard in radiation oncology. Meanwhile, improvements on linear accelerators allowed incorporation of small, mobile blocks within the machine head that were customizable to an individual patient for each radiation field, eliminating cumbersome physical blocks, and allowing the advent of intensity modulating treatments.

Radiation target PMRT targets include the chest wall, at highest risk for recurrence,[42,43] and often the regional lymphatics of the high axilla, supra/infraclavicular nodes. The lower axilla may be omitted from the target volume in patients after axillary dissection, following the practice on the EORTC and MA-20 trials, with no apparent increased risk of locoregional failure. The MA-20 and EORTC 22922 trials additionally encompassed the internal mammary node (IMN) chain in the first 3 intercostal spaces, which harbors occult disease in of 4% to 9% of node-negative patients and up to 16% to 65% of patients with involved axillary nodes.[44,45] Patients with central/medial tumors or large burden axillary disease have a higher risk of IMN involvement, so clinicians should strongly consider including these regions in the target.[44]

Modern technique A CT scan of the patient is acquired in treatment position, and from this information, the radiation oncologist delineates the target (the tumor or surgical bed) and the avoidance structures (the nearby normal structures). Virtual fields are designed using computer software, allowing the physician to encompass the target and move blocks into place to avoid critical structures. The physician then determines the dose of radiation (in Gray [Gy]), the number of treatments (fractions), and the technique most appropriate for treatment. The computer then calculates the dose, and the radiation oncologist ensures the treatment plan is safe and the objectives of tumor killing are balanced with toxicity risk.

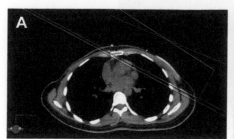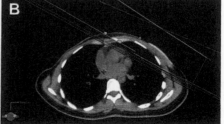

Fig. 3. Comparison of 2-D versus 3-D planning of PMRT tangent fields in a patient with bilateral mastectomy. (*A*) 2-D planning, heart (*pink*), and IMN nodes (*yellow*). (*B*) 3-D planning, heart (*pink*), note heart block (*orange translucent*) and target IMN node (*yellow*).

Current PMRT techniques utilize two tangential photon fields encompassing the involved chest wall, and a third anterior photon field treats the supra/infraclavicular nodal basins. The IMN chain, if included, is incorporated in the target volume using 1 of 2 methods: an anterior electron field, or a wider-angle tangent field (**Fig. 4**). Using CT for 3-D planning allows radiation oncologists to create custom blocks that minimize dose to the heart and lung, particularly for left breast cancers and/or when IMN radiation is indicated. The dose to the heart is further reduced by using the deep inspiratory breath hold (DIBH) technique, where patients inhale and hold their breath, effectively moving the heart posterior and medial from the chest wall. Studies evaluating the DIBH technique show heart dose reductions of 80% to 90%,[46] with relative risk of cardiac mortality reduced by 95%.[47]

Radiation toxicity Both patients and clinicians are fearful of toxicities of radiation therapy. It is important to counsel patients specifically regarding the 2 types of side effects with radiation: acute toxicity and late toxicity. In general, patients are most concerned with the acute skin changes, which are typically mild and resolve within 2 weeks to 4 weeks after completing treatment. Using modern radiation techniques, skin changes during radiation are greatly reduced compared with older studies, owing to improved equipment and dose calculations that allow consideration of modifications to reduce skin dose.

Cardiac toxicity Older studies using 2-D radiation techniques showed significant cardiac morbidity and mortality, which may have offset the survival benefits of PMRT in these studies.[3] Cardiac morbidity from radiation includes ischemic disease, congestive heart failure, cardiomyopathy, and pericarditis. Patients treated with older radiation techniques received a mean heart dose of 4.9 Gy, with an increased risk of

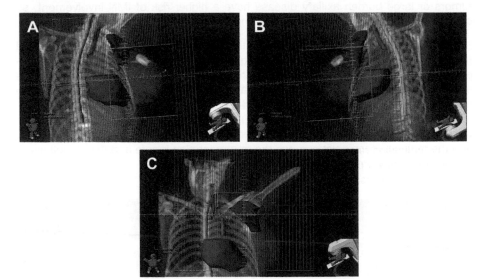

Fig. 4. Example PMRT fields of a left breast cancer, cT3N2M0, ypTisN1a, with tissue expanders in place. (*A*) Left medial partially-wide tangent field, demonstrating heart block (*blue rectangles*) and coverage of IMN chain. (*B*) Left lateral partially wide tangent field, demonstrating heart block (*blue rectangles*) and coverage of IMN chain. (*C*) Left anterior supra/infraclavicular field, demonstrating coverage of the apex of the axilla and coverage of the supra/infraclavicular lymphatics. Pink = heart; purple = axillary target volume, levels I-III; green = internal mammary (IMN) chain 1st – 3rd intercostal spaces; teal = esophagus; and blue = spinal cord.

cardiac events of 7.4% per Gy, highlighting the importance of reducing the heart dose as low as possible.[48] Recent data in patients treated from 2010 to 2015 demonstrate an increased risk of cardiac ischemia of 4.1% per Gy, or an absolute risk of 0.3% in nonsmokers. In patients who continue smoking, this risk is increased to 1%, emphasizing the importance of smoking cessation in breast cancer survivors.[49]

Analysis of more than 19,000 patients treated with radiation between 1977 to 2005 divided women into 3 groups, based on year of treatment: 1977 to 1989, 1990 to 2000, and 2001 to 2005. Women with left-sided versus right-sided breast cancer treated between 1977 and 1989 had a higher risk of heart disease; however, this risk was not significant for women treated from 1990 to 2000 ($P = .86$). The risk of heart disease increased in women treated from 2001 to 2005, corresponding to the widespread use of anthracycline and trastuzumab chemotherapy.[50] The chemotherapy regimen used in individual patients is a significant consideration, because anthracyclines and trastuzumab both cause cardiac morbidity and may increase the overall risk to the patient. To date, however, there are few data on the long-term morbidity of combined chemotherapy and PMRT.[51]

Lymphedema Surgeons have particular concern related to the elevated risk of lymphedema and the impact on breast reconstructive options with PMRT. After ALND, lymphedema rates are 13%, compared with 2% with sentinel node biopsy alone.[52] Lymphedema rates remain relatively low with chest wall only PMRT; however, with RNI, the risk of lymphedema increases to 24.3% after ALND and to 6.1% after sentinel node biopsy, with the highest risk in obese women.[53] After ALND, many radiation oncologists advocate for omitting lower axillary radiation, to minimize the risk of lymphedema.[11] Surgeons and radiation oncologists must discuss the lifelong risks of lymphedema at the time of consultation, and counsel patients appropriately.

Reconstructive outcomes Modern breast cancer therapy should emphasize cosmetic outcome, because aesthetic results play an important role in patients' quality of life as a breast cancer survivor. In consultation with a plastic surgeon, patients should discuss various materials to produce the breast contour (autologous tissue vs prosthetic implants) and optimal timing for reconstruction (immediate vs delayed). Radiation therapy has an impact on the skin and soft tissues of the chest wall, leading to fibrosis that increases risks of contracture, infection, pain, necrosis, and atrophy in reconstructed tissues.[54] Recent data demonstrate that autologous reconstruction, preferably staged reconstruction using tissue expanders has superior patient-reported satisfaction and lower complication rates in the setting of PMRT.[55,56] These risks and benefits should be discussed when patients choose their reconstruction, and women should understand potential implications, including additional surgery, if adverse events occur.

Secondary malignancies Breast radiation is shown to have a small, but increased risk of secondary malignancies of the soft tissues, lung, and esophagus; thyroid cancers were not statistically increased with PMRT.[57,58] Although modern radiation therapies specifically aim to reduce dose to the surrounding normal tissues (lung and contralateral breast), because PMRT remains an essential part of breast cancer treatment, patients must understand potential risk for second nonbreast cancers, with a relative risk of 1.2 ($P = .001$).[57] If available, patients may benefit from surveillance of late toxicities at a designated breast cancer survivorship clinic, as is common at many comprehensive cancer centers.

Looking forward: 2018 and beyond *Advancing science: personalized medicine and the abscopal effect* Breast pathology now incorporates both clinical stage (TNM) and molecular subtype, with emphasis leaning toward the molecular subtype, as shown in the updated *American Joint Committee on Cancer Staging Manual*, 8th ed.[59] Appreciating the heterogeneity of tumors and their behavior as reflected in the molecular subtype may assist with individualizing treatments in the future. The current I-SPY 2 trial (ispy2.org), is using tumor genomic profiling to identify aggressive cancer subtypes and individualize NCT in a personalized medicine approach. Initial reports from the pembrolizumab arm estimate pCR rates increased from 20% to 60% in triple negative cancers and from 13% to 35% in hormone receptor-positive/HER2-cancers.[60] These results are promising and will hopefully translate into improved patient outcomes.

Understanding of the body's immune response against tumors is also evolving. In 1953, Mole[61] described a phenomenon termed, the *abscopal effect*, where localized radiation triggers systemic antitumor effects, with treatment response outside the radiation field. Cell death caused by radiation is believed to release proimmunogenic molecules, causing up-regulation of the body's antitumor activity, which results in more tumor cell kill, even at distant sites.[62] Systemic immunotherapies are currently used in the metastatic setting; however, these drugs are likely to be introduced into the adjuvant treatments for use in high risk aggressive molecular subtypes, with radiation possibly playing a synergistic role.

Ongoing clinical trials Pertinent trials shaping current clinical guidelines are highlighted. Ongoing trials are attempting to answer remaining controversies surrounding PMRT and breast cancer treatment. A brief summary of accruing clinical trials is below:

- I-SPY 2 trial: evaluating genomics of breast tumors using the MammaPrint Assay (AgendiaUSA, Irvine, California). Patients with high-risk results on MammaPrint are then randomized to various NCT, with experimental arms investigating neoadjuvant use of systemic therapies effective in the metastatic setting. Preliminary results demonstrate increased pCR rates compared with standard chemotherapy.[60]
- NSABP B-51/RTOG 1304 trial: investigating benefit of RNI based on patient response to NCT. Patients with proven axillary metastasis at diagnosis that have ypN0 response after NCT randomize to routine postoperative therapy with or without RNI.[40] This may shift treatment recommendations if there is no significant benefit to radiation after pCRs, as suggested by results of the pooled analysis of NSABP B-18 and B-27.[34]
- SUPREMO trial: randomizing patients with intermediate-riskd isease (1–3 LN+, or N0 and high-risk features: grade 3, LVSI) after mastectomy to PMRT or observation.[63]
- Hypofractionation regional nodal radiation trials: there are several phase III trials open to recruitment investigating the safety and side-effect profile of hypofractionated radiation in the PMRT setting, and for regional nodal radiation (www.clinicaltrials.gov).
- Advanced radiation techniques: single-institution and small phase II trials are investigating the role of conformal radiation techniques, including proton therapy, which has unique dose distribution compared with conventional photon therapy.[64,65] Studies investigating intensity modulated radiation therapy are also under way, but available data suggest no improvement in late toxicity.[66] These techniques are not currently recommended or standard of care, but patient participation in clinical trials should be offered, if available.

SUMMARY

The past 10 years have demonstrated a dramatic paradigm shift in the treatment of breast cancer. As randomized, prospective, and retrospective data become available regarding PMRT, clinicians must synthesize this information to make up-to-date and appropriate recommendations for patients. At diagnosis, patients often initially consult with surgeons; therefore, it is important for surgeons to recognize high risk patients who may benefit from PMRT. Studies suggest that PMRT is underutilized, with only 77.6% of patients with strong indications receiving radiation, potentially resulting in compromised patient outcomes.[67] Surgeons often have a strong influence in patients' decision making and require a firm understanding of the pertinent data regarding PMRT.

Although the role of PMRT has evolved over the past 5 decades, the latest randomized trials continue to demonstrate a benefit of PMRT in patients with: tumors greater than 5 cm, any node-positive disease, and node-negative breast cancers with high-risk features (ER−, LVSI, grade 3). Current research may enhance understanding of tumor biology, leading to personalized treatment recommendations using tumor genomic profiling, potentially eliminating use of PMRT in patients who do not benefit, and preferentially treating those at highest risk of locoregional recurrence.

REFERENCES

1. Siegel RL, Miller KD, Jemal A. Cancer statistics, 2017. CA Cancer J Clin 2017; 67(1):7–30.
2. Howlader N, NA, Krapcho M, et al. SEER cancer statistics review, 1975-2014. Secondary SEER cancer statistics review, 1975-2014 posted to the SEER web site, April 2017. 2017.
3. Favourable and unfavourable effects on long-term survival of radiotherapy for early breast cancer: an overview of the randomised trials. Early Breast Cancer Trialists' Collaborative Group. Lancet 2000;355(9217):1757–70.
4. Overgaard M, Hansen PS, Overgaard J, et al. Postoperative radiotherapy in high-risk premenopausal women with breast cancer who receive adjuvant chemotherapy. Danish Breast Cancer Cooperative Group 82b Trial. N Engl J Med 1997;337(14):949–55.
5. Overgaard M, Christensen JJ, Johansen H, et al. Evaluation of radiotherapy in high-risk breast cancer patients: report from the Danish Breast Cancer Cooperative Group (DBCG 82) Trial. Int J Radiat Oncol Biol Phys 1990;19(5): 1121–4.
6. Overgaard M, Jensen MB, Overgaard J, et al. Postoperative radiotherapy in high-risk postmenopausal breast-cancer patients given adjuvant tamoxifen: Danish Breast Cancer Cooperative Group DBCG 82c randomised trial. Lancet 1999; 353(9165):1641–8.
7. Ragaz J, Olivotto IA, Spinelli JJ, et al. Locoregional radiation therapy in patients with high-risk breast cancer receiving adjuvant chemotherapy: 20-year results of the British Columbia randomized trial. J Natl Cancer Inst 2005;97(2):116–26.
8. Whelan TJ, Olivotto IA, Parulekar WR, et al. Regional nodal irradiation in early-stage breast cancer. N Engl J Med 2015;373(4):307–16.
9. Poortmans PM, Collette S, Kirkove C, et al. Internal mammary and medial supraclavicular irradiation in breast cancer. N Engl J Med 2015;373(4):317–27.
10. Effects of chemotherapy and hormonal therapy for early breast cancer on recurrence and 15-year survival: an overview of the randomised trials. Lancet 2005; 365(9472):1687–717.

11. Recht A, Comen EA, Fine RE, et al. Postmastectomy radiotherapy: an American Society of Clinical Oncology, American Society for Radiation Oncology, and Society of Surgical Oncology Focused Guideline Update. J Clin Oncol 2016; 34(36):4431–42.

12. Auquier A, Rutqvist LE, Host H, et al. Post-mastectomy megavoltage radiotherapy: the Oslo and Stockholm trials. Eur J Cancer 1992;28(2–3):433–7.

13. Fisher B, Slack NH, Cavanaugh PJ, et al. Postoperative radiotherapy in the treatment of breast cancer: results of the NSABP clinical trial. Ann Surg 1970;172(4):711–32.

14. Fisher B, Jeong JH, Anderson S, et al. Twenty-five-year follow-up of a randomized trial comparing radical mastectomy, total mastectomy, and total mastectomy followed by irradiation. N Engl J Med 2002;347(8):567–75.

15. Cuzick J, Stewart H, Rutqvist L, et al. Cause-specific mortality in long-term survivors of breast cancer who participated in trials of radiotherapy. J Clin Oncol 1994; 12(3):447–53.

16. Overgaard M, Nielsen HM, Overgaard J. Is the benefit of postmastectomy irradiation limited to patients with four or more positive nodes, as recommended in international consensus reports? A subgroup analysis of the DBCG 82 b&c randomized trials. Radiother Oncol 2007;82(3):247–53.

17. Davies C, Godwin J, Gray R, et al. Relevance of breast cancer hormone receptors and other factors to the efficacy of adjuvant tamoxifen: patient-level meta-analysis of randomised trials. Lancet 2011;378(9793):771–84.

18. Davies C, Pan H, Godwin J, et al. Long-term effects of continuing adjuvant tamoxifen to 10 years versus stopping at 5 years after diagnosis of oestrogen receptor-positive breast cancer: ATLAS, a randomised trial. Lancet 2013;381(9869): 805–16.

19. McGale P, Taylor C, Correa C, et al. Effect of radiotherapy after mastectomy and axillary surgery on 10-year recurrence and 20-year breast cancer mortality: meta-analysis of individual patient data for 8135 women in 22 randomised trials. Lancet 2014;383(9935):2127–35.

20. Bonadonna G, Moliterni A, Zambetti M, et al. 30 years' follow up of randomised studies of adjuvant CMF in operable breast cancer: cohort study. BMJ 2005; 330(7485):217.

21. Fisher B, Brown AM, Dimitrov NV, et al. Two months of doxorubicin-cyclophosphamide with and without interval reinduction therapy compared with 6 months of cyclophosphamide, methotrexate, and fluorouracil in positive-node breast cancer patients with tamoxifen-nonresponsive tumors: results from the National Surgical Adjuvant Breast and Bowel Project B-15. J Clin Oncol 1990;8(9): 1483–96.

22. Fisher B, Anderson S, Tan-Chiu E, et al. Tamoxifen and chemotherapy for axillary node-negative, estrogen receptor-negative breast cancer: findings from National Surgical Adjuvant Breast and Bowel Project B-23. J Clin Oncol 2001;19(4):931–42.

23. Sparano JA. Use of dexrazoxane and other strategies to prevent cardiomyopathy associated with doxorubicin-taxane combinations. Semin Oncol 1998;25(4 Suppl 10):66–71.

24. Henderson IC, Berry DA, Demetri GD, et al. Improved outcomes from adding sequential Paclitaxel but not from escalating Doxorubicin dose in an adjuvant chemotherapy regimen for patients with node-positive primary breast cancer. J Clin Oncol 2003;21(6):976–83.

25. Mamounas EP, Bryant J, Lembersky B, et al. Paclitaxel after doxorubicin plus cyclophosphamide as adjuvant chemotherapy for node-positive breast cancer: results from NSABP B-28. J Clin Oncol 2005;23(16):3686–96.

26. Romond EH, Perez EA, Bryant J, et al. Trastuzumab plus adjuvant chemotherapy for operable HER2-positive breast cancer. N Engl J Med 2005;353(16):1673–84.

27. Piccart-Gebhart MJ, Procter M, Leyland-Jones B, et al. Trastuzumab after adjuvant chemotherapy in HER2-positive breast cancer. N Engl J Med 2005; 353(16):1659–72.

28. Perez EA, Romond EH, Suman VJ, et al. Four-year follow-up of trastuzumab plus adjuvant chemotherapy for operable human epidermal growth factor receptor 2-positive breast cancer: joint analysis of data from NCCTG N9831 and NSABP B-31. J Clin Oncol 2011;29(25):3366–73.

29. Cameron D, Piccart-Gebhart MJ, Gelber RD, et al. 11 years' follow-up of trastuzumab after adjuvant chemotherapy in HER2-positive early breast cancer: final analysis of the HERceptin Adjuvant (HERA) trial. Lancet 2017;389(10075): 1195–205.

30. von Minckwitz G, Procter M, de Azambuja E, et al. Adjuvant Pertuzumab and Trastuzumab in Early HER2-Positive Breast Cancer. N Engl J Med 2017;377(2): 122–31.

31. Peto R, Davies C, Godwin J, et al. Comparisons between different polychemotherapy regimens for early breast cancer: meta-analyses of long-term outcome among 100,000 women in 123 randomised trials. Lancet 2012;379(9814): 432–44.

32. Wolmark N, Wang J, Mamounas E, et al. Preoperative chemotherapy in patients with operable breast cancer: nine-year results from National Surgical Adjuvant Breast and Bowel Project B-18. J Natl Cancer Inst Monogr 2001;(30):96–102.

33. Bear HD, Anderson S, Smith RE, et al. Sequential preoperative or postoperative docetaxel added to preoperative doxorubicin plus cyclophosphamide for operable breast cancer:National Surgical Adjuvant Breast and Bowel Project Protocol B-27. J Clin Oncol 2006;24(13):2019–27.

34. Mamounas EP, Anderson SJ, Dignam JJ, et al. Predictors of locoregional recurrence after neoadjuvant chemotherapy: results from combined analysis of National Surgical Adjuvant Breast and Bowel Project B-18 and B-27. J Clin Oncol 2012;30(32):3960–6.

35. Huang EH, Tucker SL, Strom EA, et al. Postmastectomy radiation improves localregional control and survival for selected patients with locally advanced breast cancer treated with neoadjuvant chemotherapy and mastectomy. J Clin Oncol 2004;22(23):4691–9.

36. McGuire SE, Gonzalez-Angulo AM, Huang EH, et al. Postmastectomy radiation improves the outcome of patients with locally advanced breast cancer who achieve a pathologic complete response to neoadjuvant chemotherapy. Int J Radiat Oncol Biol Phys 2007;68(4):1004–9.

37. Rusthoven CG, Rabinovitch RA, Jones BL, et al. The impact of postmastectomy and regional nodal radiation after neoadjuvant chemotherapy for clinically lymph node-positive breast cancer: a National Cancer Database (NCDB) analysis. Ann Oncol 2016;27(5):818–27.

38. Mak KS, Harris JR. Radiotherapy issues after neoadjuvant chemotherapy. J Natl Cancer Inst Monogr 2015;2015(51):87–9.

39. NCCN. Breast cancer (version 2.2017). Secondary breast cancer (version 2.2017) April 6, 2017. 2017. Available at: https://www.nccn.org/professionals/physician_gls/pdf/breast.pdf. Accessed September 1, 2017.

40. Mamounas EP, Bandos H, White JR, et al. NRG oncology/NSABP B-51/RTOG 1304: phase III trial to determine if chest wall and regional nodal radiotherapy (CWRNRT) post mastectomy (Mx) or the addition of RNRT to breast RT post

breast-conserving surgery (BCS) reduces invasive breast cancer recurrence free interval (IBCRFI) in patients (pts) with positive axillary (PAx) nodes who are ypN0 after neoadjuvant chemotherapy (NC). J Clin Oncol 2017;35(Suppl 15): TPS589.

41. Garg AK, Buchholz TA. Influence of neoadjuvant chemotherapy on radiotherapy for breast cancer. Ann Surg Oncol 2015;22(5):1434–40.

42. Strom EA, McNeese MD. Postmastectomy irradiation: rationale for treatment field selection. Semin Radiat Oncol 1999;9(3):247–53.

43. Schwaibold F, Fowble BL, Solin LJ, et al. The results of radiation therapy for isolated local regional recurrence after mastectomy. Int J Radiat Oncol Biol Phys 1991;21(2):299–310.

44. Huang O, Wang L, Shen K, et al. Breast cancer subpopulation with high risk of internal mammary lymph nodes metastasis: analysis of 2,269 Chinese breast cancer patients treated with extended radical mastectomy. Breast Cancer Res Treat 2008;107(3):379–87.

45. Veronesi U, Marubini E, Mariani L, et al. The dissection of internal mammary nodes does not improve the survival of breast cancer patients. 30-year results of a randomised trial. Eur J Cancer 1999;35(9):1320–5.

46. Remouchamps VM, Vicini FA, Sharpe MB, et al. Significant reductions in heart and lung doses using deep inspiration breath hold with active breathing control and intensity-modulated radiation therapy for patients treated with locoregional breast irradiation. Int J Radiat Oncol Biol Phys 2003;55(2):392–406.

47. Korreman SS, Pedersen AN, Aarup LR, et al. Reduction of cardiac and pulmonary complication probabilities after breathing adapted radiotherapy for breast cancer. Int J Radiat Oncol Biol Phys 2006;65(5):1375–80.

48. Darby SC, Ewertz M, McGale P, et al. Risk of ischemic heart disease in women after radiotherapy for breast cancer. N Engl J Med 2013;368(11):987–98.

49. Taylor C, Correa C, Duane FK, et al. Estimating the risks of breast cancer radiotherapy: evidence from modern radiation doses to the lungs and heart and from previous randomized trials. J Clin Oncol 2017;35(15):1641–9.

50. Rehammar JC, Jensen MB, McGale P, et al. Risk of heart disease in relation to radiotherapy and chemotherapy with anthracyclines among 19,464 breast cancer patients in Denmark, 1977-2005. Radiother Oncol 2017;123(2): 299–305.

51. Halyard MY, Pisansky TM, Dueck AC, et al. Radiotherapy and adjuvant trastuzumab in operable breast cancer: tolerability and adverse event data from the NCCTG Phase III Trial N9831. J Clin Oncol 2009;27(16):2638–44.

52. Lucci A, McCall LM, Beitsch PD, et al. Surgical complications associated with sentinel lymph node dissection (SLND) plus axillary lymph node dissection compared with SLND alone in the American College of Surgeons Oncology Group Trial Z0011. J Clin Oncol 2007;25(24):3657–63.

53. Warren LE, Miller CL, Horick N, et al. The impact of radiation therapy on the risk of lymphedema after treatment for breast cancer: a prospective cohort study. Int J Radiat Oncol Biol Phys 2014;88(3):565–71.

54. Spear SL, Onyewu C. Staged breast reconstruction with saline-filled implants in the irradiated breast: recent trends and therapeutic implications. Plast Reconstr Surg 2000;105(3):930–42.

55. Tran NV, Chang DW, Gupta A, et al. Comparison of immediate and delayed free TRAM flap breast reconstruction in patients receiving postmastectomy radiation therapy. Plast Reconstr Surg 2001;108(1):78–82.

56. Cordeiro PG, Pusic AL, Disa JJ, et al. Irradiation after immediate tissue expander/implant breast reconstruction: outcomes, complications, aesthetic results, and satisfaction among 156 patients. Plast Reconstr Surg 2004;113(3):877–81.

57. Clarke M, Collins R, Darby S, et al. Effects of radiotherapy and of differences in the extent of surgery for early breast cancer on local recurrence and 15-year survival: an overview of the randomised trials. Lancet 2005;366(9503):2087–106.

58. Grantzau T, Overgaard J. Risk of second non-breast cancer after radiotherapy for breast cancer: a systematic review and meta-analysis of 762,468 patients. Radiother Oncol 2015;114(1):56–65.

59. Giuliano AE, Connolly JL, Edge SB, et al. Breast cancer—Major changes in the American Joint Committee on Cancer eighth edition cancer staging manual. CA Cancer J Clin 2017;67(4):290–303.

60. Nanda R, Liu MC, Yau C, et al. Pembrolizumab plus standard neoadjuvant therapy for high-risk breast cancer (BC): results from I-SPY 2. Journal of Clinical Oncology 2017;35(Suppl 15):506.

61. Mole RH. Whole body irradiation; radiobiology or medicine? Br J Radiol 1953;26(305):234–41.

62. Hu ZI, McArthur HL, Ho AY. The abscopal effect of radiation therapy: what is it and how can we use it in breast cancer? Curr Breast Cancer Rep 2017;9(1):45–51.

63. Kunkler IH, Canney P, van Tienhoven G, et al. Elucidating the role of chest wall irradiation in 'Intermediate-risk' breast cancer: the MRC/EORTC SUPREMO trial. Clin Oncol (R Coll Radiol) 2008;20(1):31–4.

64. MacDonald SM, Jimenez R, Paetzold P, et al. Proton radiotherapy for chest wall and regional lymphatic radiation; dose comparisons and treatment delivery. Radiat Oncol 2013;8:71.

65. MacDonald SM, Patel SA, Hickey S, et al. Proton therapy for breast cancer after mastectomy: early outcomes of a prospective clinical trial. Int J Radiat Oncol Biol Phys 2013;86(3):484–90.

66. Pignol JP, Truong P, Rakovitch E, et al. Ten years results of the Canadian breast intensity modulated radiation therapy (IMRT) randomized controlled trial. Radiother Oncol 2016;121(3):414–9.

67. Jagsi R, Abrahamse P, Morrow M, et al. Patterns and correlates of adjuvant radiotherapy receipt after lumpectomy and after mastectomy for breast cancer. J Clin Oncol 2010;28(14):2396–403.

Breast Cancer in the Elderly

Flora Varghese, MD, MBA, Jasmine Wong, MD*

KEYWORDS

- Screening • Axillary staging • Endocrine therapy • Radiation therapy
- Chemotherapy • Surgical outcomes • Ethics

KEY POINTS

- The incidence of breast cancer in the elderly is high; with increasing life expectancy, screening and treatment methods are evolving for this population.
- Functional status, comorbidities, and treatment side effects are becoming the determining factor in deciding screening and treatment options.
- Additional research in elderly patients with breast cancer needs to determine screening recommendations, ethical considerations, and best practice treatment options.

INTRODUCTION

In 2016, the incidence of breast cancer in women older than 65 years was 436.9 per 100,000 per year.[1,2] More than 50% of breast cancers are diagnosed in patients older than 60 years (**Fig. 1**).[3] The World Health Organization and Medicare define the elderly as individuals older than 65 years.[4,5] Although the average life expectancy of women older than 65 years is 86.6 years, 1 out of 4 will live to more than 90 years of age and 1 out of 10 will live to more than 95 years of age.[2,6] This article attempts to summarize current topics pertaining to breast cancer in the elderly.

PRESENTATION

Presentation varies among the elderly population. Some elderly women are more likely to present later with breast cancer because of their lack of awareness.[7] Yet, some studies show the elderly can present at earlier stages.[8] Many patients older than 85 years self-refer because screening is not provided to them.[9] In general, the older the patients, the more likely their initial presentation of breast cancer will be a palpable mass and less likely to be screen detected.[10]

Some studies show the elderly present with a more favorable characteristic malignancy than their younger counterparts.[11] Other studies show patients with earlier-stage cancer had more poorly differentiated cancer with a higher tumor grade and Ki67 similar to their younger counterparts.[8] Recent studies show estrogen receptor

Disclosure: The authors have nothing to disclose.
Department of Surgery, University of California, San Francisco, 1600 Divisadero Street, Second Floor, Box 1710, San Francisco, CA 94115, USA
* Corresponding author.
E-mail address: jasmine.wong2@ucsf.edu

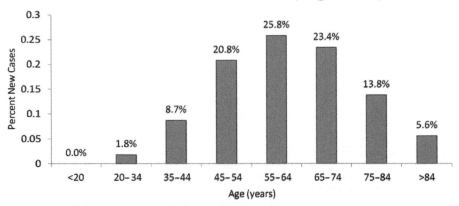

Fig. 1. Surveillance, Epidemiology, and End Results' percent of new cases of breast cancer by age. (*Data from* National Cancer Institute. SEER 18 2010–2014. Available at: https://seer.cancer.gov/statfacts/html/breast.html. Accessed October 9, 2017.)

tumors increase in occurrence with age and human epidermal growth factor receptor 2 (Her2) status decreases with age.[12,13]

Invasive ductal cancer (76%) makes up most breast cancers in the elderly. Invasive lobular carcinoma makes up 5.6%, and ductal carcinoma in situ alone was 10.0% of elderly breast pathology.[14] Overall, the most common presentation for elderly patients is higher-grade, hormone receptor–positive invasive ductal cancer.[11]

SCREENING

Among national organizations, mammography is the imaging modality of choice for screening.[15] Many randomized and case-controlled trials have evaluated the costs and benefits of screening. The Health Insurance Plan trial of New York in 1963 revealed mammographic screening reduced breast cancer mortality by 30%. Recent meta-analysis has shown a 15% to 20% relative risk reduction in mortality with breast cancer screening.[16] Yet, with about 11 trials evaluating screening, the US Preventative Services Task Force, the American Cancer Society, the American Geriatric Society, the American College of Obstetrics and Gynecology, and other organizations have not converged on a single recommendation for screening guidelines in the elderly.[17] Many of these trials did not include patients who were older than 60 years.

Critics of overscreening the elderly cite higher incidence of breast cancer in the elderly, increased risk of death from other disease, and the slow growth of most tumors.[18] The United Kingdom conducted an independent review to evaluate the benefits and harms of screening and concluded that there is an 11% to 19% overdiagnosis.[16] A Cochrane review of 7 randomized trials concluded there is a 15% reduction of breast cancer risk with screening mammogram but a 30% overdiagnosis and overtreatment. Only 6 of the 11 trials included women older than 60 years, and only the Swedish Kopparberg trial included patients older than 65 years.[19] This Swedish trial concluded that reduction in mortality was 34% in women aged 50 years and older with 0.66 odds ratio breast cancer mortality and, therefore, a greater benefit (**Table 1**).[19]

Currently, routine screening for breast cancer in patients older than 74 years is controversial. Some advocate continued clinical breast examinations over mammography in this age group.[20] The National Cancer Institute (NCI) has deferred recommendations

Table 1
Eleven trials evaluating mammography and its correlation to the odds ratio for breast cancer and overall mortality

Reference	Year	Age Group (y)	Intervention	Control	Methodologic Quality[a]	OR for Breast Cancer Mortality	OR for Overall Mortality
HIP	1963	40–64	Mammography + CE (n = 31,000)	Nothing (n = 31,000)	Less robust	0.65 (0.49–0.86)	0.95 (0.87–1.04)
Malmö 1	1976	>44	Mammography (n = 21,088)	Nothing (n = 21,195)	Sound	0.96 (0.68–1.35)	0.99 (0.93–1.05)
Kopparberg	1977	40–74	Mammography (n = 39,051)	Nothing (n = 18,846)	Less robust	0.66 (0.46–0.94)	1.03 (0.96–1.10)
Östergötland	1978	>40	Mammography (n = 39,034)	Nothing (n = 37,936)	Less robust	0.77 (0.54–1.10)	0.99 (0.94–1.05)
Malmö 2	1978	45–50	Mammography (n = 9581)	Nothing (n = 8212)	Less robust	0.75 (0.46–1.24)	1.15 (0.99–1.33)
TEDBC Edinburgh	1979	45–64	Mammography + CE (n = 22,926)	SE (n = 21,342)	Biased	0.83 (0.54–1.27)	Reduced
NBSS1	1980	40–49	Mammography + CE + SE (n = 25,214)	Initial CE + SE + SE (n = 25,216)	Sound	1.36 (0.83–2.21)	1.02 (0.82–1.27)
NBSS2	1980	50–59	Mammography + CE + SE (n = 19,711)	CE + SE (n = 19,694)	Sound	0.97 (0.62–1.52)	1.01 (0.85–1.20)
Stockholm	1981	40–64	Mammography (n = 38,525)	Nothing (n = 20,651)	Less robust	0.71 (0.47–1.07)	0.91 (0.85–0.99)
Göteborg	1982	39–59	Mammography (n = 10,821/9903)	Nothing (n = 13,101/15,708)	Less robust	0.73/0.90 (0.26–2.00/ 0.53–1.54)	1.17/0.93 (0.95–1.43/ 0.82–1.06)
UKCCR	1991	39–41	Mammography (n = 53,884)	Nothing (n = 106,956)	Sound	0.83 (0.66–1.04)	0.97 (0.89–1.04)

Abbreviation: OR, odds ratio.

From Paesmans M, Ameye L, Moreau M, et al. Breast cancer screening in the older woman: an effective way to reduce mortality? Maturitas 2010;66(3):264; with permission.

for screening to other organizations but does state the cumulative false-positive rate of mammography with clinical breast examination after 10 years of annual screening to be 50%.[21,22]

A new trial, the Wisdom trial, which looks into personalized screening of patients based on individual risks factors (breast density, family history, age, race/ethnicity, comorbidities, genomic profiling), promises to deliver the answer for how to best screen for breast cancer.[23] Patients and physicians have tools available, such as ePrognosis from the University of California San Francisco (eprognosis.ucsf.edu), which take into account patient demographics and risk factors to determine if screening is harmful or beneficial.[24] With personalized medicine in the forefront, uniformity for best practice screening methods will not only be based on age but also on risk factors and life expectancy.

SURVIVAL

By examining the NCI's Surveillance, Epidemiology, and End Results (SEER) database, the 5-year survival for breast cancer from 1975 to 2013 increased from 74.9% to 91.1%. Among patients older than 65 years, the most recent data show an 89.5% 5-year overall survival. Specifically, those between 65 and 74 years of age have a rate of 91.4% for 5-year survival. These survival rates are comparable with those from individuals aged younger than 45 years (88.1%), 45 to 54 years (90.6%), and 55 to 64 years (90.1%). When looking at survival based on the stage of breast cancer, individuals older than 50 years, stage for stage, have similar survival except for stage 4 distant disease. In this population, the survival is 24.1% for those aged 50 years and older compared with 37.1% in those aged 50 years and younger (**Fig. 2**).[25] These differences may be because, studies show, elderly patients tend to be undertreated for even early stage breast cancer compared with younger patients, which increases their breast cancer recurrence and decreases their survival. Albeit the most common reason for decreased survival may be that the elderly have more comorbidities compared with with their younger counterparts, which prohibits them from tolerating the same treatments.[26]

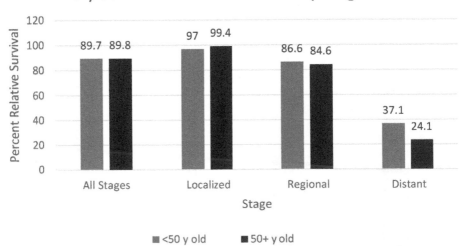

Fig. 2. SEER's 5-year relative survival for breast cancer by stage and age. (*Data from* National Cancer Institute. SEER cancer statistics: breast cancer. Available at: https://seer.cancer.gov/csr/1975_2014/results_merged/sect_04_breast.pdf. Accessed October 9, 2017.)

SURGICAL OUTCOMES

Surgery plays a central role in the treatment of breast cancer. In the elderly population, morbidity and mortality associated with surgery are increased. Even in treating early stage disease (stage 0–II) in octogenarians and nonagenarians, increased age is a significant risk factor for death.[27] Studies show surgical treatment of stage III in those 80 years old or more produces a 5-year survival of 48.5%, which is worse compared with younger patients of the same stage.[28] A multisite Breast Cancer Surgical Outcomes (BRCASO) database exists to monitor morbidity and mortality in patients with breast cancer after surgical intervention.[29] Although the study done by Pettke and colleagues[30] showed overall perioperative mortality is low, patients older than 80 years have increased mortality and systemic morbidity like cardiac arrests and pneumonias. Yet, their wound complications were equal to their younger counterparts. Certain procedures like mastectomy with immediate breast reconstruction have also increased in the elderly from 6.7% in 2004 to 18.1% in 2012, and the trend continues to increase especially in patients with larger tumors.[26,31] The main complication in this demographic is a 34% increase in 30-day readmissions even when the elderly have no comorbidities. More studies need to be conducted to evaluate surgical outcomes in the elderly so appropriate counseling can aid their decision-making for treatment.[26]

Optimal surgical treatment of breast cancer in an older patient population is not clearly defined. Difficulties in determining the optimal treatment include comorbidities, concerns about treatment effects on quality of life, shorter life expectancy, decreased mental and physical capacity, patient preference, and slower progression of disease.

ROLE OF SENTINEL LYMPH NODE BIOPSY AND AXILLARY LYMPH NODE DISSECTION

Surgical treatment of breast cancer initially included an axillary lymph node dissection regardless of lymph node status because of Halsted's theory of clearing axillary disease to prevent distant spread. Findings from National Surgical Adjuvant Breast and Bowel Project (NSABP) showed leaving positive axillary lymph nodes in the group that underwent mastectomy alone did not have an increased rate of distant recurrence or breast cancer–related mortality.[32] These findings led to the theory that axillary lymph node involvement is more likely an indicator of disease spread and that axillary clearance does not prevent distant spread. The information provided by an axillary lymph node dissection, thus, became an important part of staging to help guide adjuvant treatment recommendations. In the elderly, the role of an axillary dissection has been unclear given the morbidity associated with the procedure and shorter life expectancy. A retrospective study that included only patients older than 70 years with operable, clinically node-negative breast cancer compared patients who underwent axillary dissection with patients who did not undergo axillary dissection. Tamoxifen was prescribed for at least 2 years in this study. At a median follow-up of 15 years, there was no difference in breast cancer mortality between the two groups.[33] A meta-analysis composed of 2 randomized controlled studies with a total of 692 patients found no difference in in-breast recurrence or distant recurrence between axillary staging and no axillary staging. They also found no differences in overall survival or breast cancer–specific survival between the two groups.[34] One of the studies included in the meta-analysis looked at quality of life after an axillary lymph node dissection. The study found a significant difference in physician-reported adverse effects in the first postoperative period in terms of restriction of arm movement and arm pain among patients undergoing axillary surgery compared with the group that did not have axillary surgery.[35] Two studies by Martelli and colleagues[33,36] report the incidence of axillary disease in the groups that did not receive an axillary lymph node dissection and found only about a 6% incidence at

15 years. In patients whereby the staging information acquired from an axillary lymph node dissection is unlikely to affect the adjuvant treatment decisions, the data suggest that omission of an axillary lymph node dissection will not affect survival and results in a low rate of axillary recurrence.

The morbidities associated with an axillary lymph node dissection eventually led to the development and use of the sentinel lymph node biopsy for staging in patients with clinically node-negative disease. NSABP-32 showed that omission of the axillary lymph node dissection in patients with clinically node-negative disease had no impact on overall survival, disease-free survival, and regional control.[37] Findings in several other studies showing no survival benefit from an axillary lymph node dissection eventually led to the Society of Surgical Oncology to recommend, in 2016 as part of the Choosing Wisely campaign, that surgeons "do not routinely use sentinel lymph node biopsy in clinically node negative women older than 70 years of age with hormone receptor positive invasive breast cancer."[33,38] This recommendation raises questions about whether or not a sentinel lymph node biopsy should be eliminated for all women older than of 70 years because nodal status can affect adjuvant treatment recommendations. In a study looking at patients older than 70 years from the National Cancer Database, only 15% of the patients studied who underwent nodal evaluation had a positive lymph node. The median number of positive lymph nodes was one. The same group also did a parallel analysis using the SEER database and found that 26% of patients had a positive lymph node. Both analyses showed better overall survival in the group undergoing lymph node evaluation, but the difference was likely due to patient selection factors. The investigators concluded that following the Choosing Wisely guideline would unlikely significantly change survival in the patients who would have otherwise done well based on tumor biology or the patients who already have limited life expectancy. In a group of more high-risk patients who are healthy, lymph node evaluation may provide important information for determining their adjuvant therapy options.[39] Welsh and colleagues[40] developed a model to predict nodal positivity in women older than 70 years with hormone receptor–positive disease to help determine which group of patients has a higher risk of node positivity. They found a low-risk group of patients, those with grade 1 tumors less than 2 cm or those with grade 2 tumors less than 1 cm, had a node positivity rate of 7.8%. Patients not in the low-risk group, all grade 3 tumors, clinically T2 tumors, or grade 2 T1c tumors, were found to have a node positivity rate of 22.3%. The investigators concluded that patients identified to be in the low-risk group were ideal candidates for omission of a sentinel lymph node biopsy. Therefore, the use of sentinel lymph node biopsies in patients older than 70 years should be decided based on individual patient-specific characteristics, such as comorbidities, life expectancy, and surgical risk, as well as likelihood of having a positive node.

ROLE OF ENDOCRINE THERAPY ALONE

Surgery plays a role in standard treatment of breast cancer; but in the elderly population, multiple studies have been conducted to look at treatment with endocrine alone in patients who are not ideal surgical candidates. A retrospective study in the Netherlands looked at women older than 75 years who received primary endocrine therapy (PET) and compared those patients with patients who underwent surgical treatment. They found that women who had PET had their survival significantly compromised compared with the women who were treated with surgery. Women receiving PET had a 5-year overall survival of 27.0% compared with 62.3% for women undergoing surgery. Age and prevalence of comorbidities did differ significantly between the two groups, with the women receiving PET being older and having more comorbidities.[41] Twenty-year follow-up on a study done in Nottingham, conversely, showed no difference in overall survival or in time to distant metastases between the patients who received primary tamoxifen compared with patients who underwent a wedge mastectomy. They did find a significant difference in time to local recurrence between the two groups.[42] A Cochrane review of 7 randomized controlled trials comparing surgery versus endocrine therapy (tamoxifen) alone also showed no significant difference in overall survival but a significant difference in progression-free survival.[43] These conflicting data suggest that patient selection remains an important determinant in deciding whether or not to offer PET to elderly patients. Consideration for a breast surgery without an axillary procedure could be offered to patients who have a reasonable life expectancy and can safely undergo a surgical procedure.

ROLE OF RADIATION THERAPY

Surgical options of early stage breast cancer consist of a mastectomy or a partial mastectomy with adjuvant radiation therapy as a result of the findings from NSABP-B6. This study found breast-conserving surgery compared with mastectomy did not lead to a difference in disease-free survival, distant disease-free survival, or overall survival. The study found, however, radiation after partial mastectomy led to a decrease in in-breast recurrence.[32] Since the publication of NSABP-B6, several newer studies have looked specifically at the use of radiation therapy after breast-conserving surgery in older patients. They showed that in an older patient population, omission of radiation therapy after breast-conserving surgery also results in similar overall survival rates but with differences in local recurrence rates. Both studies randomized patients undergoing lumpectomy and endocrine therapy to either radiation or no radiation (**Table 2**). These studies found a significant difference in local regional recurrence at 5 years but no significant difference in 5-year overall survival.[38,44] However, in a study looking at radiation therapy utilization and outcomes in elderly patients, Haque and

Table 2
Trials evaluating lumpectomy, radiation and tamoxifen treatments in the elderly

	Number of Patients	Age (y)	Inclusion Criteria	Treatment Arms	Local Recurrence	5-y Survival
CALGB 9343	636	70+	T1N0 ER positive	Lumpectomy + tamoxifen + radiation vs lumpectomy + tamoxifen	1% vs 4% (P<.001)	87% vs 86% (P = .94)
PRIME II	1326	65+	Up to 3 cm clear margins, node-negative ER positive, grade 3 or lymphovascular invasion but not both	Lumpectomy + endocrine therapy, lumpectomy + endocrine therapy + whole-breast radiation	4.1% vs 1.3% (P = .0002)	Both groups 93.9% (P = .34)

Data from Hughes KS, Schnaper LA, Berry D, et al. Lumpectomy plus tamoxifen with or without irradiation in women 70 years of age or older with early breast cancer. N Engl J Med 2004;351:971–7; and Kunkler IH, Williams LJ, Jack WJL, et al. Breast-conserving surgery with or without irradiation in women aged 65 years or older with early breast cancer (PRIME II): a randomized controlled trial. Lancet Oncol 2015;16(3):266–73.

colleagues[45,46] found a survival benefit in patients with estrogen receptor (ER)–positive/Her2-negative disease using SEER data. They note in their study that they had a higher proportion of patients with grade 3 disease than the PRIME II patient cohort, which may account for the differences in findings. They also raised concerns about endocrine therapy use and compliance because SEER data are not able to provide this type of information in accounting for the possible difference in their findings compared with CALGB (Cancer and Leukemia Group B) and PRIME II patient cohorts. These studies provide definitive data to support the omission of radiation therapy in the elderly patient population.

ROLE OF ENDOCRINE THERAPY

For ER-positive breast cancers, adjuvant systemic therapy should include endocrine therapy with either tamoxifen or an aromatase inhibitor. NSABP-B14 showed the use of tamoxifen for 5 years in the adjuvant setting for ER-positive breast cancers to have a significant advantage in disease-free survival, distant disease-free survival, and overall survival at the 10-year follow-up. The study also found no advantage to more than 5 years of tamoxifen and a significant reduction in the incidence of contralateral breast cancer.[47] The development of aromatase inhibitors (AIs) led to multiple trials comparing AIs with tamoxifen. The results of a meta-analysis of these trials found a significant reduction in early recurrence with use of an AI.[48] The Breast International Group (BIG) 1-98 study at 8.1 years of median follow-up, treatment with 5 years of letrozole in postmenopausal women with estrogen-positive breast cancers results in significant improvements in disease-free survival, overall survival, distant recurrence-free interval, and breast cancer–free interval compared with tamoxifen.[49] Tamoxifen has been associated with both thromboembolic events and uterine cancer. AI use has been found to increase the odds of developing cardiovascular disease and bone fractures but decreased odds of venous thrombosis and endometrial carcinoma when compared with tamoxifen.[50] Hot flashes, arthralgia, myalgia, and alopecia are also known common side effects of treatment with an AI but seem to be tolerated by women older than 70 years. A study found no difference in toxicity or quality of life in patients treated with letrozole versus placebo-treated patients older than 70 years.[51] The role of endocrine therapy in the adjuvant setting for ER-positive breast cancers either with tamoxifen or an AI has its benefits and should be considered for patients who have a reasonable life expectancy and do not have comorbidities that preclude them from taking endocrine therapy.

CHEMOTHERAPY

Elderly patients with breast cancer are less likely to obtain chemotherapy than their younger counterparts based on reasons including comorbidities, life expectancy, and concern for chemotoxicity in the frail. Large studies are lacking that focus solely on chemotherapy in older patients in the neoadjuvant, adjuvant, and palliative settings.[52] Some studies have looked at the role of adjuvant chemotherapy in Her2-positive disease. For older women with small Her2-positive node-negative malignancy, a retrospective study from Memorial Sloan Kettering Cancer Center shows the addition of trastuzumab with adjuvant chemotherapy not only produced low cardiac events (3.2%) in patients but also had a 4-year overall survival of 99% and distant relapse-free survival of 99%.[53] Comparing the toxicity of paclitaxel (Taxol)-based treatment with doxorubicin-based treatments reveals similar rates of adverse events and 5-year breast cancer–specific survival (92% doxorubicin-based treatment vs 96% Taxol-based treatment).[54] In patients older than 65 years with triple-negative disease, adjuvant chemotherapy decreased mortality by 15% with the greatest advantage for those who had regional disease.[55]

Chemotherapeutic agents like anthracyclines are dose dependent on their cardiac and hematologic toxicity. Studies have shown increased hematoxicity in patients who are frailer, diabetic, and needing assistance at home.[56] The NCI has recommended treatment modification for high-grade toxicities, but newer studies are looking at the impact of the toxicity to activities of daily living in order to determine if modification is necessary.[57] Online Web sites like PREDICT (http://www.predict.nhs.uk/predict.html) aid in deciding chemotherapeutic regimens based on risk modeling.[58] With more trials evaluating the chemotoxicity on geriatric functionality and physiology, a better understanding of the tolerance of chemotherapy on the elderly will be assessed, so recommendations in the neoadjuvant, adjuvant, and even palliative settings may be forthcoming.

ONCOTYPE AND MAMMAPRINT

Decisions on how to best treat an aging population have in the past been reliant on multiple patient factors: comorbidities, expected life expectancy, and patient preferences. Molecular tools and genetic expression profiles can also now be incorporated into the decision-making process because these tools allow for assessment of risk. The 21-gene oncotype recurrence score has been validated in estrogen-positive, node-negative, and node-positive breast cancer in predicting the risk for both local regional recurrence and distant recurrence as well as the benefit from chemotherapy. Patients with high recurrence scores show a significant benefit from chemotherapy compared with endocrine therapy alone.[59] In patients with a low recurrence score, the findings from the TAILORx study (Trial Assigning Individualized Options for Treatment) support the use of endocrine therapy alone.[60] For patients who are candidates for chemotherapy, this recurrence score can be used to predict a benefit from chemotherapy, especially when taking into consideration the effects that chemotherapy has on the elderly population.[60]

The 70-gene Mammaprint assay has been validated to predict which patients may be at risk for recurrence. More recently, an ultralow risk threshold of the Mammaprint assay has been identified. The patients in this study who had ultralow-risk tumors had a significantly lower risk of breast specific death compared with the low-risk and high-risk tumor groups. These findings lead the authors to conclude that the ultralow risk threshold can be used to identify patients who can be safely treated with surgery alone.[61] In the elderly population, this assay could be used as another tool to risk stratify patients during the discussion of which treatments to pursue.

ETHICS AND DISPARITY

With 12% of the US population older than 70 years and increasing at a rate of 2.5% per year, the ethics of treating these patients with multiple comorbidities becomes challenging. Concerns about ageism and rationing care arise when making decisions for breast cancer treatment.[62] The average life expectancy of a 70-year-old person is 12.5 years from their initial presentation.[63] So when deciding treatment, some organizations focus on resource allocation or quality of life to decide which treatment may be fraught with discriminatory bias.[62] Some have advocated using the Comprehensive Geriatric Assessment tool to risk stratify patients in order to aid in treatment of elderly patients with breast cancer.[13,64] Ethical dilemmas for screening and treating patients with dementia have arisen with recommendations to evaluate risks and benefits, including life expectancy and quality of life of patients, to help make those complex decisions (**Fig. 3**).[65,66] The Age Gap Cohort Study in the United Kingdom is currently

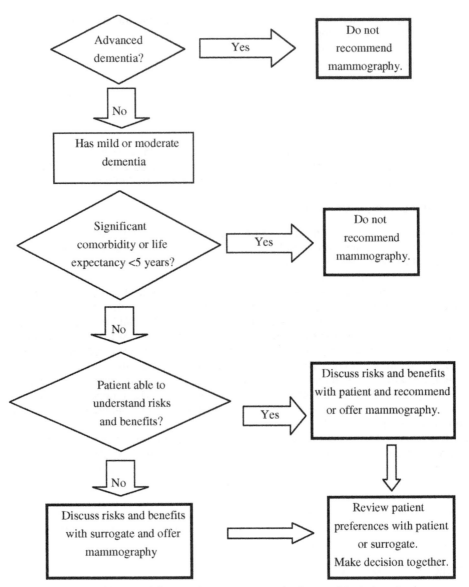

Fig. 3. Decision-making model screening mammography in cognitively impaired women. (*From* Raik BL, Miller FG, Fins JJ. Screening and cognitive impairment: ethics of forgoing mammography in older women. J Am Geriatr Soc 2004;52(3):443; with permission.)

looking into the treatment decision-making process in the elderly with breast cancer with the aim of best practice recommendations.[67]

Studies are also looking into the disparity in care of the elderly. Those with early stage breast cancer tend to die of other comorbidities; but mortality from breast cancer, nevertheless, increases with age. Still, undertreatment of the disease in the elderly is common. The discrepancy lies in adjusting the management of the cancer with the increased comorbidities of the elderly.[13] Most trials have excluded this age group in their analysis of breast cancer prevention, diagnosis, and treatment.[68] Future trials will need to investigate the best plan of action to minimize the disparity in care.

SUMMARY

With increasing life expectancy and growth of the elderly US population, it becomes paramount that breast cancer research focuses more on the prevention, screening, and treatment of these patients. Age no longer is a cutoff for managing breast cancer in the elderly. Studies have shown the current undertreatment of cancer undermines survival, but the tide is turning to provide evidence-based medicine for the elderly. More often, clinicians and surgeons look not only at tumor-specific characteristics of breast cancer but also the functionality, tolerance, comorbidities, and life expectancy of patients to determine the best treatment. The geriatric population in the twenty-first century needs appropriate assessment before managing breast cancer so individuals obtain the best practice medicine available.

REFERENCES

1. Siegel RL, Miller KD, Jemal A. Cancer statistics, 2016. CA Cancer J Clin 2016; 66(1):7–30.
2. Cancer of the breast (female) - Cancer stat facts. Available at: https://seer.cancer. gov/statfacts/html/breast.html. Accessed October 8, 2017.
3. Inwald EC, Ortmann O, Koller M, et al. Screening-relevant age threshold of 70 years and older is a stronger determinant for the choice of adjuvant treatment in breast cancer patients than tumor biology. Breast Cancer Res Treat 2017;163(1):119–30.
4. Lohr KN, editor. Medicare: A strategy for quality assurance: Volume 1. Chapter 3, The elderly population. Washington, DC: National Academies Press (US); 1990. p. 69–95. Available at: https://www.ncbi.nlm.nih.gov/books/NBK235450/. Accessed October 8, 2017.
5. WHO | Proposed working definition of an older person in Africa for the MDS Project. WHO. Available at: http://www.who.int/healthinfo/survey/ageingdefnolder/en/. Accessed October 8, 2017.
6. Calculators: life expectancy. Available at: https://www-ssa-gov.ucsf.idm.oclc.org/ planners/lifeexpectancy.html. Accessed October 9, 2017.
7. Forster AS, Forbes LJL, Abraham C, et al. Promoting early presentation of breast cancer: a preliminary evaluation of a written intervention. Chronic Illn 2014;10(1): 18–30.
8. Montroni I, Rocchi M, Santini D, et al. Has breast cancer in the elderly remained the same over recent decades? A comparison of two groups of patients 70 years or older treated for breast cancer twenty years apart. J Geriatr Oncol 2014;5(3): 260–5.
9. Richards P, Ward S, Morgan J, et al. The use of surgery in the treatment of ER+ early stage breast cancer in England: variation by time, age and patient characteristics. Eur J Surg Oncol 2016;42(4):489–96.
10. Mustacchi G, Cazzaniga ME, Pronzato P, et al. Breast cancer in elderly women: a different reality? Results from the NORA study. Ann Oncol 2007;18(6):991–6.
11. Sierink JC, de Castro SMM, Russell NS, et al. Treatment strategies in elderly breast cancer patients: is there a need for surgery? Breast 2014;23(6):793–8.
12. Dimitrakopoulos F-ID, Kottorou A, Antonacopoulou AG, et al. Early-stage breast cancer in the elderly: confronting an old clinical problem. J Breast Cancer 2015;18(3):207–17.

13. Gosain R, Pollock Y, Jain D. Age-related disparity: breast cancer in the elderly. Curr Oncol Rep 2016;18(11):69.
14. Tang S-W, Parker H, Winterbottom L, et al. Early primary breast cancer in the elderly - pattern of presentation and treatment. Surg Oncol 2011;20(1):7–12.
15. Breast cancer screening in older women. Available at: http://www.mdedge.com/clinicianreviews/article/72084/geriatrics/breast-cancer-screening-older-women. Accessed September 25, 2017.
16. Independent UK. Panel on breast cancer screening. The benefits and harms of breast cancer screening: an independent review. Lancet 2012;380(9855): 1778–86.
17. p659.pdf. Available at: http://www.aafp.org/afp/2016/0415/p659.pdf. Accessed August 21, 2017.
18. Raffin E, Onega T, Bynum J, et al. Are there regional tendencies toward controversial screening practices? A study of prostate and breast cancer screening in a Medicare population. Cancer Epidemiol 2017;50(Pt A):68–75.
19. Paesmans M, Ameye L, Moreau M, et al. Breast cancer screening in the older woman: an effective way to reduce mortality? Maturitas 2010;66(3):263–7.
20. Jatoi I. Breast cancer screening recommendations. JAMA 2013;310(19):2101–2.
21. Breast cancer screening. National Cancer Institute. Available at: https://www.cancer.gov/types/breast/hp/breast-screening-pdq. Accessed October 5, 2017.
22. Elmore JG, Barton MB, Moceri VM, et al. Ten-year risk of false positive screening mammograms and clinical breast examinations. N Engl J Med 1998;338(16): 1089–96.
23. Esserman LJ, WISDOM Study and Athena Investigators. The WISDOM study: breaking the deadlock in the breast cancer screening debate. NPJ Breast Cancer 2017;3:34.
24. ePrognosis. Available at: https://eprognosis.ucsf.edu/. Accessed October 16, 2017.
25. sect_04_breast.pdf. Available at: https://seer.cancer.gov/csr/1975_2014/results_merged/sect_04_breast.pdf. Accessed October 6, 2017.
26. Gibreel WO, Day CN, Hoskin TL, et al. Reconstruction for cancer in the elderly: a national cancer data base study. J Am Coll Surg 2017;224(5):895–905.
27. Merrill AY, Brown DR, Klepin HD, et al. Outcomes after mastectomy and lumpectomy in octogenarians and nonagenarians with early-stage breast cancer. Am Surg 2017;83(8):887–94.
28. Lee CM, Zheng H, Tan VK-M, et al. Surgery for early breast cancer in the extremely elderly leads to improved outcomes – an Asian population study. Breast 2017;36(Supplement C):44–8.
29. Aiello Bowles EJ, Feigelson HS, Barney T, et al. Improving quality of breast cancer surgery through development of a national breast cancer surgical outcomes (BRCASO) research database. BMC Cancer 2012;12:136.
30. Pettke E, Ilonzo N, Ayewah M, et al. Short-term, postoperative breast cancer outcomes in patients with advanced age. Am J Surg 2016;212(4):677–81.
31. Kummerow KL, Du L, Penson DF, et al. Nationwide trends in mastectomy for early-stage breast cancer. JAMA Surg 2015;150(1):9–16.
32. Fisher B, Jeong J-H, Anderson S, et al. Twenty-five-year follow-up of a randomized trial comparing radical mastectomy, total mastectomy, and total mastectomy followed by irradiation. N Engl J Med 2002;347(8):567–75.
33. Martelli G, Miceli R, Daidone MG, et al. Axillary dissection versus no axillary dissection in elderly patients with breast cancer and no palpable axillary nodes: results after 15 years of follow-up. Ann Surg Oncol 2011;18(1):125–33.

34. Liang S, Hallet J, Simpson JS, et al. Omission of axillary staging in elderly patients with early stage breast cancer impacts regional control but not survival: a systematic review and meta-analysis. J Geriatr Oncol 2017;8(2):140–7.

35. International Breast Cancer Study Group, Rudenstam CM, Zahrieh D, Forbes JF, et al. Randomized trial comparing axillary clearance versus no axillary clearance in older patients with breast cancer: first results of International Breast Cancer Study Group Trial 10-93. J Clin Oncol 2006;24(3):337–44.

36. Martelli G, Boracchi P, Orenti A, et al. Axillary dissection versus no axillary dissection in older T1N0 breast cancer patients: 15-year results of trial and out-trial patients. Eur J Surg Oncol 2014;40(7):805–12.

37. Krag DN, Anderson SJ, Julian TB, et al. Sentinel-lymph-node resection compared with conventional axillary-lymph-node dissection in clinically node-negative patients with breast cancer: overall survival findings from the NSABP B-32 randomised phase 3 trial. Lancet Oncol 2010;11(10):927–33.

38. Hughes KS, Schnaper LA, Bellon JR, et al. Lumpectomy plus tamoxifen with or without irradiation in women age 70 years or older with early breast cancer: long-term follow-up of CALGB 9343. J Clin Oncol 2013;31(19):2382–7.

39. Chagpar AB, Hatzis C, Pusztai L, et al. Association of LN evaluation with survival in women aged 70 years or older with clinically node-negative hormone receptor positive breast cancer. Ann Surg Oncol 2017;24(10):3073–81.

40. Welsh JL, Hoskin TL, Day CN, et al. Predicting nodal positivity in women 70 years of age and older with hormone receptor-positive breast cancer to aid incorporation of a society of surgical oncology choosing wisely guideline into clinical practice. Ann Surg Oncol 2017;24(10):2881–8.

41. Wink CJ, Woensdregt K, Nieuwenhuijzen GA, et al. Hormone treatment without surgery for patients aged 75 years or older with operable breast cancer. Ann Surg Oncol 2012;19(4):1185–91.

42. Chakrabarti J, Kenny FS, Syed BM, et al. A randomised trial of mastectomy only versus tamoxifen for treating elderly patients with operable primary breast cancer-final results at 20-year follow-up. Crit Rev Oncol Hematol 2011;78(3): 260–4.

43. Hind D, Wyld L, Reed MW. Surgery, with or without tamoxifen, vs tamoxifen alone for older women with operable breast cancer: Cochrane review. Br J Cancer 2007;96(7):1025–9.

44. Kunkler IH, Williams LJ, Jack WJL, et al. PRIME II investigators. Breast-conserving surgery with or without irradiation in women aged 65 years or older with early breast cancer (PRIME II): a randomised controlled trial. Lancet Oncol 2015;16(3):266–73.

45. Haque W, Kee Yuan DM, Verma V, et al. Radiation therapy utilization and outcomes for older women with breast cancer: impact of molecular subtype and tumor grade. Breast 2017;35:34–41.

46. Fyles AW, McCready DR, Manchul LA, et al. Tamoxifen with or without breast irradiation in women 50 years of age or older with early breast cancer. N Engl J Med 2004;351(10):963–70.

47. Fisher B, Dignam J, Bryant J, et al. Five versus more than five years of tamoxifen therapy for breast cancer patients with negative lymph nodes and estrogen receptor-positive tumors. J Natl Cancer Inst 1996;88(21):1529–42.

48. Dowsett M, Cuzick J, Ingle J, et al. Meta-analysis of breast cancer outcomes in adjuvant trials of aromatase inhibitors versus tamoxifen. J Clin Oncol 2010; 28(3):509–18.

49. Regan MM, Neven P, Giobbie-Hurder A, et al. Assessment of letrozole and tamoxifen alone and in sequence for postmenopausal women with steroid hormone receptor-positive breast cancer: the BIG 1-98 randomised clinical trial at 8·1 years median follow-up. Lancet Oncol 2011;12(12):1101–8.

50. Amir E, Seruga B, Niraula S, et al. Toxicity of adjuvant endocrine therapy in post-menopausal breast cancer patients: a systematic review and meta-analysis. J Natl Cancer Inst 2011;103(17):1299–309.

51. Muss HB, Tu D, Ingle JN, et al. Efficacy, toxicity, and quality of life in older women with early-stage breast cancer treated with letrozole or placebo after 5 years of tamoxifen: NCIC CTG intergroup trial MA.17. J Clin Oncol 2008; 26(12):1956–64.

52. Fietz T, Zahn M-O, Köhler A, et al. Routine treatment and outcome of breast cancer in younger versus elderly patients: results from the SENORA project of the prospective German TMK cohort study. Breast Cancer Res Treat 2018;167(2):567–78.

53. Cadoo KA, Morris PG, Cowell EP, et al. Adjuvant chemotherapy and trastuzumab is safe and effective in older women with small, node-negative, HER2-positive early-stage breast cancer. Clin Breast Cancer 2016;16(6):487–93.

54. Reeder-Hayes KE, Meyer AM, Hinton SP, et al. Comparative toxicity and effectiveness of trastuzumab-based chemotherapy regimens in older women with early-stage breast cancer. J Clin Oncol 2017;35(29):3298–305.

55. Elkin EB, Hurria A, Mitra N, et al. Adjuvant chemotherapy and survival in older women with hormone receptor-negative breast cancer: assessing outcome in a population-based, observational cohort. J Clin Oncol 2006;24(18):2757–64.

56. Sostelly A, Henin E, Chauvenet L, et al. Can we predict chemo-induced hemato-toxicity in elderly patients treated with pegylated liposomal doxorubicin? Results of a population-based model derived from the DOGMES phase II trial of the GI-NECO. J Geriatr Oncol 2013;4(1):48–57.

57. Extermann M, Reich RR, Sehovic M. Chemotoxicity recurrence in older patients: risk factors and effectiveness of preventive strategies-a prospective study. Cancer 2015;121(17):2984–92.

58. Karuturi M, VanderWalde N, Muss H. Approach and management of breast cancer in the elderly. Clin Geriatr Med 2016;32(1):133–53.

59. Albain KS, Barlow WE, Shak S, et al. Prognostic and predictive value of the 21-gene recurrence score assay in postmenopausal women with node-positive, oestrogen-receptor-positive breast cancer on chemotherapy: a retrospective analysis of a randomised trial. Lancet Oncol 2010;11(1):55–65.

60. Sparano JA, Gray RJ, Makower DF, et al. Prospective validation of a 21-gene expression assay in breast cancer. N Engl J Med 2015;373(21):2005–14.

61. Esserman LJ, Yau C, Thompson CK, et al. Use of molecular tools to identify patients with indolent breast cancers with ultralow risk over 2 decades. JAMA Oncol 2017;3(11):1503–10.

62. Kearney N, Miller M. Elderly patients with cancer: an ethical dilemma. Crit Rev Oncol Hematol 2000;33(2):149–54.

63. Capocaccia R, Gatta G, Dal Maso L. Life expectancy of colon, breast, and testicular cancer patients: an analysis of US-SEER population-based data. Ann Oncol 2015;26(6):1263–8.

64. Albrand G, Terret C. Early breast cancer in the elderly: assessment and management considerations. Drugs Aging 2008;25(1):35–45.

65. Yousef GM, Sovani P, Devabhaktuni S, et al. Screening mammograms in Alzheimer's disease patients. W V Med J 2012;108(3):92–5.

66. Raik BL, Miller FG, Fins JJ. Screening and cognitive impairment: ethics of forgoing mammography in older women. J Am Geriatr Soc 2004;52(3):440–4.

67. Collins K, Reed M, Lifford K, et al. Bridging the age gap in breast cancer: evaluation of decision support interventions for older women with operable breast cancer: protocol for a cluster randomised controlled trial. BMJ Open 2017;7(7): e015133.

68. Weijer C, Freedman B, Shapiro S, et al. Assessing the interpretation of criteria for clinical trial eligibility: a survey of oncology investigators. Clin Invest Med 1998; 21(1):17–26.

Evolution of Operative Technique for Mastectomy

Caroline Jones, MD, MSPH[a], Rachael Lancaster, MD[b],*

KEYWORDS

- Mastectomy • Technique • Nipple-sparing mastectomy • Breast cancer

KEY POINTS

- For the majority of the twentieth century, radical or modified radical mastectomy was the recommended mastectomy for surgical treatment of breast cancer.
- However, research has shown that extensive surgical resection does not improve survival breast cancer patients and therefore the surgical mastectomy has evolved.
- Today, the majority of patients can undergo nipple or skin sparing mastectomies, offering patients improved cosmetic results without oncologic compromise.

INTRODUCTION

Approximately 252,710 women and 2470 men in the United States were diagnosed in 2017 with invasive breast cancer. The mainstay of the treatment of breast cancer continues to be surgical: breast-conserving surgery, typically with adjuvant radiation, or mastectomy. Increasing numbers of patients eligible for breast-conserving therapy (BCT) are choosing to undergo mastectomy and breast reconstruction.[1] Today, nearly 40% of all women undergo mastectomy for breast cancer.[2] Recently, there has also been a trend of BCT-eligible patients choosing mastectomy and prophylactic mastectomy.[3] Also, as more genetic mutations have been identified that increase a woman's risk of breast cancer, mastectomy provides an opportunity for breast cancer prevention for mutation carriers.

Today, survival rates are the highest ever with more than 6 million people worldwide alive 5 years after their diagnosis.[3] Ever-increasing in number, survivors of breast cancer appropriately desire to return to a sense of normalcy as soon as possible; minimization of surgical scars and maximization of cosmetic results facilitates this return. Disfiguring surgeries are a daily reminder to patients of their struggle with breast

Disclosure: The authors have nothing to disclose.
[a] Department of Surgery, University of Alabama Birmingham, 1922 7th Avenue South KB 217, Birmingham, AL 35294, USA; [b] Department of Surgery, Division of Surgical Oncology, University of Alabama Birmingham, 510 20th Street South FOT 1153, Birmingham, AL 35233, USA
* Corresponding author.
E-mail address: rlancaster@uabmc.edu

cancer. As a consequence, surgeons have increasingly sought to maximize cosmetic results without compromising oncologic outcomes; as a result, the mastectomy has evolved over time.

HISTORICAL BACKGROUND

The Edwin Smith Papyrus, dating back to 3000 BC, contains the first known reference to breast cancer. Among 48 accounts of injuries, wounds, and tumors, it describes a case of "swellings on breast, large, spreading and hard: touching them is like touching a ball of bandages."[4] When addressing possible treatment, the investigator notes, "there is nothing."[3] In 400 BC, Hippocrates began to conjecture the causes of many medical ailments and hypothesized that breast cancer was due to having an excess of black bile. Galen of Rome promoted ridding the body of this black bile by allowing surgical wounds to bleed freely. Leonides of Alexandria, a physician of ancient Greece, performed the first operation for breast cancer using the escharotomy method, which involved alternating incision and cautery. During the Renaissance, John Hunter, the Scottish father of investigative surgery, replaced Hippocrates' black bile theory with the theory that lymph was the cause of breast cancer.[5] In the 1800s, the causes of breast cancer remained poorly understood. Surgeries were often fatal, largely because of sepsis; debate raged on whether breast cancer was an infectious disease whose spread was only quickened by surgery or whether surgery was the best hope for cure.[6] Early theories, investigations, and surgeries laid the framework for the modern era of surgical treatment of breast cancer, which was led by Dr William Halsted.

RADICAL MASTECTOMY
History

In 1882 at the Roosevelt Hospital in New York City, Dr William Stewart Halsted introduced the radical mastectomy (RM) using new techniques of anesthesia, aseptic, and antiseptic.[7] Halsted[8] went on to publish his experiences at Johns Hopkins Hospital in November 1894. Willie Meyer of the New York Graduate School of Medicine independently performed the RM in 1884 and published his technique merely 10 days after Halsted's article.[9] The Halsted mastectomy, as it became known, was an aggressive surgery aimed at achieving local control under the premise that cancer spreads centrifugally from the breast to the pectoralis muscles and regional lymph nodes first, followed by more distant sites.[10] Morbidities included large wounds that were left to heal by granulation, nearly universal lymphedema, and severely restricted arm movement, all of which led to chronic pain syndrome. However, because surgeons more than a century ago were faced with large cancers that seemed to require extreme treatment for a chance of cure, postoperative complications were of little consideration.[10] Despite this aggressive approach, survival rates improved but remained poor, ranging from 13% to 40% at 5 years.[11] RM remained the gold standard for breast cancer through much of the twentieth century and was performed on more than 90% of patients with breast cancer in the United States until the 1970s, with local and regional recurrence rates of 6% and 22%, respectively.[12,13]

Extended Radical Mastectomies

Some furthered the Halsted-Meyer theory that breast cancer disseminated through the lymphatic system by advocating for extended RMs. From 1920 Samson Handley performed an extended RM that included removing the internal mammary chain lymph nodes and placing radium needles into the anterior intercostal spaces for additional treatment. In the 1950s, Urban at New York's Memorial Sloan-Kettering Hospital performed a massive operation combining RM with resection of the internal mammary chain en bloc, costal cartilage, and intercostal muscles. These operations were based on the theory that cure rates could be increased by performing wider surgical resections.[10] After studies failed to show a survival advantage with this technique, it was abandoned.[6]

Indications

Today, RM is performed in select cases (0.05% of all mastectomies) to achieve locoregional control of the breast, axilla, and chest wall. Indications include advanced locoregional disease with fixation to the pectoralis major muscle that is refractory to chemoradiation; advanced locoregional disease with skin ulceration that is refractory to chemoradiation; recurrent, advanced locoregional disease following partial mastectomy with tumor fixated to pectoralis major muscle; recurrent, advanced locoregional disease after modified or segmental mastectomy with tumor invading the chest wall that is refractory to chemotherapy; and advanced high-lying lesions near the clavicle or sternum with muscle fixation.[14]

Operative Principles

The principles of RM include wide excision of skin, resection of both pectoral muscles, axillary dissection (levels I, II, III), resection of all tissue en bloc, and routine sacrifice of the long thoracic nerve and the thoracodorsal artery, nerve, and vein.[11]

Limits of the RM dissection are defined by clavicle superiorly, latissimus dorsi laterally, sternum medially, and aponeurosis of the rectus abdominus tendon inferiorly. The pectoralis major is transected at insertion on the humerus followed by cranial clavicular attachments. The pectoralis minor is divided at its insertion on the coracoid process of the scapula. Finally, the pectoralis major is divided from its medial origin at the costosternal junction of ribs 2 to 6 and pectoralis minor from ribs 2 to 5. Breast, muscles, and lymph nodes are removed en bloc. The large defect can be closed with a split-thickness skin graft, temporary biological dressings, or a wound vacuum with negative-pressure wound therapy.[11]

Complications

The extensive resection leads to several associated morbidities, including need for skin grafting, paresthesias, denervation of the serratus or latissimus muscles, rib cartilage damage, pneumothoraces, and lymphedema of the arm.[7]

Lymphedema is a dreaded complication of breast cancer surgery. It can lead to functional, aesthetic, and psychological problems. It also predisposes patients to infections, decreased functional ability, and potential development of malignant lymphangiosarcoma (Stewart-Treves syndrome). It adversely affects quality of life, job performance, and health care costs.[11]

MODIFIED RADICAL MASTECTOMY
History

In 1932 at the Middlesex Hospital in London, D.H. Patey first performed a mastectomy that preserved the pectoralis major muscle. This surgery improved cosmesis and was associated with less pain, lymphedema, and upper limb mobility limitation. Patey adopted this reduced mastectomy as his standard procedure in 1936. Patey and W.H. Dyson[15] described the technique in their 1948 article and reported no difference in survival or local recurrence rates between the gold standard RM and their reduced mastectomy.

In 1972, John Madden and colleagues[16] introduced the modified RM (MRM), proposing the preservation of both the pectoralis major and minor muscles.[17] Whereas Patey argued that complete axillary dissection was not possible if the pectoralis minor was preserved, Madden and colleagues[16] showed it was possible to both clear the axilla and preserve the pectoralis minor's neurovascular supply with his procedure.[16] Auchincloss[18] also advocated for the MRM and additionally suggested that level III lymph nodes only be removed when clinically involved.

The MRM became more widely accepted after the National Surgical Adjuvant Breast and Bowel B-04 clinical trial showed no survival advantage when compared with the RM in the 1970s.[19] In 1979, The Consensus Development Conference on the treatment of breast cancer stated that the MRM was the standard of treatment of women with stage I and II breast cancer.[11]

Indications

Today MRMs are performed in the setting of inflammatory breast cancer or locally advanced breast carcinoma with known axillary disease. In this setting, breast reconstruction would typically occur in a delayed manner after patients have completed adjuvant therapies.

Operative Principles

The principles of the MRM include en bloc resection of the breast, NAC, axillary lymphatics (levels I and II with preservation of level III nodes unless clinically involved), and skin overlying the tumor.[11]

The skin and breast are removed along with the pectoralis fascia, but the pectoralis muscles are spared as opposed to the RM. Level I and level II nodes are removed in a cranial to caudal fashion.[14] In select cases of clinically positive level III nodes, the pectoralis minor can be resected by dividing its attachments to the coracoid process.

Complications

MRM has less morbidity than the RM. Skin can be closed primarily. Serratus and latissimus muscles remain innervated with careful attention at identifying and preserving the long thoracic thoracodorsal and neurovascular bundles. Risk of lymphedema is reduced compared with RM, and early onset rehabilitation with range-of-motion exercises provides improvement in shoulder mobility.[14] However, lymphedema still frequently occurs after an axillary lymph node dissection. Breast reconstruction can still be performed after an MRM; however, this typically occurs in a delayed fashion. With less skin available for breast reconstruction, tissue expanders or autologous myocutaneous flaps may be used.

SIMPLE OR TOTAL MASTECTOMY

As sentinel lymph node surgery became increasingly used, the need for axillary dissection with an MRM became less frequently indicated. Therefore, when a mastectomy is performed today without axillary dissection or without immediate breast reconstruction, a simple mastectomy is typically performed. The operative resection of the breast includes the same anatomic borders as previously described with resection of the underlying pectoral fascia. The NAC is resected with surrounding breast skin with typical incisions made in an elliptical manner. Adequate breast skin should remain to facilitate skin closure.

SKIN-SPARING MASTECTOMY
History

Toth and Lappert[20] first coined the term *skin-sparing mastectomy* (SSM) in 1991. Instead of removing a large ellipse of skin, the SSM procedure removes the breast while preserving the skin envelope.[21] The skin incision includes the nipple-areola complex (NAC) and should be amenable for axillary dissection.[20] This technique allows better breast shape after reconstruction, reduces the area of skin necessary on myocutaneous flaps, and reduces the need for contralateral breast surgery to achieve symmetry.[22] SSM has become increasingly popular by facilitating immediate breast reconstruction.[23]

Indications and Contraindications

Indications for SSM include multicentric disease; invasive carcinoma associated with an extensive intraductal component; extensive ductal carcinoma in situ (DCIS) not amenable to breast conservation; invasive disease not amenable to breast conservation because of size; tumor that extends to and involves the NAC; breast cancer prevention in high-risk patients; or women with breast cancer or DCIS who are ineligible for radiation therapy. Furthermore, if nipple preservation cannot be performed because of breast ptosis, large breast size, then SSM offers a viable option for mastectomy in these patients.

Skin involvement with tumor that cannot be resected with small extension of the SSM incision would be a contraindication. Other considerations and possible contraindications include previous breast or chest irradiation, adjuvant radiation, smoking, high body mass index (BMI), and delayed reconstruction.[24]

Operative Considerations

SSM's skin incision is more limited compared with MRM or simple mastectomy and typically involves a circular incision at the areola border, thereby excising the NAC. Skin flaps are created with excision of the underlying breast tissue, and skin flap viability is important to facilitate breast reconstruction. Preservation of the skin envelope facilitates preservation of the inframammary fold and enhanced overall breast shape. Furthermore, the circular scar at the areolar border ultimately becomes more hidden in the future with nipple reconstruction or nipple tattooing. The incision can allow access to the axilla for lymph node biopsy or dissection. At times the incision may require extension to facilitate exposure to the axilla.

Complications of SSM include infection, hematoma, and skin flap necrosis. Risk factors for skin flap necrosis include smoking, previous or adjuvant breast irradiation, diabetes, and high BMI.

NIPPLE-SPARING MASTECTOMY
History

Nipple preservation in the setting of mastectomy was described in 1990.[25] However, widespread acceptance of nipple-sparing mastectomy (NSM) by surgeons was prolonged because of initial concerns regarding local recurrence and procedure complications. In 2003, Gerber and colleagues[26] showed that SSM with conservation of the NAC was an oncologically safe procedure in patients with tumors distant from the nipple. Initially patients with tumors to 2 cm or greater away from the nipple by mammogram or ultrasound were considered eligible for this procedure.[26] However, with extension of eligibility criteria for NSM for patients, NSMs have increased in popularity significantly in recent years. Analysis of Surveillance, Epidemiology, and End

Results (SEER) data shows an almost 7-fold increase in the number of NSM mastectomies performed.[27] Although many refer to this procedure as NSM, many surgeons prefer calling this procedure a total SSM (TSSM) because the entirety of the breast skin envelope is preserved, including the nipple areolar skin, whereas the underlying breast tissue including ductal tissue extending into the nipple is excised.

Indications and Contraindications

Contraindications to NSM include clinical or imaging evidence of tumor or disease involvement of the NAC, locally advanced tumors with skin involvement, and inflammatory breast cancer.[28] Additional concerns and possible contraindications include large ptotic breasts, active smokers, uncontrolled diabetes, or other immunosuppressive therapy that could complicate wound healing.

However, many women without nipple involvement with disease are eligible for this procedure. Women who have axillary involvement with invasive disease have a history of breast radiation or who will require postoperative radiation are still candidates for nipple preservation. Women who initially present with stage II or III breast cancer who undergo NAC with a good response are increasingly eligible for TSSM. There is no specific tumor size that is a contraindication. Furthermore, previous requirements of a certain distance from tumor to nipple are no longer relevant.[28,29] However, obtainment of a negative tumor margin at the nipple remains key.

Operative Considerations

An NSM or TSSM involves the removal of the entirety of the breast tissue, including ductal tissue at the NAC, but with preservation of the nipple-areolar dermal layer. Therefore, the skin envelope of the breast is left intact and facilitates breast reconstruction. Incisions for NSM vary among surgical practices but include crescentic mastopexy, inframammary fold, peri-areolar with or without a radial extension, vertical, or inferolateral. Peri-areolar incisions should be maintained to less than one-third of the circumference of the NAC to decrease the risk of nipple loss.[30] Inframammary or inferolateral incisions are frequently approximately 10 cm in length but can be less to facilitate adequate exposure.[31]

NSMs are more technically challenging because the surgeon needs to complete the same oncologic procedure through a smaller incision or a more peripheral incision. Surgeon fatigue and strain has been reported to be greater with NSM compared with SSM due to the inherent increase in technical challenges with this procedure,.[32] Exposure of the breast tissue in this small and deep space can be challenging. A light source (whether lighted retractor or headlight), retractors, and other low-profile instruments with sufficient length are crucial in the success of this technique.[31]

Dissection of the retro-areolar ductal tissue from the areolar skin is a key step. Many perform dissection of the breast tissue both medial and lateral to the NAC before dissection of the nipple tissue at the ductal dermal junction to facilitate optimal exposure. The nipple margin, frequently excised sharply, should be labeled to enable pathologic evaluation of this margin. Histologic evaluation of the nipple margin can be accomplished by frozen section; however, many prefer permanent section for this assessment.[31] Frozen section is known to be less accurate than permanent section. Furthermore, although nipple or areolar resection in the setting of a positive margin would require an additional operation, this operation is relatively minor and can be accomplished without general anesthesia.

Skin flap and nipple viability relies on adequate blood supply. Because the nipple skin vascular supply will be limited to breast skin cutaneous branches, preservation of these branches is important in ensuring nipple and skin flap viability. Dissection in the correct anatomic plane within the Cooper ligaments is critical and will yield skin flaps of varying thickness between patients and even within a single breast. Minimizing tension on skin flaps is also key, as persistent tension can lead to flap compromise.

Oncologic Safety

Previously, the surgical field had concerns regarding the oncologic safety of the NSM. However, as patients undergoing prophylactic mastectomy or mastectomy for early stage breast cancers began having NSM with increasingly good outcomes, the eligibility for NSM increased. Previously discussed contraindications to NSM certainly remain; however, the previously required tumor-to-nipple distance seems to be decreasing, with many surgeons now considering the nipple another surgical margin. Many surgeons now consider a negative nipple margin as adequate.[28,33] Certainly, a tumor present at the nipple margin requires resection of the nipple.[31]

High-risk patients with BRCA mutations frequently desire prophylactic mastectomy for breast cancer risk reduction, and evaluating the NSM within this population has been shown to be oncologically safe. Although the follow-up was at short intervals at 34 and 56 months, BRCA1 and BRCA2 carriers were shown to have persistent risk reduction in breast cancer events after NSM across multiple institutions.[34] A systemic review, again with limited follow-up to 2 years, showed a risk of locoregional recurrence rate of 2.8% when evaluating 3331 NSMs.[35] A single-institution study evaluated the risk of local recurrence in a high-risk population (N = 210, 49% underwent neoadjuvant chemotherapy; N = 78, 18.2% underwent adjuvant chemotherapy), and the observed risk of locoregional recurrence was shown to be 2.4% in patients with at least a 3-year follow-up.[33] Using the SEER database from 1998 to 2013, those who underwent NSM for breast cancer showed a 5- and 10-year overall survival of 94.1% and 88.0%, respectively. The 5- and 10-year cancer-specific survival for this group was 96.9% and 94.9%, respectively.[27] Certainly, continued follow-up of this patient population will prove insightful; but thus far the NSM does not show evidence of oncologic compromise.

Complications

Ischemic complications involving the NAC can occur in varying degrees, with complete necrosis leading to nipple loss occurring in about 2.0% of cases and partial nipple necrosis occurring in 9.1% of cases.[35] Partial-thickness necrosis of the nipple can be treated conservatively with topical agents and will typically heal without complication. Complete nipple loss due to necrosis can lead to infection and implant loss.[31] Radiation therapy either administered adjuvantly or a history of previous breast or chest radiation certainly increases the risk of ischemic complications.[36] However, the treatment with radiation therapy should not be a contraindication to NSM; but knowledge of this increased risk should inform the surgical preoperative discussion with patients. Necrosis of the skin flap occurs in just less than 10% of cases.[35] Positive nipple margin is an additional risk of this procedure and should result in nipple resection. If the nipple resection is positive for carcinoma, then areolar resection typically follows.[31] Risk of infection is also present with this procedure; certainly infection in the setting of implant increases the risk of implant loss.

CONTRALATERAL PROPHYLACTIC MASTECTOMY
History

In 1991, the National Cancer Institute Consensus Conference endorsed BCT for early stage breast cancer based on results from prospective randomized trials showing equivalent survival rates when compared with mastectomy.[37] In spite of this endorsement, contralateral prophylactic mastectomy (CPM) rates doubled for all stages of breast cancer in the United States from 1998 through 2003. This trend continued, and by 2005 the rate of CPM was 24%.[38] Rates of BCT also increased, indicating that patients are choosing minimal surgery (lumpectomy) and more aggressive surgery (bilateral mastectomies) over unilateral mastectomy.[39]

Indications

Indications for CPM include risk reduction of contralateral breast cancer; reconstructive considerations, including symmetry and balance; and patients with difficult surveillance due to a mammographically occult cancer, dense breasts, or cystic breasts that are difficult to examine.[40]

Factors Associated with Decision for Contralateral Prophylactic Mastectomy

Women who choose to undergo CPM are younger, have higher levels of education and private health insurance, and are more likely to be treated at comprehensive cancer centers or teaching facilities. They are more likely to have undergone genetic testing, even if that testing is negative.[38] When asked why they choose CPM, many women cite emotional reasons. They desire peace of mind and freedom from recurrence. Without CPM, the risk of contralateral breast cancer at 10 years is 4% to 5% in all patients and 40% in patients who are BRCA positive.[41,42] CPM decreases the risk by about 90%.[42] However, it is important for the surgeon to educate patients that the risk is not eliminated. In addition, improvements in disease-specific survival have been inconclusive; the 2010 Cochrane Database Review was unable to conclude that CPM improved survival.[43]

Complications and Pitfalls

Surgery is one form of risk reduction, but bilateral mastectomies do not offer absolute protection against the development of breast cancer. Discussion should address alternative approaches, including close surveillance and other risk-reduction strategies. In addition, full disclosure of risks is important. The overall complication rate of bilateral mastectomies with reconstruction is 20%.[42] These complications include increased risk of superficial nipple necrosis, wound breakdown, and implant exposure.[44]

SUMMARY

The mastectomy technique has evolved from Halsted's morbid RM to the technically more demanding NSM. These new mastectomy techniques offer results that are oncologically equivalent to older operations but allow for immediate breast reconstruction with good aesthetic results.

REFERENCES

1. Kummerow KL, Du L, Penson DF, et al. Nationwide trends in mastectomy for early-stage breast cancer. JAMA Surg 2015;150(1):9–16.
2. Habermann EB, Abbott A, Parsons HM, et al. Are mastectomy rates really increasing in the United States? J Clin Oncol 2010;28(21):3437–41.
3. Tauxe W. A tumour through time. Nature 2015;527(7578):S102–3.
4. Muller T, Baratte A, Bruant-Rodier C, et al. Oncological safety of nipple-sparing prophylactic mastectomy: a review of the literature on 3716 cases. Ann Chir Plast Esthet 2017. https://doi.org/10.1016/j.anplas.2017.09.005.

5. Lakhtakia R. A brief history of breast cancer: part I: surgical domination reinvented. Sultan Qaboos Univ Med J 2014;14(2):e166–9.
6. Borgen P. Breast cancer in the 20 century: quest for the ideal therapy. Ochsner J 2000;2(1):5–9.
7. Plesca M, Bordea C, El Houcheimi B, et al. Evolution of radical mastectomy for breast cancer. J Med Life 2016;9(2):183–6.
8. Halsted WS. I. The results of operations for the cure of cancer of the breast performed at the Johns Hopkins Hospital from June, 1889, to January, 1894. Ann Surg 1894;20(5):497–555.
9. Staunton MD, Melville DM, Monterrosa A, et al. A 25-year prospective study of modified radical mastectomy (Patey) in 193 patients. J R Soc Med 1993;86(7): 381–4.
10. Zurrida S, Bassi F, Arnone P, et al. The changing face of mastectomy (from mutilation to aid to breast reconstruction). Int J Surg Oncol 2011;2011:980158.
11. Bland KI, Copeland EM, Klimberg VS, et al. The breast: comprehensive management of benign and malignant diseases. 5th edition. Philadelphia: Elsevier; 2018.
12. Consensus statement: treatment of early-stage breast cancer. National Institutes of Health Consensus Development Panel. J Natl Cancer Inst Monogr 1992;(11):1–5.
13. Halsted WS. I. The results of radical operations for the cure of carcinoma of the breast. Ann Surg 1907;46(1):1–19.
14. Bland KI, Klimberg VS. Breast surgery. Master techniques in general surgery. Philadelphia: Wolters Kluwer Health/Lippincott Williams & Wilkins; 2011. p. 555, xv.
15. Patey DH, Dyson WH. The prognosis of carcinoma of the breast in relation to the type of operation performed. Br J Cancer 1948;2(1):7–13.
16. Madden JL, Kandalaft S, Bourque RA. Modified radical mastectomy. Ann Surg 1972;175(5):624–34.
17. Scanlon EF, Caprini JA. Modified radical mastectomy. Cancer 1975;35(3):710–3.
18. Auchincloss H. Modified radical mastectomy: why not? Am J Surg 1970;119(5): 506–9.
19. Fisher B, Jeong JH, Anderson S, et al. Twenty-five-year follow-up of a randomized trial comparing radical mastectomy, total mastectomy, and total mastectomy followed by irradiation. N Engl J Med 2002;347(8):567–75.
20. Toth BA, Lappert P. Modified skin incisions for mastectomy: the need for plastic surgical input in preoperative planning. Plast Reconstr Surg 1991;87(6):1048–53.
21. Carlson GW. Skin sparing mastectomy: anatomic and technical considerations. Am Surg 1996;62(2):151–5.
22. Patani N, Mokbel K. Oncological and aesthetic considerations of skin-sparing mastectomy. Breast Cancer Res Treat 2008;111(3):391–403.
23. Cunnick GH, Mokbel K. Skin-sparing mastectomy. Am J Surg 2004;188(1):78–84.
24. Carlson GW, Bostwick J 3rd, Styblo TM, et al. Skin-sparing mastectomy. Oncologic and reconstructive considerations. Ann Surg 1997;225(5):570–5 [discussion: 575–8].
25. Bishop CC, Singh S, Nash AG. Mastectomy and breast reconstruction preserving the nipple. Ann R Coll Surg Engl 1990;72(2):87–9.
26. Gerber B, Krause A, Reimer T, et al. Skin-sparing mastectomy with conservation of the nipple-areola complex and autologous reconstruction is an oncologically safe procedure. Ann Surg 2003;238(1):120–7.
27. Li M, Chen K, Liu F, et al. Nipple sparing mastectomy in breast cancer patients and long-term survival outcomes: an analysis of the SEER database. PLoS One 2017;12(8):e0183448.

28. Coopey SB, Tang R, Lei L, et al. Increasing eligibility for nipple-sparing mastectomy. Ann Surg Oncol 2013;20(10):3218–22.

29. Wang F, Peled AW, Garwood E, et al. Total skin-sparing mastectomy and immediate breast reconstruction: an evolution of technique and assessment of outcomes. Ann Surg Oncol 2014;21(10):3223–30.

30. Garwood ER, Moore D, Ewing C, et al. Total skin-sparing mastectomy: complications and local recurrence rates in 2 cohorts of patients. Ann Surg 2009;249(1):26–32.

31. Coopey SB, Mitchell SD. Nipple-sparing mastectomy: pitfalls and challenges. Ann Surg Oncol 2017;24(10):2863–8.

32. Jackson RS, Sanders T, Park A, et al. Prospective study comparing surgeons' pain and fatigue associated with nipple-sparing versus skin-sparing mastectomy. Ann Surg Oncol 2017;24(10):3024–31.

33. Warren Peled A, Foster RD, Stover AC, et al. Outcomes after total skin-sparing mastectomy and immediate reconstruction in 657 breasts. Ann Surg Oncol 2012;19(11):3402–9.

34. Jakub JW, Peled Aw, Gray RJ, et al. Oncologic safety of prophylactic nipple-sparing mastectomy in a population with BRCA mutations: a multi-institutional study. JAMA Surg 2018;153(2):123–9.

35. Piper M, Peled AW, Foster RD, et al. Total skin-sparing mastectomy: a systematic review of oncologic outcomes and postoperative complications. Ann Plast Surg 2013;70(4):435–7.

36. Tang R, Coopey SB, Colwell AS, et al. Nipple-sparing mastectomy in irradiated breasts: selecting patients to minimize complications. Ann Surg Oncol 2015;22(10):3331–7.

37. NIH consensus conference. Treatment of early-stage breast cancer. JAMA 1991;265(3):391–5.

38. King TA, Sakr R, Patil S, et al. Clinical management factors contribute to the decision for contralateral prophylactic mastectomy. J Clin Oncol 2011;29(16):2158–64.

39. Tuttle TM, Habermann EB, Grund EH, et al. Increasing use of contralateral prophylactic mastectomy for breast cancer patients: a trend toward more aggressive surgical treatment. J Clin Oncol 2007;25(33):5203–9.

40. Giuliano AE, Boolbol S, Degnim A, et al. Society of Surgical Oncology: position statement on prophylactic mastectomy. Approved by the Society of Surgical Oncology Executive Council, March 2007. Ann Surg Oncol 2007;14(9):2425–7.

41. Early Breast Cancer Trialists' Collaborative, Peto R, Davies C, Godwin J, et al. Comparisons between different polychemotherapy regimens for early breast cancer: meta-analyses of long-term outcome among 100,000 women in 123 randomised trials. Lancet 2012;379(9814):432–44.

42. Burke EE, Portschy PR, Tuttle TM. Prophylactic mastectomy: who needs it, when and why. J Surg Oncol 2015;111(1):91–5.

43. Lostumbo L, Carbine NE, Wallace J. Prophylactic mastectomy for the prevention of breast cancer. Cochrane Database Syst Rev 2010;(11):CD002748.

44. Wang F, Amara D, Peled AW, et al. Negative genetic testing does not deter contralateral prophylactic mastectomy in younger patients with greater family histories of breast cancer. Ann Surg Oncol 2015;22(10):3338–45.

Breast Reconstruction

Hani Sbitany, MD

KEYWORDS

- Breast reconstruction • Oncoplastic breast surgery • Breast implants
- Autologous free flap • Fat grafting • Acellular dermal matrix
- Nipple-sparing mastectomy

KEY POINTS

- Many options exist for postmastectomy and postlumpectomy breast reconstruction.
- Surgeons must present all options to safely offer reconstruction, based on patient preferences and adjuvant treatment effects.
- Postmastectomy reconstruction outcomes have been enhanced, in terms of aesthetics and outcomes, by nipple-sparing mastectomy, autologous fat grafting, acellular dermal matrices, and prepectoral breast reconstruction.
- Reconstructive outcomes are heavily influenced by postmastectomy radiation therapy; in such cases, autologous reconstruction or breast conservation and oncoplastic reconstruction may be preferable.

 Video content accompanies this article at http://www.surgical.theclinics.com.

An estimated 253,000 women in the United States will be diagnosed with invasive breast cancer in 2017, and another 63,000 with in situ breast cancer. Since the federal enactment of the Women's Health and Cancer Right Act in 1998, mandating that all women will have insurance coverage for breast reconstruction, the rates of women seeking these options has increased significantly.[1] In 2016, there were 109,256 breast reconstruction procedures performed in the United States, representing approximately 40% of women undergoing mastectomies, and a 39% increase from 2000.[2]

Breast reconstruction after either mastectomy or breast conservation offers well-documented benefits regarding body image, quality of life, and patient satisfaction.[3–5] This is in large part owing to the advances in surgical techniques, and the multitude of available options for women seeking breast reconstruction after either mastectomy or lumpectomy.

Disclosure Statement: Dr H. Sbitany is a consultant for Allergan, Inc. He received no compensation or support for this article.
Division of Plastic and Reconstructive Surgery, University of California, San Francisco, 505 Parnassus Avenue, Suite M-593, San Francisco, CA 94143, USA
E-mail address: hani.sbitany@ucsf.edu

Surg Clin N Am 98 (2018) 845–857
https://doi.org/10.1016/j.suc.2018.03.011
0039-6109/18/© 2018 Elsevier Inc. All rights reserved.

POSTMASTECTOMY BREAST RECONSTRUCTION

After mastectomy, implant-based breast reconstruction is the most commonly performed option. Either through the traditional 2-stage approach with tissue expansion, or through the single-stage (direct to implant) approach, these options produce highly aesthetic breasts in a multitude of sizes (**Fig. 1**).[6,7]

The immediate placement of a tissue expander or permanent implant at the time of mastectomy is preferable, owing to the ability to use the shape of the breast skin envelope and achieve an improved aesthetic outcome. However, delayed breast reconstruction, after a previously performed mastectomy, is also possible and routinely performed (**Fig. 2**). Tissue expanders and implants, when placed for postmastectomy reconstruction, can be placed in different anatomic planes: fully submuscular (underneath pectoralis major muscle and serratus anterior muscle or fascia), dual plane (under a combination of pectoralis major muscle and acellular dermal matrix [ADM]), or prepectoral (completely covered with ADM).

The major benefits of prosthetic breast reconstruction are the ability for patients to choose the size of their reconstructed breasts, with rapid recovery and return to life/work, owing to avoidance of incorporating other parts of the body as surgical sites. However, for those women looking to avoid foreign bodies, or use a more natural approach to breast reconstruction, autologous breast reconstruction is also an option for most patients. This involves using a combination of skin, fat, and muscle to reconstruct and replace the missing breast tissue and skin.[8] This option most commonly involves tissue harvest from the abdomen (deep inferior epigastric perforator, transverse rectus abdominis flaps), inner or outer thighs (transverse upper gracilis, profunda artery perforator flaps), gluteal area (superior gluteal artery perforator, inferior gluteal artery perforator flaps), or back (latissimus dorsi flap).

The majority of these autologous procedures are now performed using microvascular (free tissue transfer) techniques, because this procedure allows for the harvest of little to no donor site muscle (less donor site morbidity), and enhanced perfusion once these flaps are reanastomosed to a vascular supply in the breast.

Both prosthetic and autologous breast reconstruction are highly successful techniques, allowing for reconstruction of reproducible and desirable breasts, after mastectomy. However, certain considerations and techniques must be taken into account when selecting the safest option; furthermore, recent advances have added

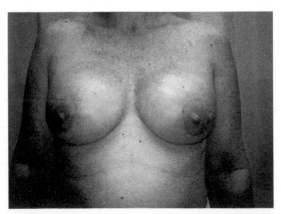

Fig. 1. Postoperative photograph of a 52-year-old woman, 4 years after bilateral nipple-sparing mastectomies, and bilateral 2-stage prosthetic breast reconstruction.

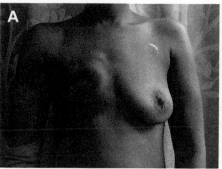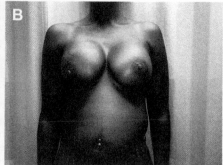

Fig. 2. (A) Preoperative and (B) 2-year postoperative photographs of a 48-year-old woman after undergoing delayed right breast 2-stage prepectoral breast reconstruction. The patient also underwent left breast augmentation for symmetry.

to efficacy of these techniques in more challenging clinical situations, based on patient factors or adjuvant treatments.

NIPPLE-SPARING MASTECTOMY

In recent years, the frequency of nipple-sparing mastectomy being offered has increased significantly, owing to expanding indications and inclusion criteria.[9] Equivalent locoregional recurrence rates to skin sparing mastectomy, in patients with stages 1 through 3 tumors, and no preoperative nipple skin involvement, has resulted in many more patients being offered this option. This factor has enhanced the appearance of breast reconstructive outcomes, because retention of the native nipple/areola complex results in greater patient satisfaction and quality of life scores on validated patient surveys.[10]

When considering nipple-sparing mastectomy, the preoperative size and breast ptosis must be assessed, to ensure that excellent aesthetic outcomes will be attainable. This step is of high importance, given that with nipple-sparing mastectomy, little can be done to tighten or lift the skin envelope in the immediate setting, owing to the risk of disrupting central nipple perfusion. Thus, this technique is recommended for patients with a breast mass of less than 800 g, and grade 1 or 2 ptosis preoperatively.[11] When adhering to these criteria, nipple and skin necrosis rates are also minimized.

For those patients in whom a nipple-sparing mastectomy is desired, but preoperative breast size or ptosis are too great, a multistage approach to nipple-sparing mastectomy can be offered. In the first stage, a premastectomy breast reduction or mastopexy can be offered, to reduce the breast size, lift the nipple/areola complex, and tighten the skin envelope. In patients with ductal carcinoma in situ or stage 1 invasive cancer, this can be accompanied by a partial mastectomy at the time of reduction/mastopexy. Then, after healing, a nipple-sparing mastectomy can be performed at a second stage, on a now smaller, lifted breast with the nipple/areola complex in the correct position. At that time, the breast reconstruction can be started or performed completely.

This approach has been proven safe from an oncologic standpoint when performed on the appropriately selected patients. Furthermore, nipple-sparing mastectomy on a patient with a previous circumareolar incision has been shown to be safe, with maintained nipple/areola complex perfusion, when performed at least 5 months after the reduction/mastopexy.[12] Using this approach, many more patients can be offered nipple preservation and breast reconstruction, even if they are not ideal candidates at the outset (**Fig. 3**).

The incisional approach to nipple-sparing mastectomy is critical in determining clinical and aesthetic outcomes. The inframammary fold incision is most commonly used,

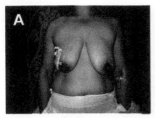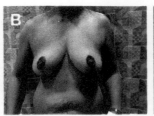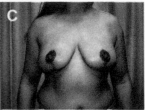

Fig. 3. (A) Preoperative view of a 50-year-old patient with right breast stage 1 cancer, initially not a candidate for nipple-sparing mastectomy, undergoing right partial mastectomy and bilateral oncoplastic breast reduction; after healing, patient seen preoperatively (B) before bilateral nipple-sparing mastectomies and prepectoral tissue expander placement. After complete expansion, patient underwent exchange of bilateral expanders for bilateral deep inferior epigastric perforator free flaps, and is seen 1 year after this operation (C).

and this works well, especially in patients with smaller breasts and minimal preoperative breast ptosis (Fig. 4). However, for patients with grade 2 preoperative ptosis, a perieareolar incisional approach has been used with success, because this procedure allows for a crescent mastopexy pattern that will also allow for correction of 1 to 2 cm of nipple/areola complex ptosis with the mastectomy (see Fig. 1). This process must be designed in such a way that not more than 2 cm of elevation is planned, or the areola will develop an elliptical shape. Furthermore, as long as the periareolar portion of the incision involves at most 25% of the areola circumference, then nipple/areola complex necrosis is not a concern (Fig. 5).[13]

POSTMASTECTOMY RADIATION

Breast reconstruction in the setting of postmastectomy radiation therapy (PMRT) represents a particular challenge, owing to higher reported rates of incisional dehiscence, infection, and capsular contracture. Reported rates of overall complications in this setting range from 15% to 40%. This challenge occurs frequently with rates of PMRT in some centers reported at rates of 30% to 40%.[14]

When planning prosthetic reconstruction with PMRT, the surgeon must first decide whether radiation will be delivered to the tissue expanders or permanent implants. Reported rates of infection are lower with radiation of permanent implants, because all operations have been performed on the breast before radiation.[15] However, rates of capsular contracture are higher with this option, because the radiated implant remains in place permanently, without the option for capsulectomy after radiation completion. Radiation delivery to tissue expanders offers the opportunity for capsulectomy and

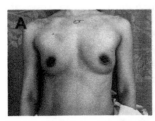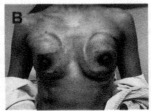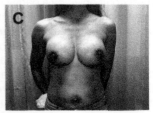

Fig. 4. (A) Preoperative view of a 37-year-old woman undergoing bilateral nipple-sparing mastectomy and bilateral prepectoral tissue expander placement. (B) Photo taken 3 weeks after mastectomy showing thin mastectomy skin flaps over tissue expanders. (C) Postoperative view, 18 months after completion of prepectoral breast reconstruction.

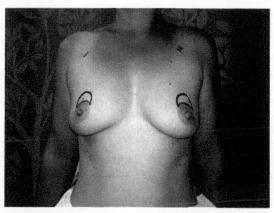

Fig. 5. Preoperative view of periareolar approach design for nipple-sparing mastectomy, diagrammed as a crescent mastopexy, providing excellent exposure for both mastectomy and placement of prosthesis.

contracture reduction, and modification of any displacement or deformity that occurred during radiation. For this reason, radiation of tissue expanders remains the most common approach in this setting.

Even in the setting of desired radiation delivery to the permanent implant, many patients undergoing 2-stage reconstruction will not be candidates, owing to the need to begin radiation around 4 weeks after mastectomy.[16] Thus, the timeline will not allow sufficient for the second stage expander to implant exchange to be performed before radiation delivery.

Given these risks and constraints, many strategies have been developed to decrease the complication rates after mastectomy and prosthetic reconstruction in the setting of PMRT, especially as frequency of nipple-sparing mastectomy has increased. In these patients, radiation increases rates skin necrosis and infection, but not necessarily rates of nipple necrosis, relative to nonradiated breasts.[17] Thus, nipple-sparing mastectomy can be safely performed when PMRT is anticipated (**Fig. 6**).

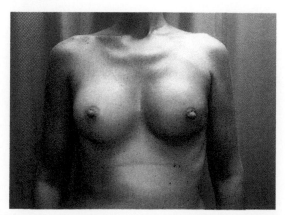

Fig. 6. Postoperative photo of a 41-year-old woman with left breast cancer taken 2 years after undergoing left nipple-sparing mastectomy and prepectoral breast reconstruction, with left postmastectomy radiation therapy. The right native breast underwent augmentation for symmetry.

Incision location has also been shown to be critical in decreasing complications in the setting of PMRT. The periareolar, radial, or any other incision on the anterior face of the breast results in lower complication rates compared with the inframammary fold mastectomy incision, when radiation follows.[18] Regardless of the incision type used for nipple-sparing mastectomy and immediate tissue expander placement, the second stage exchange operation for permanent implant, after radiation, should always be performed through a new incision. After radiation, the original incision consists of radiated scar tissue, and thus it is significantly devascularized. Instead, a new incision should be planned in an area without previous scars (**Fig. 7**). This strategy decreases wound dehiscence rates after PMRT significantly.

Another important consideration is the duration of time after radiation completion and before the second stage expander to implant exchange operation is performed. Although there remains no absolute consensus on this factor, there are data to suggest that waiting at least 6 months after radiation completion significantly reduces complication rates with the second operation.[19] This waiting period will allow many of the acute effects of radiation fibrosis to have dissipated, including the acute inflammation of the skin envelope, likely allowing for improved healing. During this time period, many surgeons will perform autologous fat grafting on the acutely radiated breast skin, because this procedure has been shown to decrease some of the damaging symptoms of radiation fibrosis.[20]

The increased use of ADM in breast reconstruction has also helped to decrease the complication rates in the setting of PMRT. Multiple centers have published similar findings that prosthetic devices with ADM coverage experience significantly lower rates of all complications, including extrusion, in the setting of PMRT, relative to those breasts with full submuscular coverage.[17,21,22] Thus, the use of ADM to support and cover prosthetic breasts with known need for radiation is encouraged. Other benefits of ADM include greater control over the aesthetic boundaries of the reconstructed breast, less implant movement, and reduced rates of capsular contracture.[23,24]

The use of autologous breast reconstruction in the setting of radiation results in lower reported rates of infection, given the vascularized nature of these reconstructions. However, certain considerations are also necessary in these patients. Radiation of autologous flaps results in higher reported rates fat necrosis and partial flap loss.

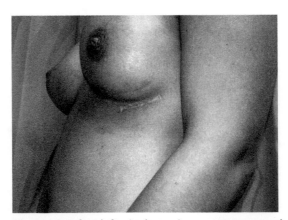

Fig. 7. A 38-year-old woman after left nipple-sparing mastectomy and prosthetic reconstruction, and postmastectomy radiation therapy. Separate incisions were made for mastectomy (upper inframammary fold incision) and exchange operation after radiation therapy (lower inframammary fold incision).

Thus, for this reason, many centers delay the autologous flap reconstruction until after completion of radiation, instead proceeding with temporary tissue expander placement at time of mastectomy, to maintain the shape of the skin envelope.[25]

However, some highly specialized centers have experienced high degrees of success performing immediate autologous reconstruction, and then radiating these flaps.[26] In their experience, the rates of revision surgeries to treat PMRT induced complications with flaps are the same as with nonradiated flaps, giving merit to performing the entire procedure in 1 operation, before radiation. They have also found that flaps with enhanced perforator blood supply (muscle-sparing transverse rectus abdominis myocutaneous flaps) offer lower complications and better outcomes when radiated, compared with more poorly perfused single or double perforator (deep inferior epigastric perforator) flaps. Thus, muscle-sparing transverse rectus abdominis myocutaneous flaps are preferentially performed when radiation is anticipated in this setting.

For those patients undergoing microsurgical autologous reconstruction after radiation, as is more common, waiting longer periods after radiation completion will result in improved free flap outcomes. This finding is due to recovery of the internal mammary or thorocodorsal vessels over this time, from the damaging effects of radiation. This step in turn will result in improved anastomotic patency and improved vascularity. Studies have shown that waiting 1 year after radiation completion before microvascular breast reconstruction results in significantly decreased total flap loss rates, relative to proceeding within 1 year.[27]

Regardless of the exact procedure planned, both pedicle and autologous flaps result in excellent outcomes in the setting of radiation. Their vascularized, autologous nature makes them well-suited to resist the damaging effects of radiation, and specifically to offer lower infection rates.

PREPECTORAL BREAST RECONSTRUCTION

Traditionally, prosthetic breast reconstruction after mastectomy has involved placing a tissue expander or permanent implant not only under the preserved breast skin, but also underneath the pectoralis major muscle. This was also assisted in coverage by incorporating the serrauts anterior muscle or fascia, or more recently, ADM for additional coverage.[28] The purpose of such submuscular placement of prosthetic devices is the belief that this results in lower rates of capsular contracture, relative to subcutaneous placement.[29]

For years, this submuscular approach has become the most common technique for postmastectomy breast reconstruction. However in recent years, with the advent of ADM, there has been an increase in the incidence of prepectoral breast reconstruction being performed. This method involves full avoidance of any pectoralis or serratus muscle dissection or elevation, and instead uses only ADM for soft tissue coverage of the tissue expanders or implants, which are placed anterior to the pectoralis major muscle (**Fig. 8**).

The prepectoral approach has resulted in numerous benefits for patients, including decreased levels of pain, and elimination of animation deformity.[30,31] Furthermore, without involvement of the pectoralis major muscle in the reconstructive process, women experience enhanced aesthetic definition of the reconstructed breast (because implant position is no longer inhibited by pectoralis muscle anatomy), and no loss of upper body strength (owing to full muscle preservation).

The outcomes of prepectoral breast reconstruction, with the use of ADM for soft tissue coverage and support, have been shown to be equivalent to those of subpectoral reconstruction.[31,32] This finding also stands true in the setting of PMRT (see **Fig. 6**). Many of the initial concerns surrounding this procedure were due to the increased

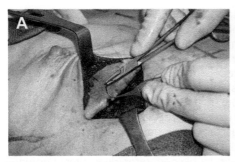
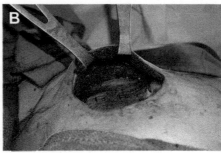

Fig. 8. Intraoperative view (*A*, *B*) of a prepectoral tissue expander placed at time of nipple-sparing mastectomy. Full soft tissue support with acellular dermal matrix allows for full preservation of the pectoralis major muscle, making this procedure less invasive and more form preserving.

risk of rippling and upper pole aesthetic deformities without the pectoralis major muscle covering the upper pole of these implants. However, with autologous fat grafting of this area for volume restoration, and cohesive implants, such concerns are no longer an issue.[33,34] These advances in breast reconstruction nicely eliminate the need for the pectoralis major muscle sacrifice just to provide an improved upper pole aesthetic outcome (**Fig. 9**). Thus, the frequency of prepectoral reconstruction techniques in the United States is now growing rapidly.

When planning a prepectoral reconstruction, the surgeon must keep in mind certain contraindications. This technique is reserved for patients in whom the mastectomy skin flaps are viable and well-perfused. Thin skin flaps can still undergo tissue expander–based prepectoral breast reconstruction, as long as they are seen to be viable and well-perfused. Furthermore, this technique is not promoted in patients with uncontrolled diabetes, an active smoking habit, or in morbidly obese patients. From an oncologic standpoint, contraindications for prepectoral reconstruction include those patients with deep breast tumors that come to within 0.5 cm of the chest wall, or those with inflammatory breast cancer. All these factors are essential for consideration when planning this approach.

AUTOLOGOUS FAT GRAFTING

Of all advances in breast reconstruction in the last 10 years, perhaps that with the greatest impact has been the advent of autologous fat grafting. With this technique,

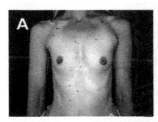
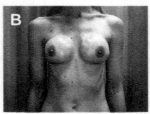
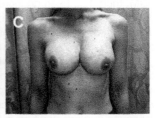

Fig. 9. (*A*) Preoperative view of a 42-year-old woman undergoing bilateral nipple-sparing mastectomy and bilateral prepectoral tissue expander placement. (*B*) After completion of tissue expansion, patient has thin upper pole skin, indicating a need for fat grafting at the time of exchange to prevent rippling and contour deformity of upper pole. (*C*) Postoperative view, 2 years after completion of prepectoral breast reconstruction, showing no clinical rippling, owing in part to autologous fat grafting.

autologous fat can be harvested from a patient's body using liposuction techniques. The fat is then washed, to remove blood and oil, and immediately reinjected into the breast for volume restoration, soft tissue augmentation, and masking of contour deformities.

In the setting of prosthetic breast reconstruction, this technique is valuable for injection into the upper pole skin flaps, which are often thin, over the prosthetic implant.[35] This fat will thicken the upper pole skin flaps, and help to prevent clinically noticeable rippling or implant palpability. In the setting of prepectoral breast reconstruction, fat grafting has been especially valuable at adding upper pole volume over the implant that is no longer provided by an elevated pectoralis major muscle because it was in submuscular reconstruction (**Fig. 10**).

An added benefits of autologous fat grafting is its ease of performance. It is most commonly performed at the time of tissue expander to implant exchange in 2-stage reconstructions. When performed properly, complications specific to overinjection of fat (fat necrosis and oil cysts) are rare, and up to 80% reported permanent survival rates of injected fat can be achieved once the fat revascularizes from the surrounding tissue bed.

Human adipocytes are a rich source of autologous stem cells, and thus when injected as fat graft have a notable improvement on tissue quality. This finding has been clearly illustrated in the setting of postmastectomy radiation breast envelopes, where autologous fat grafting has reversed some of the deleterious effects of radiation fibrosis, including abnormal collagen deposition and microvascular depletion.[20] The

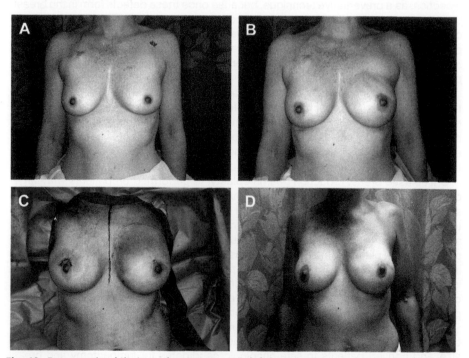

Fig. 10. Preoperative (*A*) view of a patient with left breast cancer. Postreconstruction view (*B*) after left nipple-sparing mastectomy and prepectoral breast reconstruction without fat grafting, and right augmentation for symmetry. Patient (*B*) exhibits left breast upper and medial pole rippling and volume hollowing, owing to lack of fat grafting. This is treated (*C*) with left breast fat grafting over the existing prepectoral implant. Postoperative (*D*) view at 6 months shows aesthetic correction of the left breast volume deficiency and rippling.

key to achieving such results is the injection of high-quality fat cells, whose viability has been maintained through intraoperative washing and processing. To ensure such outcomes, minimal processing should be used, most commonly through filtration (light washing and decanting).[36] This step will result in healthy fat for reinjection, and high rates of graft survival (Video 1).

The other benefit of autologous fat grafting, and the use of adipocytes as a filler, lies in the oncologic safety of this procedure. Even with the high stem cell concentration of autologous fat cells, because these stem cells are not purified and directed down a specific stem cell growth lineage, this technique has been shown to be safe in patients with breast cancer.[37]

ONCOPLASTIC (POSTLUMPECTOMY) BREAST RECONSTRUCTION

Although postmastectomy breast reconstruction remains the most commonly performed oncologic reconstruction technique, the rise of oncoplastic breast reconstruction, performed alongside partial mastectomy (breast conservation) procedures, has been rapid. This finding is due to the potential severity of postlumpectomy breast defects, and the desire to avoid them. As such, 2 oncoplastic techniques are now commonly employed used the time of partial mastectomy: local tissue rearrangement and oncoplastic reduction mammoplasty.

The desire is to perform such techniques simultaneous to the oncologic tissue resection, as a preventative technique, because once these defects form in the breast, they are very challenging to repair and reconstruct secondarily. This finding is especially true if such patients proceed to radiation therapy. When techniques for oncoplastic reconstruction have been compared for morbidity, those performed before radiation therapy result in significantly lower operative complications, relative to those performed after radiation therapy.[38]

Local tissue rearrangement is often performed in patients with small breasts, small tumors, and minimal preoperative breast ptosis. With this technique, after completion of the partial mastectomy, the remaining healthy surrounding breast parenchyma is mobilized as vascularized parenchyma flaps, and advanced and inset into the lumpectomy cavity.[39] This process allows for the obliteration of the open space, reducing the risk of contour deformities or cavities, as well as seroma and infection.

Oncoplastic breast reduction (mammoplasty) is performed on patients with larger preoperative breast size (C to D cup), who have grade 2 or 3 ptosis, and require a large skin resection. This procedure is performed on both breasts, including the nonlumpectomy breast, to maintain postoperative symmetry. This technique is performed as a standard breast reduction, with either a Wise or vertical pattern technique. The nipple pedicle can be placed with any location, based on tumor location, such that this tissue is safely preserved.[39,40] This technique is powerful, because it allows for planning a lumpectomy as a standard breast reduction, with removal of the necessary quadrant of the breast. The final result is thus a very aesthetic breast mound, with correction of ptosis, and avoidance of any contour deformities.

In many cases, preoperative tumor size may be too large to safely allow for breast conservation. However, neoadjuvant chemotherapy may be used to shrink the tumor size, and convert patients to safe oncologic candidates for lumpectomy and breast conservation. Furthermore, when postoperative radiation therapy is required, this option can result in lower complication rates, compared with patients who undergo mastectomy with whole breast reconstruction, followed by adjuvant radiation therapy.[41]

Thus, oncoplastic reduction mammoplasty allows for conservation of the breasts with an improved aesthetic outcome, and reduction in postoperative complication rates in some cases. Similarly, this option can be safer in the setting of complete axillary lymph node dissection, where mastectomy and complete reconstruction is known to have higher complication rates, specifically infection.[42]

SUPPLEMENTARY DATA

Supplementary data related to this article can be found online at https://doi.org/10.1016/j.suc.2018.03.011.

REFERENCES

1. Albornoz CR, Bach PB, Mehrara BJ, et al. A paradigm shift in U.S. breast reconstruction: increasing implant rates. Plast Reconstr Surg 2013;131(1):15–23.
2. American Society of Plastic Surgeons. 2016 procedural statistics. Arlington Heights (IL). Available at: https://www.plasticsurgery.org/documents/News/Statistics/2016/plastic-surgery-statistics-full-report-2016.pdf. Accessed September 9, 2017.
3. Alderman AK, McMahon L Jr, Wilkins EG. The national utilization of immediate and early delayed breast reconstruction and the effect of sociodemographic factors. Plast Reconstr Surg 2003;111(2):695–703.
4. Wilkins EG, Alderman AK. Breast reconstruction practices in North America: current trends and future priorities. Semin Plast Surg 2004;18(2):149–55.
5. Eltahir Y, Werners LL, Dreise MM, et al. Quality-of-life outcomes between mastectomy alone and breast reconstruction: comparison of patient-reported BREAST-Q and other health-related quality-of-life measures. Plast Reconstr Surg 2013;132(2):201e–9e.
6. Sbitany H, Amalfi AN, Langstein HN. Preferences in choosing between breast reconstruction options: a survey of female plastic surgeons. Plast Reconstr Surg 2009;124(6):1781–9.
7. Colwell AS, Damjanovic B, Zahedi B, et al. Retrospective review of 331 consecutive immediate single-stage implant reconstructions with acellular dermal matrix: indications, complications, trends, and costs. Plast Reconstr Surg 2011;128(6):1170–8.
8. Macadam SA, Bovill ES, Buchel EW, et al. Evidence-based medicine: autologous breast reconstruction. Plast Reconstr Surg 2017;139(1):204e–29e.
9. Peled AW, Wang F, Foster RD, et al. Expanding the indications for total skin-sparing mastectomy: is it safe for patients with locally advanced disease? Ann Surg Oncol 2016;23(1):87–91.
10. Bailey CR, Ogbuagu O, Baltodano PA, et al. Quality-of-life outcomes improve with nipple-sparing mastectomy and breast reconstruction. Plast Reconstr Surg 2017;140(2):219–26.
11. Wang F, Alvarado M, Ewing C, et al. The impact of breast mass on outcomes of total skin-sparing mastectomy and immediate tissue expander-based breast reconstruction. Plast Reconstr Surg 2015;135(3):672–9.
12. Alperovich M, Tanna N, Samra F, et al. Nipple-sparing mastectomy in patients with a history of reduction mammaplasty or mastopexy: how safe is it? Plast Reconstr Surg 2013;131(5):962–7.
13. Wang F, Peled AW, Garwood E, et al. Total skin-sparing mastectomy and immediate breast reconstruction: an evolution of technique and assessment of outcomes. Ann Surg Oncol 2014;21(10):3223–30.
14. Sbitany H, Wang F, Peled AW, et al. Tissue expander reconstruction after total skin-sparing mastectomy: defining the effects of coverage technique on nipple/areola preservation. Ann Plast Surg 2016;77(1):17–24.

15. Cordeiro PG, Albornoz CR, McCormick B, et al. What is the optimum timing of post-mastectomy radiotherapy in two-stage prosthetic reconstruction: radiation to the tissue expander or permanent implant? Plast Reconstr Surg 2015;135(6):1509–17.
16. Nava MB, Pennati AE, Lozza L, et al. Outcome of different timings of radiotherapy in implant-based breast reconstructions. Plast Reconstr Surg 2011;128(2):353–9.
17. Sbitany H, Wang F, Peled AW, et al. Immediate implant-based breast reconstruction following total skin-sparing mastectomy: defining the risk of preoperative and postoperative radiation therapy for surgical outcomes. Plast Reconstr Surg 2014; 134(3):396–404.
18. Peled AW, Foster RD, Ligh C, et al. Impact of total skin-sparing mastectomy incision type on reconstructive complications following radiation therapy. Plast Reconstr Surg 2014;134(2):169–75.
19. Peled AW, Foster RD, Esserman LJ, et al. Increasing the time to expander-implant exchange after postmastectomy radiation therapy reduces expander-implant failure. Plast Reconstr Surg 2012;130(3):503–9.
20. Garza RM, Paik KJ, Chung MT, et al. Studies in fat grafting: part III. Fat grafting irradiated tissue–improved skin quality and decreased fat graft retention. Plast Reconstr Surg 2014;134(2):249–57.
21. Seth AK, Hirsch EM, Fine NA, et al. Utility of acellular dermis-assisted breast reconstruction in the setting of radiation: a comparative analysis. Plast Reconstr Surg 2012;130(4):750–8.
22. Spear SL, Seruya M, Rao SS, et al. Two-stage prosthetic breast reconstruction using AlloDerm including outcomes of different timings of radiotherapy. Plast Reconstr Surg 2012;130(1):1–9.
23. Sbitany H, Sandeen SN, Amalfi AN, et al. Acellular dermis-assisted prosthetic breast reconstruction versus complete submuscular coverage: a head-to-head comparison of outcomes. Plast Reconstr Surg 2009;124(6):1735–40.
24. Sbitany H, Serletti JM. Acellular dermis-assisted prosthetic breast reconstruction: a systematic and critical review of efficacy and associated morbidity. Plast Reconstr Surg 2011;128(6):1162–9.
25. Kronowitz SJ. Delayed-immediate breast reconstruction: technical and timing considerations. Plast Reconstr Surg 2010;125(2):463–74.
26. Mirzabeigi MN, Smartt JM, Nelson JA, et al. An assessment of the risks and benefits of immediate autologous breast reconstruction in patients undergoing post-mastectomy radiation therapy. Ann Plast Surg 2013;71(2):149–55.
27. Baumann DP, Crosby MA, Selber JC, et al. Optimal timing of delayed free lower abdominal flap breast reconstruction after postmastectomy radiation therapy. Plast Reconstr Surg 2011;127(3):1100–6.
28. Sbitany H, Langstein HN. Acellular dermal matrix in primary breast reconstruction. Aesthet Surg J 2011;31(7 Suppl):30S–7S.
29. Serletti JM, Fosnot J, Nelson JA, et al. Breast reconstruction after breast cancer. Plast Reconstr Surg 2011;127(6):124e–35e.
30. Lentz RB, Piper ML, Gomez-Sanchez C, et al. Correction of breast animation deformity following prosthetic breast reconstruction. Plast Reconstr Surg 2017; 140(4):643e–4e.
31. Sbitany H, Piper M, Lentz R. Pre-pectoral breast reconstruction: a safe alternative to submuscular prosthetic reconstruction following nipple-sparing mastectomy. Plast Reconstr Surg 2017;140(3):432–43.
32. Sigalove S, Maxwell GP, Sigalove NM, et al. Pre-pectoral implant-based breast reconstruction: rationale, indications, and preliminary results. Plast Reconstr Surg 2017;139(2):287–94.

33. Sbitany H. Important considerations for performing prepectoral breast reconstruction. Plast Reconstr Surg 2017;140(6S Prepectoral Breast Reconstruction): 7S–13S.
34. Vidya R. Prepectoral breast reconstruction or muscle-sparing technique with the Braxon porcine acellular dermal matrix. Plast Reconstr Surg Glob Open 2017; 5(6):e1364.
35. Khouri RK Jr, Khouri RK. Current clinical applications of fat grafting. Plast Reconstr Surg 2017;140(3):466e–86e.
36. Fisher C, Grahovac TL, Schafer ME, et al. Comparison of harvest and processing techniques for fat grafting and adipose stem cell isolation. Plast Reconstr Surg 2013;132(2):351–61.
37. Kronowitz SJ, Mandujano CC, Liu J, et al. Lipofilling of the breast does not increase the risk of recurrence of breast cancer: a matched controlled study. Plast Reconstr Surg 2016;137(2):385–93.
38. Kronowitz SJ, Feledy JA, Hunt KK, et al. Determining the optimal approach to breast reconstruction after partial mastectomy. Plast Reconstr Surg 2006; 117(1):1–11.
39. Kronowitz SJ, Kuerer HM, Buchholz TA, et al. A management algorithm and practical oncoplastic surgical techniques for repairing partial mastectomy defects. Plast Reconstr Surg 2008;122(6):1631–47.
40. Piper M, Peled AW, Sbitany H. Oncoplastic breast surgery: current strategies. Gland Surg 2015;4(2):154–63.
41. Peled AW, Sbitany H, Foster RD, et al. Oncoplastic mammoplasty as a strategy for reducing reconstructive complications associated with postmastectomy radiation therapy. Breast J 2014;20(3):302–7.
42. Wang F, Peled AW, Chin R, et al. The impact of radiation therapy, lymph node dissection, and hormonal therapy on outcomes of tissue expander-implant exchange in prosthetic breast reconstruction. Plast Reconstr Surg 2016;137(1):1–9.

Role of Operative Management in Stage IV Breast Cancer

Mediget Teshome, MD, MPH

KEYWORDS

- De novo metastatic breast cancer
- Locoregional management of metastatic breast cancer
- Surgery for stage IV breast cancer

KEY POINTS

- Surgery for the intact breast primary in stage IV breast cancer traditionally has been reserved for palliation.
- Survival advantage with surgery for the intact breast primary in stage IV breast cancer has been demonstrated in several retrospective studies.
- Randomized trials evaluating survival outcome after surgery in stage IV breast cancer are ongoing with two early trials reporting conflicting survival outcomes.
- Stage IV NED (no evidence of disease) is associated with improved survival particularly in limited de novo metastatic disease and after local therapy for the breast primary.
- Comprehensive local therapy in Stage IV inflammatory breast cancer may improve locoregional control outcomes.

INTRODUCTION

Stage IV breast cancer accounts for approximately 6% of all breast cancer diagnoses in the United States and is defined by metastasis from the breast and axilla to distant sites, most commonly the bone, brain, liver, and lung.[1] It is estimated that in 2017 approximately 155,000 women will have stage IV breast cancer in the United States, approximately one-quarter of whom were diagnosed with de novo disease, characterized by metastasis present at diagnosis. Although associated with a poor prognosis, survival rates of women with de novo stage IV breast cancer have improved over the past 3 decades.[2,3]

Traditionally considered incurable, the primary therapeutic focus in stage IV breast cancer is systemic therapy to reduce disease progression and support quality of life. In this context, surgery for the breast primary historically has been reserved for palliation

The author has nothing to disclose.
Department of Breast Surgical Oncology, University of Texas M.D. Anderson Cancer Center, 1400 Pressler Street, Unit 1434, Houston, TX 77030, USA
E-mail address: mteshome@mdanderson.org

of symptoms. In the setting of de novo stage IV disease, locoregional management with surgery for the breast primary and axillary disease with or without radiation therapy is generally not recommended given no clear survival benefit.

However, there is growing evidence that aggressive local therapy improves survival in stage IV disease in other malignancies. With respect to breast cancer, although retrospective studies have suggested improved survival with resection of the breast primary, prospective analysis has not yet demonstrated a clear survival difference in patients treated with neoadjuvant systemic therapy. Currently, the National Clinical Cancer Network (NCCN) guidelines promote individualized decision making for consideration of local therapy in de novo stage IV disease, suggesting such intervention may be reasonable in patients with a response to systemic therapy, whereas further studies are pending.[4]

This article examines the role of operative management in de novo stage IV breast cancer, including insights from retrospective and prospective trials and populations wherein considerations for local regional therapy despite distant metastatic disease may provide maximum benefit, including achieving no evidence of disease (NED) status and inflammatory breast cancer (IBC).

RATIONALE FOR OPERATIVE THERAPY IN STAGE IV BREAST CANCER

Inherently, the approach to treatment of metastatic breast cancer is with palliative intent. Given this, therapies offering benefit with minimal toxicity or morbidity are favored, and traditionally, operative management has been limited to palliation of symptoms. With respect to the breast primary, symptoms may include protracted pain, bleeding, ulceration, and presence of a fungating mass. In the setting of symptomatic metastases, surgical intervention may be considered for palliation of secondary complications, including spinal cord compression, pathologic fracture, pleural or pericardial effusions, and localized bony pain.[4] Similarly, surgery for the breast primary may provide local control and decrease future morbidity associated with locally progressive disease. This approach may be particularly beneficial in the setting of extensive locoregional disease, such as IBC.[5] The impact of resection of the breast primary on survival in the setting of stage IV disease is debated, with conflicting survival outcomes described in the literature, which are further explored in this review. Although a survival advantage has not yet been clearly demonstrated in prospective studies, selected populations with metastatic breast cancer suggested to benefit from local therapy include those with limited oligometastatic disease, those with a significant response to systemic therapy, and those who achieve stage IV NED.

THE IMPACT OF SURGERY IN STAGE IV BREAST CANCER ON SURVIVAL OUTCOME
Retrospective Studies

Several retrospective single-institution and population-based studies have suggested improved survival with surgery in stage IV breast cancer (**Table 1**). The largest among these is an analysis of the National Cancer Database from 1990 to 1993 by Khan and colleagues,[6] who evaluated 16,023 patients with stage IV breast cancer. Fifty-seven percent of these patients received surgery for the breast primary (38.3% treated with segmental mastectomy and 61.7% treated with mastectomy), and 43% did not have surgical intervention. The observed 3-year survival was 24.9% overall, 17.3% without surgery, 27.7% with segmental mastectomy, and 31.8% with mastectomy ($P<.0001$). Negative surgical margin was associated with improved 3-year survival despite surgery type. Independent prognostic factors included surgical resection of

Table 1
Retrospective studies evaluating survival outcome after surgery for stage IV breast cancer

		n	Survival Outcome	
Khan[6]			3-y survival	Median survival
2002	Total	16,023	24.9%	
	No surgery	6861 (43%)	17.3%	19.3 mo
	Surgery	9162 (57%)		
	BCS	3513 (38.3%)	27.7%	26.9 mo
	TM	5649 (61.7%)	31.8%	31.9 mo
	Negative margin	1410 (69.5%)	35.7%	25.3 mo
	Positive margin	1817 (30.5%)	26.1%	20 mo
Babiera[9]			Trend to improved OS, Metastatic	
2006	Total	224	progression-free survival, HR 0.54	
	No surgery	142 (63%)	95% CI (0.38–0.77) with surgery	
	Surgery	82 (37%)		
Rapiti[8]			5-y overall	5-y disease-specific
2006			survival	survival
	Total	300	16%	
	No surgery	173 (58%)		12%
	Surgery	127 (42%)		
	Negative margin	61 (48%)		27%
	Positive margin	33 (26%)		16%
	Unknown margin	33 (26%)		12%
Gnerlich[7]			Overall survival	
2007	Total	9734		
	No surgery	5156 (53%)	21 mo	
	Surgery	4578 (47%)	36 mo	
Fields[31]	Total	409	Median survival	
2007	No surgery	222 (54%)	12.6 mo	
	Surgery	187 (46%)	26.8 mo	
Bafford[32]			Median survival	
2008	Total	147		
	No surgery	86 (59%)	2.36 y	
	Surgery	61 (41%)	3.52 y	
Blanchard[33]			Median survival	
2008	Total	395		
	No surgery	153 (39%)	16.8 mo	
	Surgery	242 (61%)	27.1 mo	
Ruiterkamp[34]			5-y survival	Median survival
2009	Total	728		
	No surgery	440 (60.4%)	24.5%	14 mo
	Surgery	288 (39.6%)	31.1%	31 mo
Lang[11]			Median survival	
2013	Total	208	44.4 mo	
	No surgery	134 (64.4%)	37.2 mo	
	Surgery	74 (35.6%)	56.1 mo	
Thomas[3]			Overall survival	
2016	Total	21,372	23 mo	
	No surgery	13,042 (61%)	19 mo	
	Surgery	8330 (39%)	28 mo	

Abbreviations: BCS, breast-conserving surgery; CI, confidence interval; HR, hazard ratio; mo, month; n, number; OS, overall survival; TM, total mastectomy; y, year.

the tumor, including margin status, receipt of systemic therapy, the number of metastatic sites, and type of metastatic disease.

Similarly, an analysis of the Surveillance, Epidemiology, and End Results database from 1998 to 2003 by Gnerlich and colleagues[7] of 9734 patients with stage IV breast cancer found an improved median survival with surgery as compared with no surgery. Improved survival was demonstrated in patients alive at the completion of the study period (36 months vs 21 months, P<.001) and among those who died within the study period (18 months vs 7 months, P<.001). After adjusting for possible confounding factors, patients treated with surgery were 37% less likely to die during the study period as compared with those who did not have surgery.

These findings were further supported by an analysis of the Geneva Cancer Registry from 1977 to 1996 by Rapiti and colleagues[8] evaluating 300 patients with stage IV breast cancer. Five-year breast cancer–specific survival was 16% overall, 27% with surgery with negative margins, 16% with surgery with positive margins, 12% with surgery and unknown margins, and 12% without surgery. This accounted for a 40% reduced risk of death with negative margins as compared with those who did not have surgery or who had surgery with a positive margin. Furthermore, bone-only disease was associated with improved survival outcome with surgery as compared with other metastatic sites.

The University of Texas MD Anderson Cancer Center has published outcomes in 224 patients treated from 1997 to 2002 with stage IV breast cancer on presentation or diagnosed within 3 months of presentation.[9] Eighty-two patients (37%) received surgery for the breast primary compared with 142 (63%) treated with systemic therapy alone. At 32.1 months median follow-up, the authors found no improvement in overall survival; however, there was a trend toward improved metastatic progression-free survival in patients treated with surgery. Patients who received surgery were more likely to have a single site of metastatic disease, neoadjuvant chemotherapy, younger age, and decreased nodal disease burden. They were also more likely to have bone and liver disease as compared with brain and lung metastasis and more likely to be HER2-positive. Further analysis of this cohort found improved progression-free survival when surgery was performed 3 or more months after diagnosis; however, the timing of surgery did not have a significant impact on overall survival.[10] All patients received systemic therapy, which may have influenced the selection of patients for surgery and survival advantage in timing of surgery described. Furthermore, when reevaluated after a longer median follow-up of 74.2 months, a similar institutional cohort found surgery to be associated with improved median overall survival (56.1 months with surgery vs 37.2 months without surgery, P = .002) and progression-free survival (P<.0001).[11]

In contrast, matched analysis of the NCCN Breast Cancer Outcomes Database from 1997 to 2007 of 551 patients with data available, survival outcome was similar between the patients treated with surgery and without surgery (3.5 years vs 3.4 years, respectively).[12] In addition, a similar matched pair analysis of 622 patients with stage IV disease and intact primary found improved overall survival with surgery; however, this finding did not persist after case-matched control analysis.[13]

These retrospective studies collectively suggest improved outcome with surgical resection of the breast primary in the setting of stage IV disease. However, these studies are confounded by selection bias whereby patients selected for surgical therapy may have been healthier, with decreased metastatic disease burden and appropriate response to systemic therapy, which may have influenced the findings. The potential impact of selection bias is further suggested by matched analysis cohorts, which have not demonstrated improved survival outcome. Given this, prospective studies were developed to determine the impact of surgery on survival in stage IV breast cancer.

Prospective Studies

The Translational Breast Cancer Research Consortium 013 is a multi-institutional prospective registry study evaluating the role of surgery in stage IV breast cancer. From 2009 to 2012, 128 patients with stage IV disease at presentation (group A, n = 112) or stage IV within 3 months of diagnosis (group B, n = 16) were enrolled. The groups were similar with the exception of increased clinical nodal burden in group A. Early analysis showed a 2-year overall survival of 86% in both groups with 96% in those treated with surgery compared with 74% in those not treated with surgery (P = .002).[14] At a median follow-up of 54 months, 3-year overall survival was 70%. Eighty-five percent of patients were responders to systemic therapy, and 3-year overall survival in this group was superior as compared with nonresponders (78% vs 24%, respectively, P<.001). Among responders, surgery did not impact 3-year overall survival as compared with no surgery (77% vs 76%, respectively), consistent among breast cancer subtypes. Those treated with surgery were more likely to have larger tumors, single-organ metastatic disease, and first-line chemotherapy.[15] These findings suggest that improved survival may be driven by response to systemic therapy rather than surgical intervention.

Interestingly, this trial also evaluated the impact of the 21-gene recurrence score (RS) on outcome in 101 patients in which the RS could be determined. The 21-gene RS independently predicted both time to progression and 2-year overall survival such that low- (RS <18) and intermediate- (RS 18–30) risk scores were associated with improved outcome. Furthermore, in patients with estrogen receptor (ER)-positive HER2-negative disease and high-risk score (RS ≥31), treatment with endocrine therapy resulted in shorter overall survival and time to progression, whereas treatment with chemotherapy showed no difference in survival outcome. Although additional validation is necessary, this raises the potential for the RS to assist in clinical decision making in patients with de novo ER-positive HER2-negative metastatic breast cancer to determine appropriate systemic therapy.[16]

Two international randomized trials evaluating surgery for the breast primary in stage IV breast cancer have been reported (**Table 2**). Investigators at Tata Memorial Centre in India randomized 350 patients to receive locoregional treatment (n = 173) or no locoregional treatment (n = 177). They reported no difference in overall survival at 2 years between the groups (42% vs 43%, respectively). Subgroup analysis did not identify a population in which surgery provided a survival benefit by menopausal status, metastatic disease burden, or tumor subtype. On multivariate analysis, overall survival was associated with ER positivity and less than 3 distant metastases on presentation, although not associated with initial site of metastasis.[17] Of note, the systemic therapy regimens used departed from contemporary practice in the United States because they did not uniformly include taxanes, and most patients (92%) with HER2-positive breast cancer did not receive trastuzumab therapy.

MF07-01, a multicenter trial conducted in Turkey, randomized 274 patients to surgery followed by systemic therapy (n = 138) or systemic therapy alone (n = 136). At 36 months, there was no difference in overall survival. At 5 years, overall survival was improved for the surgery group at 41.6% as compared to 24.4% in the no surgery group. Subgroups with higher overall survival following surgery included ER-positive, HER2-negative, solitary bone metastasis and age less than 55 years.[18] The groups differed such that the surgery group had fewer patients with triple-negative subtype and visceral metastasis, and more patients with bone only or solitary bone metastasis. Local progression in the surgery group was 1% compared with 11% in the systemic therapy alone group. In this trial, patients received surgery before systemic therapy, thus limiting evaluation of response to therapy in predicting outcome.

Table 2
Randomized control trials evaluating survival outcomes after surgery for stage IV breast cancer

n		Survival Outcome			
Badwe,[17] 2015 Total	350	Median overall survival	2-y survival	Locoregional progression	
No surgery	177 (51%)	20.5 mo	43%	10.6%	
Surgery	173 (49%)	19.2 mo	41%	5.3%	

Randomized after response to neoadjuvant endocrine therapy or chemotherapy.
Limited receipt of Taxanes, Tamoxifen, and trastuzumab.
Improved survival if ER-positive/PR-positive, fewer distant metastasis at diagnosis.

Soran,[18] 2016 Total	274	3-y survival	5-y survival	Locoregional progression	
No surgery	136 (50%)	51%	24.4%; 37 mo	11%	
Surgery	138 (50%)	60%	41.6%; 46 mo	1%	

Randomized and received upfront surgery followed by adjuvant systemic therapy.
Surgery group had more ER-positive and less TNBC.
Improved survival if ER-positive, HER2-negative, solitary bone metastasis, age <55 y.

Abbreviations: ER, estrogen receptor; n, number; PR, progesterone receptor; TNBC, triple-negative breast cancer; y, years.

Limitations withstanding, these randomized trials suggest there is no early survival benefit to surgery in patients who present with stage IV breast cancer, although this is suggested after 5 years in one study. However, these limitations make it challenging to extrapolate to standard practice in the United States, where patients with advanced disease typically receive neoadjuvant treatment with anthracycline-taxane based chemotherapy and anti-HER2-directed therapy with trastuzumab and pertuzumab if indicated. It is unclear if this discrepancy would have an impact on the findings.

Further insights will be provided by findings of ongoing international clinical trials, including in the United States and Canada, Japan, Austria, and the Netherlands.[19] One such trial is the Eastern Cooperative Oncology Group E2108, a phase III prospective multicenter study evaluating the role of surgery in patients with de novo stage IV breast cancer with stable or improved response after neoadjuvant systemic therapy. All patients are planned to receive neoadjuvant systemic therapy followed by randomization to (1) continued systemic therapy with local therapy for palliation only or (2) aggressive locoregional therapy with surgery to negative margins and radiation therapy if indicated. The primary objective is to evaluate if early local therapy will result in prolonged survival as compared with local therapy for palliation in this population. Secondary objectives are to compare time with uncontrolled chest wall disease, quality-of-life outcomes, and absolute value of circulating tumor cell burden at 6 months.[20] This trial is now closed, and the results are eagerly awaited to better inform the impact of surgery in stage IV breast cancer on survival, locoregional outcomes, and quality of life.

LOCAL THERAPY TO ACHIEVE NO EVIDENCE OF DISEASE STATUS IN STAGE IV BREAST CANCER

Metastatic breast cancer represents a heterogeneous group of patients: some with extremely aggressive disease unresponsive to systemic therapies and others with an indolent course that may remain controlled for many years. The majority of patients develop metastatic disease following initial breast cancer treatment. In these patients, with limited metastatic disease burden, there is evidence that multimodality therapy where appropriate can achieve stage IV NED and improve outcomes.

Investigators at the University of Texas MD Anderson Cancer Center evaluated patients with breast cancer with solitary distant metastasis treated with surgical resection, radiation if indicated, and adjuvant chemotherapy. In this cohort, disease-free survival was improved in the short and long term when compared with historical controls treated with local therapy alone (36% vs 7% at 5 years, 26% vs 4% at 10 years, 24% vs 3% at 15 years, and with only 2 additional events after 26 years).[21,22] Improved survival is also demonstrated after definitive surgery to the metastatic site particularly in patients with complete surgical resection, limited metastatic disease, adequate performance status, and long disease-free interval after initial treatment.[23] These findings suggest that there may be a subset of patients with metastatic breast cancer who may attain a long-term durable outcome and effectively be cured.

Retrospective institutional analysis of a contemporary cohort of 570 patients with metastatic breast cancer from 2003 to 2005 found 16% achieved NED. Overall survival at 3 and 5 years was 96% and 78% if NED compared with 44% and 24% overall. Achieving NED was associated with de novo stage IV disease, a single metastatic site, local treatment of the breast primary, whereas negatively associated with overweight or obese body mass index and triple-negative disease. Median time to NED was 11 months, and most patients continued on maintenance therapy. Furthermore, among those with NED, 34% persisted without evidence of relapse.[24]

These studies suggest that there are selected patients with metastatic breast cancer who will develop a durable long-term response and improved survival outcome with multimodality therapy, including local therapy. Currently, the NRG BR002 trial is accruing patients with limited metastatic disease treated with systemic therapy, and definitive local therapy to the breast primary to evaluate whether local therapy (surgery or radiation) to the metastatic site influences progression-free survival and overall survival in oligometastatic breast cancer.[25]

LOCOREGIONAL THERAPY IN STAGE IV INFLAMMATORY BREAST CANCER

IBC is an aggressive breast malignancy characterized by clinical findings of edema, skin thickening, peau d'orange, and erythema involving at least one-third of the breast typically with rapid onset of symptoms. Systemic staging is indicated in IBC with approximately 30% of patients diagnosed with de novo stage IV disease.[26] Overall survival in metastatic IBC is worse when compared with metastatic non-IBC with shorter median survival of 2.27 years as compared with 3.4 years ($P = .0128$).[27]

The University of Texas MD Anderson Cancer Center has reviewed the institutional experience in 172 patients with stage IV IBC at presentation and within 3 months of diagnosis treated between 1997 and 2002. The investigators found 29% 5-year overall survival and 17% 5-year distant progression-free survival. Overall survival was 47% with surgery compared with 10% without surgery, and distant progression-free survival was 30% versus 3%, respectively. Furthermore, receipt of both surgery and radiation showed increased overall survival of 50% as compared with 25% for surgery alone and 14% for radiation alone. Distant progression-free survival was also improved with surgery and radiation at 32% compared with 18% for surgery alone and 15% for radiation alone. These findings were noted despite response to systemic therapy. Independent predictors of improved survival and distant progression-free survival included surgery (with or without radiation) and response to chemotherapy. Local control was significantly improved with surgery with or without radiation at 81% as compared with no locoregional therapy at 8%. Selection bias in determination of surgical candidacy may have impacted the findings. Furthermore, sufficient information was not available to determine the impact of surgical margin status on the outcome.[28]

In metastatic IBC, local failure is less common after receipt of local therapy as compared with systemic therapy alone (17% vs 57%, respectively).[29] A follow-up analysis from the MD Anderson investigators evaluated 36 patients with metastatic IBC treated from 2006 to 2011 with aggressive multimodality therapy with contemporary neoadjuvant chemotherapy, modified radical mastectomy, and postmastectomy radiation therapy to the chest wall, ipsilateral nodal basins, and sites of metastatic disease when feasible. The locoregional control rate at 5 years was 86%, and the overall survival was 54%.[30] These outcomes suggest value in comprehensive local therapy in the setting of metastatic IBC for locoregional control independent of potential survival benefit.

SUMMARY

Metastatic breast cancer represents a heterogeneous group of patients some with aggressive disease unresponsive to systemic therapies and others with an indolent course for many years. The population of patients with metastatic breast cancer is increasing with modest improvements in survival outcome. Considered incurable, surgery for the breast primary was historically offered for palliation in the setting of stage IV breast cancer. Several retrospective analyses, although limited by selection bias, have challenged this dogma, suggesting aggressive local therapy in stage IV breast cancer may also offer survival benefit and local control in IBC. Prospective and randomized trials have not shown a clear survival advantage in early analysis; however, further studies are maturing data. The addition of local therapy, when appropriate, may provide an effort to facilitate a personalized approach to therapy for metastatic breast cancer. Future areas of inquiry include identification of selected patient populations with maximum benefit and evaluation of quality-of-life outcomes particularly given the potential long-term impact of side effects from surgery and radiation, including lymphedema.

REFERENCES

1. Siegel RL, Miller KD, Jemal A. Cancer statistics, 2017. CA Cancer J Clin 2017; 67(1):7–30.
2. Mariotto AB, Etzioni R, Hurlbert M, et al. Estimation of the number of women living with metastatic breast cancer in the United States. Cancer Epidemiol Biomarkers Prev 2017;26(6):809–15.
3. Thomas A, Khan SA, Chrischilles EA, et al. Initial surgery and survival in stage IV breast cancer in the United States, 1988-2011. JAMA Surg 2016;151(5):424–31.
4. National Comprehensive Cancer Network (NCCN) Clinical Care Guidelines. Breast Cancer Version 4.2017. 2017. Available at: https://www.nccn.org/professionals/physician_gls/pdf/breast.pdf. Accessed March 5, 2018.
5. Woodward WA. Should surgery referral be standard practice in metastatic inflammatory breast cancer? Ann Surg Oncol 2015;22(8):2466–7.
6. Khan SA, Stewart AK, Morrow M. Does aggressive local therapy improve survival in metastatic breast cancer? Surgery 2002;132(4):620–6 [discussion: 626–7].
7. Gnerlich J, Jeffe DB, Deshpande AD, et al. Surgical removal of the primary tumor increases overall survival in patients with metastatic breast cancer: analysis of the 1988-2003 SEER data. Ann Surg Oncol 2007;14(8):2187–94.
8. Rapiti E, Verkooijen HM, Vlastos G, et al. Complete excision of primary breast tumor improves survival of patients with metastatic breast cancer at diagnosis. J Clin Oncol 2006;24(18):2743–9.

9. Babiera GV, Rao R, Feng L, et al. Effect of primary tumor extirpation in breast cancer patients who present with stage IV disease and an intact primary tumor. Ann Surg Oncol 2006;13(6):776–82.

10. Rao R, Feng L, Kuerer HM, et al. Timing of surgical intervention for the intact primary in stage IV breast cancer patients. Ann Surg Oncol 2008;15(6):1696–702.

11. Lang JE, Tereffe W, Mitchell MP, et al. Primary tumor extirpation in breast cancer patients who present with stage IV disease is associated with improved survival. Ann Surg Oncol 2013;20(6):1893–9.

12. Dominici L, Najita J, Hughes M, et al. Surgery of the primary tumor does not improve survival in stage IV breast cancer. Breast Cancer Res Treat 2011; 129(2):459–65.

13. Cady B, Nathan NR, Michaelson JS, et al. Matched pair analyses of stage IV breast cancer with or without resection of primary breast site. Ann Surg Oncol 2008;15(12):3384–95.

14. King TA, Lyman JP, Gonen M, et al. TBCRC 013: a prospective analysis of the role of surgery in stage IV breast cancer. Cancer Res 2013;73(24 Suppl) [abstract P2-18-09].

15. King TA, Lyman JP, Gonen M, et al. A prospective analysis of surgery and survival in stage IV breast cancer (TBCRC 013). J Clin Oncol 2016;34(Suppl 15):1000–6.

16. King TA, Lyman JP, Gonen M, et al. Prognostic impact of 21-gene recurrence score in patients with stage IV breast cancer: TBCRC 013. J Clin Oncol 2016; 34(20):2359–65.

17. Badwe R, Hawaldar R, Nair N, et al. Locoregional treatment versus no treatment of the primary tumour in metastatic breast cancer: an open-label randomised controlled trial. Lancet Oncol 2015;16(13):1380–8.

18. Soran A, Ozmen V, Ozbas S, et al. A randomized controlled trial evaluating resection of the primary breast tumor in women presenting with de novo stage IV breast cancer: Turkish Study (Protocol MF0701). J Clin Oncol 2016;34(Suppl 15):1005.

19. Khan SA. Surgery for the intact primary and stage IV breast cancer…lacking "robust evidence". Ann Surg Oncol 2013;20(9):2803–5.

20. Eastern Cooperative Oncology Group. Early surgery or standard palliative therapy in treating patients with stage IV breast cancer. 2010. Available at: https://clinicaltrials.gov/ct2/show/NCT01242800. Accessed March 5, 2018.

21. Hortobagyi GN. Can we cure limited metastatic breast cancer? J Clin Oncol 2002;20(3):620–3.

22. Rivera E, Holmes FA, Buzdar AU, et al. Fluorouracil, doxorubicin, and cyclophosphamide followed by tamoxifen as adjuvant treatment for patients with stage IV breast cancer with no evidence of disease. Breast J 2002;8(1):2–9.

23. Singletary SE, Walsh G, Vauthey JN, et al. A role for curative surgery in the treatment of selected patients with metastatic breast cancer. Oncologist 2003;8(3):241–51.

24. Bishop AJ, Ensor J, Moulder SL, et al. Prognosis for patients with metastatic breast cancer who achieve a no-evidence-of-disease status after systemic or local therapy. Cancer 2015;121(24):4324–32.

25. NRG oncology. Standard of care therapy with or without stereotactic radiosurgery and/or surgery in treating patients with limited metastatic breast cancer. 2015. NRG-BR002. Available at: https://clinicaltrials.gov/ct2/show/NCT02364557. Accessed March 5, 2018.

26. Wingo PA, Jamison PM, Young JL, et al. Population-based statistics for women diagnosed with inflammatory breast cancer (United States). Cancer Causes Control 2004;15(3):321–8.

27. Fouad TM, Kogawa T, Liu DD, et al. Overall survival differences between patients with inflammatory and noninflammatory breast cancer presenting with distant metastasis at diagnosis. Breast Cancer Res Treat 2015;152(2):407–16.

28. Akay CL, Ueno NT, Chisholm GB, et al. Primary tumor resection as a component of multimodality treatment may improve local control and survival in patients with stage IV inflammatory breast cancer. Cancer 2014;120(9):1319–28.

29. Warren LE, Guo H, Regan MM, et al. Inflammatory breast cancer: patterns of failure and the case for aggressive locoregional management. Ann Surg Oncol 2015;22(8):2483–91.

30. Takiar V, Akay CL, Stauder MC, et al. Predictors of durable no evidence of disease status in de novo metastatic inflammatory breast cancer patients treated with neoadjuvant chemotherapy and post-mastectomy radiation. Springerplus 2014;3:166.

31. Fields RC, Jeffe DB, Trinkaus K, et al. Surgical resection of the primary tumor is associated with increased long-term survival in patients with stage IV breast cancer after controlling for site of metastasis. Ann Surg Oncol 2007;14(12):3345–51.

32. Bafford AC, Burstein HJ, Barkley CR, et al. Breast surgery in stage IV breast cancer: impact of staging and patient selection on overall survival. Breast Cancer Res Treat 2009;115(1):7–12.

33. Blanchard DK, Shetty PB, Hilsenbeck SG, et al. Association of surgery with improved survival in stage IV breast cancer patients. Ann Surg 2008;247(5): 732–8.

34. Ruiterkamp J, Ernst MF, van de Poll-Franse LV, et al. Surgical resection of the primary tumour is associated with improved survival in patients with distant metastatic breast cancer at diagnosis. Eur J Surg Oncol 2009;35(11):1146–51.

Sarcomas of the Breast

Mallory A. Duncan, MD[a], Meeghan A. Lautner, MD, MSc[b],*

KEYWORDS

- Breast sarcoma • Angiosarcoma • Radiation-associated sarcoma
- Radiation-induced sarcoma

KEY POINTS

- Sarcoma of the breast is very rare.
- Diagnosis of breast sarcoma is similar to that of invasive or in situ breast cancer, but treatment is very different with fewer options.
- Angiosarcoma of the breast after radiation treatment of invasive or in situ carcinoma is also rare, but incidence may begin to increase with increasing use of breast-conservation therapy.

INTRODUCTION

Sarcomas of the breast are a rare and diverse group of mesenchymal-derived malignancies with unique natural history, treatment, and prognosis compared with the more common carcinoma-type malignancies of the breast. Primary breast sarcomas account for less than 1% of all breast malignancies and less than 5% of all sarcomas.[1] The estimated incidence is 4.6 new cases per million women per year.[2] Because of the rarity of this disease and the inherently small number of cases, no prospective randomized controlled studies have been feasible. Instead, the knowledge and common clinical practices relating to this rare and potentially aggressive disease process are largely guided by small population retrospective studies, case reports, and extrapolated data from larger prospective studies on extremity soft tissue sarcomas.[3] This article highlights the unique considerations in clinical presentation, diagnosis, treatment, and prognosis of breast sarcoma.

CAUSE AND RISK FACTORS

Breast sarcomas are nonepithelial tumors arising from the mesenchymal tissue of the breast.[4] Sarcomas of the breast comprise a variety of subtypes and can be a challenge to diagnose initially because they mimic benign breast disease or benign

Disclosure Statement: The authors have nothing to disclose.
[a] Department of General Surgery, UT Health San Antonio, 7703 Floyd Curl Drive, Mail Code 7737, San Antonio, TX 78229, USA; [b] Department of Surgery, University at Buffalo, 100 High Street, C317, Buffalo, NY 14203, USA
* Corresponding author.
E-mail address: meeghanl@buffalo.edu

Surg Clin N Am 98 (2018) 869–876
https://doi.org/10.1016/j.suc.2018.03.013
0039-6109/18/© 2018 Elsevier Inc. All rights reserved.

cutaneous disease. Most primary breast sarcomas present in women in their fourth to sixth decade of life as a unilateral, large, painless, solitary, mass that grows rapidly and may be difficult to differentiate from a fibroadenoma.[5] The size of the mass at the time of diagnosis is on average from 3 to 5 cm, but it can range from 1 to 20 cm. There is no known predisposition for laterality or quadrant of the breast. Other concerning signs, such as nipple discharge, nipple inversion, and skin retraction or dimpling (excluding angiosarcomas), are rarely seen.[5] Unlike epithelial carcinomas of the breast, which metastasize via lymphatic spread, breast sarcomas demonstrate hematologic metastasis most commonly to the lungs, bones, and liver.

TYPES OF SARCOMA OF THE BREAST

Primary breast sarcomas arise from the hormone-responsive periductal stroma and are referred to as stromal sarcomas.[6,7] The other subtypes of primary breast sarcomas are named based on their type of cell origin and include angiosarcoma, fibrosarcoma, leiomyosarcoma, osteosarcoma, liposarcoma, chondrosarcoma, malignant histiocytoma, and Kaposi sarcoma. Of the primary breast sarcomas, angiosarcoma is the most common subtype.[8] Therefore, this article provides a review of primary breast sarcomas with specific emphasis on angiosarcoma. The overall most common type of breast sarcoma is secondary breast sarcoma, particularly secondary angiosarcoma, which is closely associated with previous high doses of radiation, particularly adjuvant radiation therapy for breast carcinoma and mantle radiation for treatment of Hodgkin lymphoma.[9] The risk of secondary angiosarcoma increases with higher dose of radiation, radiation therapy concurrent with chemotherapy, radiation exposure in childhood, and genetic conditions like BRCA-1.[10] BRCA mutations may result in a genetic predisposition to radiation-associated sarcoma development because BRCA-1 and -2 are DNA repair genes, and high doses of radiation in mutation carriers would allow a rare escape from cell death and formation of secondary tumors.[11]

ANGIOSARCOMA

Angiosarcomas are malignant vascular neoplasms of the breast that can have an aggressive clinical course with higher recurrence rates and lower overall survival that the other sarcoma subtypes.[5] Angiosarcoma of the breast is very rare with an overall incidence of 0.002% to 0.05% and can be divided into 2 types. Primary breast angiosarcoma arises from the breast parenchyma, but its cause is not well known. Secondary breast angiosarcoma, whose incidence is 0.01% to 0.02% per year, is thought to arise as a result of the breast radiation component of treatment of ductal carcinoma in situ or invasive carcinoma.[12] These lesions arise from the dermis, are less likely to involve the underlying breast tissue, and are often confused with benign cutaneous cause.[13,14] The cause is related to double-stranded DNA damage caused by radiation, which then results in genome instability that may lead to sarcoma development.[11]

   Primary angiosarcoma of the breast typically occurs in young women aged 30 to 40 and will present as an ill-defined breast mass within the parenchyma, which is usually high grade.[5,14] Diagnosis is made by an abnormal mammogram, ultrasound, or MRI resulting in a core biopsy. A single-institution retrospective review performed by the MD Anderson Cancer Center identified that radiation therapy–naive angiosarcoma of the breast occurred in younger patients who were more likely to have distant metastasis at presentation. The early outcomes for these patients were more favorable compared with the patients who had received prior radiation therapy; however, the late overall survival was not statistically different.[12] Treatment modalities for the patients with primary angiosarcoma varied among type of surgery and adjuvant therapy with some radiation-naive patients receiving external-beam radiation after breast-conserving surgery. Over the study period of 14 years, 30% of radiation-naive patients developed recurrence with disease-free survival being lowest in those with tumors greater than 5 cm in size, similar to soft tissue sarcomas in other anatomic sites.[12]

Radiation-associated angiosarcoma of the breast has been expected to increase in incidence as the use of breast-conserving therapy (breast-conserving surgery combined with whole breast radiation) increases.[13] This type of angiosarcoma often presents in older women as multifocal reddish/blue discolored macules and is widely distributed within the previous radiation therapy field.[5,13] In a review of the Surveillance, Epidemiology, and End Results database by Yap and colleagues,[15] the median latent period for the development of the radiation-associated sarcoma was 6 years (range 1–21 years). Mammography may not have any suspicious findings, and ultrasound findings are nonspecific in one-third of patients.[5] The most common treatment is radical surgical excision without lymph node dissection. As most patients who develop radiation-associated angiosarcoma have undergone breast conserving therapy, total mastectomy with radical resection of all previously radiated skin is the recommended surgical treatment. This includes radiated skin even outside the borders of the breast.[13] In a single-institution retrospective review, improved disease-specific survival and lower local recurrence rates were seen in patients who underwent a more radical skin resection as opposed to a more conservative resection.[13] In many cases, this resection will require a split-thickness skin graft or other form of chest wall coverage. Tumor grade is essential to prognosis as in other sarcomas mentioned above. Angiosarcomas are graded by the appearance of histologic behavior of the endothelial cells based on nuclear atypia, mitotic activity, papillary formations, and presence of blood lakes.[5]

There is a paucity of data to suggest a survival benefit of chemotherapy in radiation-associated angiosarcoma; however, a multidisciplinary approach should be taken with each case. In another retrospective review from the MD Anderson Cancer Center, Torres and colleagues[14] found that the risk of local recurrence was lower in patients who received chemotherapy, but this did not translate into a survival benefit. Reirradiation of the chest wall is controversial without strong data to support its use.[13] Prognosis is still very poor for radiation-associated angiosarcoma because most patients are diagnosed many years after radiation treatment, which often means in the elder years. The range of overall survival for angiosarcoma of the breast is 1.1 to 2.8 years.[12] As such, index of suspicion should be high at the development of skin lesions of the breast particularly after radiation treatment.

STEWART-TREVES SYNDROME

Angiosarcoma of the breast that arises after radiation treatment is a distinctly different disease from Stewart-Treves syndrome, which is angiosarcoma that arises in the breast and upper extremity affected by lymphedema from an axillary lymphadenectomy.[16] Although there is some association with radiation treatment, the main cause for Stewart-Treves syndrome is long-standing lymphedema as a result of axillary lymph node dissection. It is usually a late presentation as a purple-colored, multifocal maculopapular rash that may progress to ulceration.[16] Treatment may include chemotherapy, radiation, and radical surgical resection with amputation, but prognosis remains poor because the disease is very aggressive and often presents with distant metastasis.[16]

DIAGNOSIS AND STAGING

The usual diagnostic pathway initiated after a patient presents with a breast mass includes evaluation with standard diagnostic imaging with mammography, ultrasound, or MRI, depending on the patient's age and clinical history. There are no known patho-gnomonic features of primary breast sarcoma on imaging, and commonly the findings may mimic invasive carcinomas of the breast. On mammogram, primary breast sarcoma can either manifest as a noncalcified, irregular or oval mass with indistinct margins, or as architectural distortion. Ultrasound evaluation generally shows an irregular, hypoechoic mass with indistinct or spiculated margins. MRI similarly reveals lesions with irregular or spiculated margins and a variety of different internal enhancement behaviors.[17] The most recent retrospective studies report that 58.1% of the time these mammographic characteristics when associated with a primary sarcoma were documented as a Breast Imaging Reporting and Data System (BI-RADS) 4 or 5, and 41.9% of the time as BI-RADS 3, which means that breast sarcomas are typically not missed on breast imaging.[10]

Definitive diagnosis is made histologically, and core needle biopsy is the procedure of choice in order to better appreciate the morphology of the tumor.[10] Immunohisto-chemistry studies of the tissue are also essential, not only for distinguishing sarcomas from carcinomas but also for classifying sarcomas further into the array of different subtypes. Sarcomas will lack the diffuse reactivity for cytokeratin and myoepithelial markers that would be seen in epithelial tumors, like carcinomas.[7] An accurate histo-logic diagnosis is paramount, because the pathways of treatment and clinical decision making are quite different, not only between carcinomas and sarcomas but also among the various subtypes of sarcomas. From a technical standpoint regarding core needle biopsy, it is important to obtain the biopsy in such a way that the biopsy tract is able to be well incorporated into the tissue resection at the time of surgery, because the malignant cells are known to seed along this tract.[18] At gross inspection, sarcomas of the breast are usually fleshy, firm tumors with some amount of hemor-rhage and necrosis.[5]

Breast sarcoma staging is based on the American Joint Committee on Cancer (AJCC) for soft tissue sarcomas rather than AJCC staging criteria for breast epithelial carcinomas. While staging for breast epithelial carcinomas accounts for tumor size, node status and distant metastasis, AJCC staging for breast sarcomas considers his-tologic grade which is based on tumor differentiation, mitotic index, and necrosis and plays an important role in prognosis.[5] Because of the nature of hematologic metas-tasis seen with breast sarcomas, as opposed to nodal metastasis in breast carci-nomas, nodal status in breast sarcoma is not as useful for staging; therefore, sentinel lymph node biopsy is not routinely performed. Instead, imaging studies such as computed tomographic scan are used to evaluate the lungs, bones, and liver, which are the most common sites of distant metastasis via hematogenous spread.[19] At minimum, a preoperative chest radiograph should be performed in all patients before surgical resection given the risk of lung metastasis.[5]

TREATMENT

The treatment of breast sarcomas mirrors the treatment of other soft tissue sarcomas, with the main goal being surgical resection with wide margins, and inclusion of the bi-opsy site in the specimen.[10] Tumor size and adequate resection margins are the most important prognostic factors, with adequate resection margin being the most impor-tant determinant of long-term survival.[10] The standard recommendation is to obtain a 1-cm clear margin for all resected breast sarcomas, with the exception of angiosar-comas by which a 3-cm clear resection margin is recommended.[10] These margin widths are in stark contrast to the margins required in the surgical treatment of breast epithelial carcinomas, which do not require as wide a margin. Based on current recommendations, if a breast sarcoma is small in size and appropriate clear resection margins can be obtained with an acceptable cosmetic outcome, breast-conserving excision should be adequate.[10] There is no additional benefit in patients who undergo mastectomy.[5] Of note, some caution against breast-conserving excision, even with small tumor size, if the tumor is high grade or if it is an angiosarcoma. Breast-conserving surgery in patients with angiosarcoma has been associated with high levels of local recurrence—up to 30% of patients in a single-institution study.[12,20] There is no clear evidence on the benefit of adjuvant radiotherapy in the treatment of breast sarcomas, and in the case of radiation-associated angiosarcoma, needs to be considered with caution. There have been studies dedicated to analyze the effect of postoperative radiotherapy on the clinical outcome of patients with breast sarcomas; however, there has not been enough evidence to warrant a change in the standard of care for treatment.[10]

As previously discussed, sarcomas demonstrate hematologic metastasis, and lymph node metastasis is not common. Therefore, no sentinel lymph node sampling or axillary lymph node dissection is indicated unless there is clinically palpable axillary lymphadenopathy, which is exceedingly rare.[19]

ADJUVANT THERAPY

Studies have demonstrated improved local control of recurrence and prolonged disease-free survival with adjuvant radiotherapy after breast-conserving resection, especially if the resection margin is marginal or inadequate. Adjuvant radiotherapy is recommended after a positive margin resection because of the high risk of recurrence, especially if reexcision is not feasible.[5] It is also recommended for any negative resection margin in a tumor larger than 5 cm or with any high-grade sarcoma because of the high recurrence of local recurrence. One study recommends postoperative radiation should deliver microscopic tumoricidal dose to the whole breast, and at least 60 Gy to the tumor bed.[21] Adjuvant radiation for radiation-associated angiosarcomas should be considered in a multidisciplinary setting given the healthy tissue radiation limits even years after the initial radiation therapy and remains controversial without a well-defined complication profile.[4,13]

The role of chemotherapy for breast sarcomas has remained controversial. Some studies have suggested that neoadjuvant chemotherapy and/or radiation may be warranted to decrease tumor size to allow for a negative margin of resection. However, responses to chemotherapy are highly variable; thus prolonging the time to surgical resection could render the patient unresectable if the patient does not have an acceptable response to neoadjuvant chemotherapy.[10] As for adjuvant chemotherapy, it has not been associated with better overall survival in any histologic subgroup, although there may be an advantage to recurrence-free survival. One study, dealing in general with soft tissue sarcomas, concluded that an ifosfamide plus doxorubicin regimen gave a marginal benefit in operable soft tissue sarcomas with respect to overall survival and local and distant recurrence.[22] Because breast sarcomas are characteristically hormone receptor negative, adjuvant endocrine therapy is not a therapeutic option.[7]

ONCOPLASTIC RECONSTRUCTION

With a 5-year survival as high as 67% for most primary breast sarcomas, and with the advancement in oncoplastic reconstruction, breast reconstruction should be considered appropriate. Oncoplastic reconstruction has widened the population of patients that may be candidates for breast-conserving therapy, because wider margins can be resected with acceptable cosmetic outcomes. Because the natural progression of breast sarcoma is an eventual poor oncologic outcome, the timing of reconstruction should be immediate whenever possible to aid in preserving quality of life.[23] Oncoplastic reconstruction with parenchymal rearrangement or reconstruction with local flap, namely an intercostal artery, long thoracic artery, or thoracodorsal perforator flap, is acceptable for patients who have undergone a partial mastectomy, regardless of their previous history of radiation or their risk for requiring adjuvant radiation.[23] Patients who undergo a total mastectomy for sarcoma, who have no previous history of radiation and whose tumor is low risk for requiring adjuvant radiation (small tumor with low-grade features), are good candidates for immediate reconstruction with tissue expanders or implants, abdominal flap, gluteal flap, or latissimus dorsi flap. Patients who undergo total mastectomy who have a previous history of radiation are also considered to be candidates for immediate reconstruction.

OUTCOMES

It is difficult to generalize meaningful data to such a heterogeneous group of tumors, but in general, breast sarcomas share prognostic factors similar to that of other soft tissue sarcomas. Prognostic factors include tumor size >5 cm, high-grade disease, positive resection margins, and histologic subtype of angiosarcoma.[10] In one series, the 10-year overall survival of breast sarcomas was 62%, and in another series, the 5-year and 10-year recurrence-free survival was 47% and 42% in breast sarcomas, which did not have distant metastasis at presentation.[10] In radiation-associated angiosarcoma with cutaneous origin, historically local recurrence rates are high, and long-term survival is poor.[13]

Similar to patients with invasive or in situ breast carcinoma, patients with breast sarcoma should be followed closely. However, given the difference in the biology of the disease as well as staging and prognosis, patients with breast sarcoma should be followed according to National Comprehensive Cancer Network (NCCN) Guidelines for Soft Tissue Sarcoma, including frequent visits for a history and physical examination as well as local imaging and chest imaging.[24]

SUMMARY

Because of the rarity of breast sarcomas, there are no randomized trials to guide standardized treatment. Instead, there have been numerous small retrospective studies and case reports that currently guide the management of this potentially aggressive disease. For this reason, a multidisciplinary approach is important for expert clinical protocol-driven care as well as for standardization of data, and the opportunity for patients to participate in clinical trials. In general, treatment of breast sarcomas necessitates adequate resection margins. If adequate resection margins and satisfactory cosmetic outcome can be obtained with breast-conserving resection, mastectomy can be avoided. Adjuvant radiation, especially if there are inadequate margins, demonstrates a trend toward improved local control and possibly improved overall survival in select studies. However, this treatment modality may not be an option for patients with radiation-associated angiosarcoma depending on the amount of prior radiation received. Sentinel lymph node and axillary lymph node dissections are not generally indicated, because breast sarcomas demonstrate hematologic metastasis. The role of chemotherapy remains unclear, and more research is warranted in this area. Close surveillance is indicated for all patients with sarcoma in accordance with the NCCN Guidelines for Soft Tissue Sarcoma. Last, with the widely accepted use of breast radiation to complete breast-conservation therapy for invasive and in situ breast carcinoma, the incidence of radiation-associated angiosarcoma is expected to increase. Patients who have undergone breast conserving therapy should therefore undergo a thorough skin examination at surveillance visits with a low threshold for biopsy or excision of cutaneous lesions in order to identify the disease at its earliest stage. All patients with breast sarcoma should be considered for multidisciplinary treatment so that prognosis may be optimized.

REFERENCES

1. Surov A, Holzhausen HJ, Ruschke K, et al. Primary breast sarcoma: prevalence, clinical signs, and radiological features. Acta Radiol 2011;52(6):597–601.
2. McGowan TS, Cummings BJ, O'Sullivan B, et al. An analysis of 78 breast sarcoma patients without distant metastases at presentation. Int J Radiat Oncol Biol Phys 2000;46(2):383–90.
3. Sheth GR, Cranmer LD, Smith BD, et al. Radiation-induced sarcoma of the breast: a systematic review. Oncologist 2012;17(3):405–18.
4. Voutsadakis IA, Zaman K, Leyvraz S. Breast sarcomas: current and future perspectives. Breast 2011;20(3):199–204.
5. Kuerer HM. Kuerer's breast surgical oncology. The McGraw Hill Companies, Inc; 2010.
6. Adem C, Reynolds C, Ingle JN, et al. Primary breast sarcoma: clinicopathologic series from the Mayo Clinic and review of the literature. Br J Cancer 2004;91(2): 237–41.
7. Krings G, Rabban JT, Shin SJ. In: Dabbs D, editor. Breast pathology. 2nd edition. Philadelphia: WB Sauders; 2012. p. 663–717.
8. Smith TB, Gilcrease MZ, Santiago L, et al. Imaging features of primary breast sarcoma. AJR Am J Roentgenol 2012;198(4):W386–93.
9. Guibout C, Adjadj E, Rubino C, et al. Malignant breast tumors after radiotherapy for a first cancer during childhood. J Clin Oncol 2005;23(1):197–204.
10. Lim SZ, Ong KW, Tan BK, et al. Sarcoma of the breast: an update on a rare entity. J Clin Pathol 2016;69(5):373–81.
11. Kadouri L, Sagi M, Goldberg Y, et al. Genetic predisposition to radiation induced sarcoma: possible role for BRCA and p53 mutations. Breast Cancer Res Treat 2013;140(1):207–11.
12. Vorburger SA, Xing Y, Hunt KK, et al. Angiosarcoma of the breast. Cancer 2005; 104(12):2682–8.
13. Li GZ, Fairweather M, Wang J, et al. Cutaneous radiation-associated breast angiosarcoma: radicality of surgery impacts survival. Ann Surg 2017;265(4): 814–20.
14. Torres KE, Ravi V, Kin K, et al. Long-term outcomes in patients with radiation-associated angiosarcomas of the breast following surgery and radiotherapy for breast cancer. Ann Surg Oncol 2013;20(4):1267–74.
15. Yap J, Chuba PJ, Thomas R, et al. Sarcoma as a second malignancy after treatment for breast cancer. Int J Radiat Oncol Biol Phys 2002;52(5):1231–7.
16. Roy P, Clark MA, Thomas JM. Stewart-Treves syndrome–treatment and outcome in six patients from a single centre. Eur J Surg Oncol 2004;30(9):982–6.
17. Wienbeck S, Meyer HJ, Herzog A, et al. Imaging findings of primary breast sarcoma: results of a first multicenter study. Eur J Radiol 2017;88:1–7.
18. Schwartz HS, Spengler DM. Needle tract recurrences after closed biopsy for sarcoma: three cases and review of the literature. Ann Surg Oncol 1997;4(3):228–36.

19. Al-Benna S, Poggemann K, Steinau HU, et al. Diagnosis and management of primary breast sarcoma. Breast Cancer Res Treat 2010;122(3):619–26.
20. Thorton K. Sarcomas of the breast with a spotlight on angiosarcoma and cystosarcoma phyllodes. Surg Oncol Clin N Am 2016;25(4):713–20.
21. Gutman H, Pollock RE, Ross MI, et al. Sarcoma of the breast: implications for extent of therapy. The M. D. Anderson experience. Surgery 1994;116(3):505–9.
22. Pervaiz N, Colterjohn N, Farrokhyar F, et al. A systematic meta-analysis of randomized controlled trials of adjuvant chemotherapy for localized resectable soft-tissue sarcoma. Cancer 2008;113(3):573–81.
23. Crosby MA, Chike-Obi CJ, Baumann DP, et al. Reconstructive outcomes in patients with sarcoma of the breast. Plast Reconstr Surg 2010;126(6):1805–14.
24. National Comprehensive Cancer Network. Clinical Practice Guidelines in Oncology Soft Tissue Sarcoma 2017. Version 1.2018. Available at: https://www.nccn.org/professionals/physician_gls/pdf/sarcoma.pdf. Accessed November 6, 2017.

Moving?

Make sure your subscription moves with you!

To notify us of your new address, find your **Clinics Account Number** (located on your mailing label above your name), and contact customer service at:

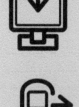

Email: **journalscustomerservice-usa@elsevier.com**

800-654-2452 (subscribers in the U.S. & Canada)
314-447-8871 (subscribers outside of the U.S. & Canada)

Fax number: 314-447-8029

Elsevier Health Sciences Division
Subscription Customer Service
3251 Riverport Lane
Maryland Heights, MO 63043

ELSEVIER

Printed and bound by CPI Group (UK) Ltd, Croydon, CR0 4YY

07/10/2024

01040502-0005